Applied Behavior Analysis fc
with Autism Spectrum Disorders

Johnny L. Matson

Editor

Applied Behavior Analysis for Children with Autism Spectrum Disorders

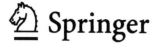 Springer

Editor
Johnny L. Matson
Department of Psychology
Louisiana State University
Baton Rouge, LA 70803
USA
johnmatson@aol.com

ISBN 978-1-4419-0087-6 (hardcover)   ISBN 978-1-4419-0088-3 (eBook)
ISBN 978-1-4419-8132-5 (softcover)
DOI 10.1007/978-1-4419-0088-3
Springer New York Dordrecht Heidelberg London

Library of Congress Control Number: 2009933463

Printed on acid-free paper

Springer is part of Springer Science+Business Media (www.springer.com)

Contents

Contributors

Lauren Brookman-Frazer, Ph.D.
Assistant Professor of Psychiatry, University of California-San Diego,
Child and Adolescent Services Research Center (CASRC), 3020 Children's Way,
MC 5033, San Diego, CA 92123, USA
lbrookman@ucsd.edu

Dennis Dixon, Ph.D.
Manager, Research and Development, Center for Autism and Related
Disorders, Inc., 19019 Ventura Blvd. #300, Tarzana, CA 91356, USA
D.Dixon@centerforautism.com

Frederick Furniss, Ph.D.
Professor, The Hesley Group, School of Psychology, University of Leicester,
Mallard House, Sidings Court, Doncaster DNS 5NV, UK
fred.furniss@hesleygroup.co.uk

Linda LeBlanc, Ph.D.
Associate Professor, Co-Director, WMU Center for Autism,
Department of Psychology, Western Michigan University,
1903 W. Michigan Avenue, Kalamazoo, MI 49008-5439, USA
linda.leblanc@wmich.edu

James K. Luiselli, Ed.D., A.B.P.P., B.C.B.A.
May Institute, 41, Pacella Park Drive, Randolph, MA 02368, USA
jluiselli@mayinstitute.org

Johnny L. Matson, Ph.D.
Professor and Distinguished Master, Department of Psychology,
Louisiana State University, Baton Rouge, LA 70803, USA

Oliver Mudford, Ph.D., B.C.B.A.
Director of Applied Behavior Analysis Program, Department of Psychology
(Tamaki Campus), University of Auckland, Private Bag 92019, Auckland,
New Zealand
o.mudford@auckland.ac.az

Nozomi Naoi, Ph.D.
Department of Psychology, Keio University, 2-15-45 Mita, Minato-Ku, Tokyo
108-8345, Japan
nnaoi@psy.flet.keio.ac.jp

Joel Ringdahl, Ph.D.
Department of Pediatrics, Division of Pediatric Psychology,
Children's Hospital of Iowa, Center for Disabilities and Development,
100 Hawkins Drive, Iowa City, IA 52224-27011, USA
joel-ringdahl@uiowa.edu

Jeff Sigafoos, Ph.D.
Professor, School of Education, The University of Tasmania, Private Bag 166,
Hobart, TAS 7001, Australia
Jeff.Sigafoos@utas.edu.au

Naomi Swiezy, Ph.D.
Clinical Psychology in Psychiatry, Clinical Director, Christian Sarkine
Autism Treatment Center, Riley Hospital for children, 702 Barnhill Drive,
Rm. 4300, Indianapolis, IN 46202-5000, USA
nswiezy@iupui.edu

Jeffrey H. Tiger, Ph.D.
Department of Psychology, Louisiana State University, Baton Rouge, LA 70803, USA
jtiger@lsu.edu

Tim Vollmer, Ph.D.
Professor, Department of Psychology, P.O. Box 112250, University of Florida,
Gainesville, FL 32611-2250, USA
vollmera@ufl.edu

Mary Jane Weiss, Ph.D., B.C.B.A.
Professor, Douglas Developmental Disabilities Center, Rutgers,
The State University of New Jersey, 25 Gibbons Circle, New Brunswick,
NY 08901-8528, USA
weissnj@rci.rutgers.edu

Chapter 1
History and Overview

Johnny L. Matson and Daniene Neal

This chapter will present developments that have resulted in the current state of applied behavior analysis (ABA). Initial parts of the chapter will be on ABA and its history with autism. The chapter will conclude with a rationale for the book and potential further developments in the future.

Beginning

According to John B. Watson (1919), the history of psychology began "as soon as there were two individuals on the earth living near enough for the behavior of one to influence the behavior of the other" (p. 2). Thus, it could be argued that the beginnings of applied behavior analysis (ABA) date to the beginnings of civilization. The origins of ABA and its applications to the autism spectrum disorders (ABA) would best be described as rooted in the early foundations of experimental psychology. Gustav Fechner (1801–1887) is credited with being the first modern day experimental psychologist with his research on the measurement of sensations Boring (1950) in his classic book on the history of experimental psychology attributes the beginning of scientific psychology to "Fechner and other Germans." But, others have suggested that John Locke (1632–1704) is the true "father" of modern day empiricism.

Regardless of one's view on this point, the German school certainly provided the critical mass of researchers and profoundly affected American psychology. G. Stanley Hall worked in the first experimental

psychology laboratory in Leipzig, Germany, which was established by Wilhelm Wundt (1832–1920). Their work involved the systematization of measurement procedures for psychological process. Also influential was Hermann Ebbinghaus and his groundbreaking book, *Memory: A Contribution to Experimental Psychology*. Perhaps the key points to be derived from these developments was that the experimental method has value for establishing some of the basic mechanisms by which people learn and the notion that developments in science tend to be evolutionary. Furthermore, from the very +beginning, psychology has had a strong empirically based foundation.

Watson

The facts behind the history of modern day ABA as we see it practiced are less contested. John B. Watson (1878–1958) is generally considered the first person to formulate a science of applied behavior, a claim supported by B.F. Skinner who was heavily influenced by Watson's ideas (1989). Watson's book, *Psychology from the Standpoint of a Behaviorist* (Watson, 1919) was one of the earliest pieces of scientific writing to use the term behaviorism in the title. Furthermore, he also used terms such as "psychology, a science of behavior" which are still in common usage among professionals who endorse ABA today. This data based approach was particularly important in tying together basic experimental psychology principles to applied work. Such a development was revolutionary at the time. Remember that Freud and associates and their theories of human behavior held sway in applied psychology at the time. And, his conditioning experiments with simple phobias with a small child are still frequently quoted in

J.L. Matson (✉)
Department of Psychology, Louisiana State University,
Baton Rouge, LA, 70803, USA
e-mail: johnmatson@aol.com

J.L. Matson (ed.), *Applied Behavior Analysis for Children with Autism Spectrum Disorders*,
DOI 10.1007/978-1-4419-0088-3_1, © Springer Science+Business Media, LLC 2009

ABA, psychology, and special education textbooks today (Cover Johnes, 1924; Watson & Rayner, 1920). The classical conditioning paradigm established then is still a foundation for the treatment of fear and phobias today.

Skinner

The individual in the ABA field generally considered to be most linked to codifying and popularizing ABA is B.F. Skinner (1904–1990; Labrador, 2004). Despite developments in experimental psychology and the efforts of Watson and associates, most of the "science" of human behavior was practiced in university laboratories prior to Skinner's work. As noted, in applied settings, psychodynamic theories and practices dominated as a result of Freud, Jung, and their colleagues and adherents. Furthermore, popular books at the time which dealt with mental health issues focused on patient rights vs. efforts to develop effective data based interventions. Clifford Beers, a Yale law student who developed schizophrenia and was hospitalized for an extended time is particularly notable. The book he wrote following his hospitalization, *A Mind That Found Itself* (Beers, 1908), described the terrible state of mental hospitals at the time. This book helped launch the mental hygiene movement. Through his efforts, and with the assistance of prominent professionals at the time –psychiatrist Adolph Meyer and psychologist William James, he was able to establish the National Committee for mental hygiene in 1909. This point has particular relevance for ABA and ASD, since parent advocacy groups have been instrumental in promoting and advocating ABA interventions. Thus, Beers helped establish a model for patient/parent advocacy that thrives today.

B.F. Skinner, then, was the right person, with the right ideas, at the right time. He earned a B.A. from Hamilton College in 1926. Beginning a career as a writer, he read and was influenced by Watson, as just noted, and also by the Russian physiologist, Pavlov. He returned to school after his adventures in the literary world and received a Ph.D. in psychology from Harvard University. Skinner then began his academic career at the University of Minnesota where he conducted a number of operant studies with pigeons. One particularly memorable one, Project Pigeon, which was conducted

during WWII, involved conditioning pigeons to peck at a set of cross hairs to be used as a guidance system for bombs. The military never adopted the idea. He then accepted the position as the chair of the Department of Psychology at Indiana University in 1945. Skinner's final academic move involved his return to Harvard in 1948 as a professor of psychology.

Skinner courted the popular press using an innovative strategy that caught the fancy of the general public. One of the most publicized of these inventions was the "baby tender," a plexiglass enclosed heated crib. The invention was described in some detail in the *Ladies Home Journal*, a very popular outlet that reached millions of homes and helped educate the public on the science of human behavior. Another effort that received a good deal of press was a fictional book entitled *Walden Two* (Skinner, 1948). Skinner described a communal life style, where tokens were used as a form of barter that would be used to obtain services vs. money. Skinner describes a small rural community of 1,000 people where "members" are happy, creative and productive. The head of the town is T.E. Frazier (presumably Skinner's alter ego) who along with managers, planners and scientists, runs the community. The concepts of self-sufficiency harkens to Thoreau's original Walden but was placed in the context of a community vs. a single person. Furthermore, the use of reinforcement principles to promote a well ordered society was seen as a means of promoting ABA methods and procedures. The book was so popular that actual Walden communities patterned on the volume were started. Some of these were the New Haven, Connecticut group led by Arthur Gladstone (1955), the Twin Oaks Community in Lousia, Virginia (1967), Walden House, a student collective later renamed The Sunflower House in Lawrence, Kansas (1969), Lake Village in Michigan (1971), Los Horcones in Hermosillo, Mexico (1971), and East Wind in Missouri (1979). Twin Oaks is still in operation, and while it maintains some of the management principles described in *Walden Two*, it is no longer considered a "Walden project." Thus, these experimental communities appear to have run their course, although, the book itself is still read. Further evidence of *Walden Two*'s popularity was the fact that Skinner wrote a sequel, *Walden Revisited* (Skinner, 1976).

These efforts as a whole were largely successful at engaging the culture with respect to ABA. Thus, the application of ABA to positively impact the society was a major development and the mainstream publicity these projects generated were a major springboard for establishing ABA. While large scale societal applications of ABA never really caught on, popular attention to the field did spark the imagination of many researchers. Applications largely became the purview of specific clinical populations. Additionally, ABA rapidly became multidisciplinary. Methods and procedures that began as the purview of experimental psychology, rapidly spread to clinical, rehabilitation and school psychology, special education, general education, social work and other human service disciplines.

Timing Is Everything

Labrador (2004) does an excellent job of describing a series of setting events which resulted in the development and widespread application of ABA. Most behaviorally oriented professionals would, we believe, like to think that these gains were based almost exclusively on the value of ABA. However, timing is a critical factor in any large scale endeavor of this sort. ABA is no exception. Psychodynamic models which were the dominant theories up until the 1960s are lengthy in terms of the number of treatment sessions required, they are costly, and despite arguments of proponents, largely ineffective. Little research was done to demonstrate the utility of the procedures. As mental health and special education services expanded from the almost exclusive purview of private providers who largely catered to wealthy consumers, the issues changed. This much more expansive and democratic service model put greater emphasis on cost and demonstrated efficacy since most of the expense was being shouldered by third party payers such as district schools and insurance companies. Because cost was and remains a major issue, training parent, and professionals with less credentialing than the doctorate, paired with the need for rapid effects, took on greater importance as well. Thus, health providers were looking for an alternative treatment model. All these social forces thus gave additional credibility and impetus to ABA. Labradore (2004) summarizes these points as "the demand to cover a large number of people with behavior problems, along with the inability of existing psychotherapies to satisfy demand, and the availability of a body of knowledge which would permit alternative solutions."

Another fortunate happenstance for ABA was the rapid development and requests for child mental health and developmental disability services at approximately the same time that ABA principles were being fostered. Thus, a "new" population of potential consumers presented itself, and there were no entrenched treatments for children, unlike the status quo in the adult field. With respect to the latter, numerous articles and books have been written describing how existing therapies such as various psychodynamic treatments, Gestalt Therapy and Client Centered Therapy were superior to learning based methods. These entrenched methods were defended by attacking behavioral methods as simplistic and shallow. Treating a set of observable behaviors vs. core symptoms, it was argued, would merely result in the client developing other maladaptive behaviors (symptom substitution). Furthermore, behavior modification and behavior therapy (these methods along with ABA can be seen as variants of empirically based learning methods) were attacked as mechanistic and controlling. The popular movie *Clockwork Orange* further played on this theme. Conversely, children had received little formal treatment when reviewed from an overarching national level. Thus, ABA filled a treatment vacuum, and developed more rapidly because of less resistance from other professional groups.

Child Treatment

By far, the childhood developmental disabilities that are most frequent and which have been most frequently studied are autism, now ASD, and intellectual disabilities (ID). Furthermore, estimates are that ASD and ID overlap by as much as 70% (Fombonne, 1999; Magnusson & Saemundsen, 2001). In addition, there is a long history, to the extent that one would describe psychology's history as long, for the identification and the recognition of treatment of these children. Alfred Binet (1857–1911) and the development of the I.Q. testing movement, was a direct result of efforts to identify children with ID in Paris. This line of research continued and expanded under the supervision of Lewis Terman (1877–1956) who normed the Binet-Simon test on an American sample. The resulting Stanford-Binet test is still in widespread use today. Furthermore, this became a major research area for applied psychology which still continues, and spawned a huge commercial test industry.

Lightner Witner (1867–1956) was the first American psychologist to emphasize modern mental health treatment services for children. Initially, he was a doctoral student of James McKeen Cattell at the University of Pennsylvania. However, when Cattell relocated to Columbia University, Witmer traveled to Leipzig, Germany and obtained his Ph.D. with Wilhelm Wundt. In 1907, Witmer coined the term *clinical psychology*. In his article by the same name (Witmer, 1907) he described a laboratory at the University of Pennsylvania that he had been running for 10 years which he referred to as psychological clinic. Witmer noted that parents or teachers brought children to the clinic due to "moral defects" or poor school performance. All the children seen by Witmer and his team were initially assessed with the help of physical and mental examinations. Witmer, in the course of this paper, also went on to emphasize his particularly strong interest in ID. (He served as a consulting psychologist at the Pennsylvania Training School for Feeble-Minded Children in Elwyn, Pennsylvania.) Furthermore, he set the stage for ABA by linking applied clinical work to basic research, much as Watson and Skinner were to do later. Witmer noted the scientific advances of Helmholtz and Fechner in the measurement of physiological processes and sensation respectively. He emphasized that without them "clinical psychology could never have developed. The pure and the applied sciences advance in a single front." While many years passed before the field of ABA could develop, it is both interesting and illustrative to see that much of the DNA for data based psychological methods goes back to the beginnings of the fieldof?

Autism and the Spectrum

The definition of autism has changed a great deal since it was first described by Leo Kanner (1943). The core symptoms of the 11 children he initially described are relatively the same: language and social impairments, rituals, routines, and cognitive rigidity. However, autism is now a spectrum of like conditions, not one disorder. The high prevalence disorders are autism, Pervasive Developmental Disorder, Not Otherwise Specified (PDDNOS) which has autism features but where all the criteria for autism are not met, and Asperger's Syndrome

Very rare (ASD) that includes Rett Syndrome and Disintegrative Childhood Disorder (CDD).

Heller

The first ASD to be described was CDD by Theodor Heller (1869–1938) in 1908. Heller, an Austrian psychiatrist, was born in Vienna. His family had a history of serving the blind, but Heller wished to not only help these individuals, but all handicapped children as well. He observed this rare condition with onset at 3–10 years of age, leading to what he referred to as progressive dementia. Heller reported that these children, who were somewhat delayed initially, as developing a host of devastating deficits. These could include tics, mutism, stereotypies, withdrawn helplessness, immature behavior and challenging behaviors. Heller called the condition *dementia infantilis*, since it appeared that these children were developing dementia. Also, referred to as Heller Syndrome, CDD has only been officially reorganized as disorder in the last two decades. This situation is most likely due to the paucity of studies on the topic, which can be attributed to its rarity.

Kanner

Autism is the ASD which, according to the United States Center for Disease Control, is now believed to occur in 1–150 children. This rate makes it one of the most frequently diagnosed of all childhood conditions and one of the most devastating. Furthermore, it is one of the most researched, based on publications in scientific journals and discussed in the popular press perhaps more often than any other mental health concern. This situation is largely due to the snowball effect initiated by Leo Kanner, who is credited with defining this most popular of the ASD. In a recent study, for example, the number of published studies from 1973 to 2008 on autism was nearly five times greater than all four of the other ASD combined.

Until 1943, when Leo Kanner from Klekotov, Austria entered the field, autism as a clinical entity was unknown (Kanner, 1943). He attended the University of Berlin but did not receive his MD until 1921 due to World War I and his service in the Austrian army.

In 1924, he migrated to the United States to take a position as an "Assistant Physician" at the state hospital in Yankton County, South Dakota. In 1930, he was hired to develop the child psychiatry program at Johns Hopkins University Medical School where he continued the rest of his career. He was the first person in America to be identified as a child psychiatrist and his textbook, *Child Psychiatry*, published in 1935, was the first English language book devoted to developmental disabilities and mental health problems of childhood. Kanner's classic 1943 paper describes 11 children who had no apparent affect and who seemed to draw into a shell and live within themselves. As a result, he chose the word autism from the Greek self to describe the disorder. And, as people say, the rest is history.

Asperger

As fate would have it, Hans Asperger (1906–1980) was exploring a similar avenue of nosology and diagnosis in Vienna at the same time that Kanner was conducting his research on autism in Baltimore. Asperger's first paper on the topic appeared in 1944 in a German language scientific journal. Interestingly, he also used the term autism in his diagnosis (autistic psychopathy). Asperger described four boys he had observed as "little professors" since they were deeply absorbed in highly specific topics on which they were extremely knowledgeable. He also noted that the children used one sided communication, had few friends, evinced clumsy motor skills, and lacked empathy. However, as noted, his work was written in German and was published during the final stages of World War II and the ensuing chaos that occurred in post war Germany. Thus, for many years people knew of Kanner's discoveries but not Asperger's. Asperger's work was rediscovered and translated into English in the early 1980s. With the rediscovery of Asperger's syndrome has faced some controversy. The last two decades have seen a debate about whether Asperger's Syndrome was separate from persons with autism but without ID, also referred to as high functioning autism (HFA) in the literature. The general consensus, although some prominent experts disagree, is that the two disorders are distinct. Asperger's Syndrome appears to have a much later onset, and there is some variation in symptom patterns between the disorders.

The fifth of the five ASD is Rett Syndrome, named after the man who identified the disorder, Andreas Rett (1924–1997). He attended medical school at the University of Innsbruck, but did not finish until 1949 because of a stint in German navy during World War II. A pediatrician by training, he became a lecturer in neurology and pediatrics at the University of Vienna in 1967. At that point, he also became the head of the Ludwig Boltzmann Institute for Research in Brain Disordered Children. Prior to that, he ran a hospital for disabled children and, in 1954, he noticed two young girls in his waiting room engaged in a number of ritualistic hand washing behaviors. Upon further review of his case load, four other girls with similar physical features and motor behaviors were identified. His first paper on the topic was published in 1966 but, as with Asperger's work, was little noticed at the time because it appeared in German. The disorder received its name, Rett Syndrome, in 1983 when a Swedish physician named Bengt Hagberg, published the first paper in English. He used Rett Syndrome to honor the person who discovered the disorder. In 1999, Rett Syndrome became the first ASD to have its genetic code broken. A research team from Baylor University found $MECP^2$, the gene which causes Rett Syndrome when it mutates. The gene is located on the Xq28 site of the X chromosome. This finding further underscored the neurodevelopmental origins of ASD. This etiology is in stark contrast to the psychodynamic formulations of Bruno Bettelheim, an Austrian trained art historian who directed a home for emotional and developmentally impaired children associated with the University of Chicago. Bettelheim argued that cold and emotionally detached parents were the cause of the disorder. Of course the data does not support these claims. Furthermore, the success of ABA as an intervention, has further discredited these theories.

ABA and ASD

Witmer stressed the fact that clinical psychology was based on the foundations established in experimental psychology. In much the same way, the ABA has built upon the experimental analysis of behavior. The proliferation of journals and research in general makes it nearly impossible to select just one journal which has popularized ABA. ABA has been so successful that many journals now devote all or a large portion of their space to ABA articles (e.g., *Behavior Modification, Behaviour Research and Therapy, Behavior Therapy, Behavioral Interventions, Journal of Child and Adolescent Behavior Therapy, Education and Treatment of Children, Journal of Applied Behavior Analysis, Journal of Positive Behavioral Supports, Research in Developmental Disabilities,* and *Research in Autism Spectrum Disorders*). This trend is particularly true for developmental disabilities, communication disorders, special education and rehabilitation psychology. For example, the major journal publishing companies such as Elsevier and Springer list 51 journals in the rehabilitation field alone.

JEAB

The 1950s and 1960s were a simpler time with regard to the proliferation of journals. Therefore,s, it is easier to establish one journal that was the precursor of EBA, much in the way that Watson and Skinner are considered as individual researchers who influenced the field. The journal was the *Journal of the Experimental Analysis of Behavior* (JEAB). This publication was started as a private enterprise. The Society for the Experimental Analysis of Behavior (SEAB) was formed out of the legal necessity for a journal to be owned by an agency or business (Hineline & Laties, 2006). As these authors note, behaviorally oriented researchers lamented the lack of acceptance f of their research methods and theories. The senior author of this chapter had similar first hand experiences of this sort. He recalls having an article submitted to a prominent journal in developmental disabilities being returned without review. The editor simply noted that "you behaviorists should have your own journals."

C.B. Ferster, a Ph.D., who received his training in psychology at Columbia University and who later worked for 5 years in Skinner's lab at Harvard became the first editor of JEAB. Ferster is credited by many as the one person most responsible for the establishment of the journal. On April 2, 1957 at the Eastern Psychological Association annual convention, he and a number of colleagues, including Peter Dews, Nat Schoenfeld and Murray Sidman, began the launch of JEAB. Seed money to start the journal ironically came from nine pharmaceutical companies who were interested in further

developing the new field of behavioral pharmacology (see Laties, 2008 for a more detailed description of those developments). The new journal was very crucial for the soon to develop field of ABA. The notion of small N research, with no inferential statistics, operationally defined target behaviors (overtly observable), multiple sessions for each organism tested, and a focus on the further development of rules of learning were just some of the benefits. Furthermore, the initiation of JEAB gave legitimacy to the fledgling field, a great opportunity for dissemination of information on the experimental analysis of behavior, and gave encouragement to young investigators interested in the topic.

JEAB was an immediate success and within a few years had 2,000 subscribers. Originally, the journal was published at the Department of Psychology at Indiana University (remember Skinner had been department chair there) and later moved to the University of Rochester. For many years, JEAB published primarily animal research. Rats and pigeons were largely the object of these studies. In recent years, a mix of human and animal studies has been reported., Animal labs are becoming increasingly more expensive. This factor is largely a result of increasing regulations that require external support for such research. National funding agencies such as the National Institute of Health, Institute of Mental Health and National Institute of Child Health and Human Development have traditionally and to this day been tending to fund basic and applied researchers in the biological sciences. These agencies are operated almost exclusively by physicians, who favor research in pharmacology, genetic and other medical subfields. The bias against EAB research by these agencies has made obtaining external funding difficult. This situation may also explain the inordinate amount of funding for research and the disproportionate number of publications of papers in ASD on medical topics (i.e., genetics, physiology) despite the fact that the greatest treatment breakthroughs for ASD to date have involved ABA (Matson & LoVullo, 2008).

Ferster and DeMeyer

While basic behavioral research was, and continues to be, a viable interest area for investigators, the bulk of the published studies rapidly shifted to ABA research. Ferster and DeMeyer (1961) reported on one of the first ABA studies on autism with children. Their stated goal was to extend the range of appropriate skills of these children from what they described as a very restrictive repertoire. They hypothesized that complex tasks could be taught by gradually increasing task complexity as more rudimentary skills were acquired. Furthermore, they note that "durable" reinforcers would need to be identified if this goal was to be achieved. What they describe would later be labeled by various terms. Pivotal responses is one of the more commonly used terms today. Ferster and DeMeyer note that skills once taught in a controlled laboratory setting could then be used to "investigate many aspects of the autistic repertoire which have heretofore been inaccessible" (p. 313). Ferster and DeMeyer taught four children, an 8 year old boy and a 9.5 year old girl with autism, and two matched regularly developing controls. Reinforcers used were foods of various types including candy, and trinkets in the initial stages of treatment. Later in the study, coins were substituted. These coins could then be exchanged for preferred items. The authors chose key pressing as the target behavior. Their rationale was that the response took little time or effort to execute (presumably making the skill easier to teach and, because key pressing could be done quickly, allowing for many learning trials in a short period of time). Furthermore, they lay stress on the reliability of data recording and note that they were able to connect the key to an automated tabulating device. This approach resulted in highly accurate frequency counts. The study proved to be a success. Ferster and DeMeyer's (1961) study was soon followed by the rapid establishment of ABA as a credible treatment and assessment technology.

BRAT

As noted, considerable frustration began to develop as more and more researchers started producing research papers on behavioral methods. The obvious outcome of this pressure was the impetus to establish more outlets devoted specifically to the topic. The first journal to appear was a British journal, *Behaviour Research and Therapy* (BRAT) based at the Maudsley Clinical of the University of London. The first volume appeared in 1963. Notable papers for those interested in ABA, which were published that first year were: (1) A.J. Yates

paper *Recent Empirical and Theoretical Approaches to the Experimental Manipulation of Speech in Normal Subjects and in Stammerers*; (2) S.H. Lovibond on *Intermittent Reinforcement in Behaviour Therapy*; (3) D.H. Neale's *Behaviour Therapy and Encopresis in Children*; (4) M. Wolf, T. Risley and H. Mees work entitled *Application of Operant Conditioning Procedures to the Behaviour Problems of an Autistic Child*; and (5) C.G. Costello on *Behavioural Therapy: Criticisms and Confusions*.

Wolf, Risley, and Mees

Wolf , Risley, and Mees (1964) in their BRAT article start by noting that in the decade preceding this particular paper, experimental analysis of behavior had produced powerful and reliable methods to change behavior. They use cumulative graphs on tantrums, severe self-destruction, and bedtime problems of an autistic 3.5 year boy. Treatment included extinction and a mild punisher in the form of time-out. The child in the study, Dicky, did not eat normally, according to the authors, and lacked social and verbal repertoires. Head-banging, hair-pulling, face slapping and face scratching characterized his tantrums, and resulted in large surface areas that were black and blue. Further complicating the picture was his third target behavior, bedtime problems. This behavior pattern consisted of his inability to sleep at night, resulting in one or both parents having to remain by his bed at night. Previous interventions included sedative and tranquilizing drugs, and restraint As a result of all these difficulties, he had been placed in a mental hospital.

Goals of intervention included decelerating the three main problem behaviors just described and teaching him to wear his glasses. According to Wolf et al. (1964), Dick's ophthalmologist predicted that failure to begin wearing his glasses within the next 6 months would result is the child losing his macular vision. For tantrums, the authors rightly pointed out that extinction alone would likely be ineffective since ward staff of the hospital were not trained in the methods and would have difficulty in carrying out the methods of treatment.. Thus, treatment involved putting Dicky in his room when tantrums erupted, and his door was kept closed until the tantrum stopped. By month 3 of the intervention, tantrums of 5 min duration or less were common, leading to a policy of time-outs that were, at a minimum, 10 min in length to offset the social reinforcement associated with staff escorting him to his room. Parents then began to assist in training at the hospital, on early recognition for the need to promote generalization. These visits started as 1 h per week but rapidly accelerated in frequency.

For bedtime problems, Dicky was cuddled briefly, and then put to bed with the door open. If Dicky got out of bed, he was prompted to return and told if he did not do so his door would be closed. According to the authors, when the door was closed it was re-opened after a "short time," or after a tantrum subsided.

Generalization was also part of moving him back home once marked improvement in his challenging behaviors was noted. For a number of days prior to hospital discharge, Dicky made short home visits alone with hospital staff. His first night at home, an attendant stayed to assist his parents. Wolf et al. (1964) report that after being put to bed, Dicky was heard humming to himself. When Mom started for Dicky's room, the attendant stopped her. The authors report that within the next 15 min, Dicky had fallen asleep and no further nighttime issues occurred. An increasing number of nights were spent at home until discharge 3 months later.

Shaping was used as a primary means to teach Dicky to wear his glasses. To condition the click of a toy noisemaker, the sound was paired with bites of candy or fruit during two or three daily 20 min sessions. Soon, Dicky learned that when the clicker was detonated to go on his own and take an edible from the fruit/candy bowl. Training started with frames for the glasses only as the authors conjectured that the change in visual stimuli from the glasses might be mildly be aversive. Five weeks of this treatment with various modifications proved ineffective. Finally, after modifying prescription glasses and withholding breakfast and lunch, then using bites of the meal at about 2:00pm, they got cooperation. After this, progress occurred rapidly, and very soon, Dicky began to wear his glasses all the time during meals. After wearing his glasses was established, the researchers were able to maintain the behavior without resorting to a reinforcement schedule. If however, he removed his glasses during meals, snacks, automobile rides, walks, outdoor play or other activities, the activity was terminated. By discharge, he was wearing his glasses all the time. The authors conclude their article by stating that

6 months after discharge, Dicky continues to wear his glasses, has no tantrums or destruction, or sleep problems. Additionally, it is noted that he was becoming increasingly verbal.

We have spent a good deal of space on this paper because we believe it helps establish that investigators were seeing the value of ABA in the treatment of multiple behaviors of ASD children. Furthermore, this article highlights the important role BRAT has played in the early beginnings of ABA. Finally, food deprivation at the time described here would not be acceptable today. However, for a paper that is now 45 years old, many of the features of their training are still remarkable up to date. The focus on decelerating and teaching multiple behaviors at once, involving parents in training, programming for generalization, and the use of shaping, reinforcement and mild punishers such as time-out in the child's room are still relevant today.

Costello

In *Behavioural Therapy: Criticisms and Confusions*, Costello takes on what traditional therapy advocates had been contending to be the downfall of behavioral methods, symptom substitution. As briefly mentioned earlier in the chapter, the argument that behavioral treatments were superficial and did not address the underlying disorder was made by ABA opponents. Thus, if a symptom or maladaptive behavior was eliminated, then another symptom or maladaptive behavior would pop up. Looking back from the vantage point of many years and thousands of successful behavioral treatment studies, this argument seems quite out of step with current practices and theories. However, in the 1960s and 1970s there were many heated exchanges on the subject. Costello quotes the editor of BRAT Hans Eysenck at the time in his article.. Eysenck famously pointed out the behavioral position in the bluntest of terms. "There is no neurosis underlying the symptoms but merely the symptom itself. Get rid of symptoms and you have eliminated the neurosis" (Eysenck, 1960). Another of Eysenck's positions was that traditional therapy was not any better than no therapy at all. He asserted that 1/3 would get better, 1/3 would get worse and 1/3 would see no change with psychotherapy or with nothing.

Eysenck

Hans Eysenck (1916–1997) was something of a character, and a prolific scholar as well, with over 900 publications. Till he time of his death, he was the most cited psychologist, living.. Born Hans Jürgen Eysenck in Berlin to German film and stage celebrities, he migrated to England in the 1930s during the rise of Nazi, Germany. He received his Ph.D. in psychology from the University College London under the mentorship of Cyril Burt. He was once punched in the nose during a talk he was giving at the London School of Economics. Very opinionated, he could bring out the best and the worst in people, as this punching incident shows. In his autobiography, *Rebel with a Cause* (Eysenck, 1997) he wrote the following:

> I always felt that science owes the world only one thing, and that is the truth as he sees it. If the truth contradicts deeply held beliefs, that is too bad. Tact and diplomacy are fine in international relations, in politics, perhaps even in business; in science only one thing matters, and that is the facts (p. 119).

He had a sense of humor that is displayed in the title of some of his works: *Decline and Fall of the Freudian Empire, ...I Do! Your Happy Guide to Marriage, Suggestion and Suggestibility, Crime and Personality* (Obviously he liked to play off titles of popular books and movies: *Rebel without a Cause, Decline and Fall of the Roman Empire, Sense and Sensibility, Crime and Punishment,* etc.). Clearly, however, he caught people's attention, and he did a great deal to advance the cause of behaviorally based assessments and treatments.

JABA

For many in the field of ABA, the journal they are most familiar with is the *Journal of Applied Behavior Analysis* (JABA). Nathan H. Azrin, a graduate of Harvard who received his Ph.D. under the direction of B.F. Skinner, was commissioned to determine if an applied journal on behavior analysis would be feasible and popular. Azrin was a significant transition figure in the move from the laboratory to applied settings. Trained in the experimental analysis of behavior, he shifted his work to applied issues largely in the area of developmental disabilities. Also, he had just served as

editor of JEAB when he began his "needs evaluation" for an ABA journal in 1967. Montrose W. Wolfe, a professor in the Department of Human Development at the University of Kansas, was named the first editor of JABA. Wolfe co-authored one of the first papers on ABA with autism as previously discussed.

Azrin

Azrin was a major supporter of the new journal, publishing many ground breaking studies on the developmentally disabled population (primarily adults) at Anna State Hospital in Anna, Illinois. Many of these persons would now be classified as ASD based on current diagnostic criteria. Azrin developed treatment methods such as overcorrection, and with Ted Ayllon, developed successful token economy systems for this population. A variety of skills were taught including toileting, dressing and slowing rapid eating. Other papers were written, which reported on ABA methods to decelerate aggression, nail biting, floor sprawling, habitual vomiting, stuttering, stealing, and stereotypies. It is hard to overstate the importance or value of these studies conducted by Azrin and associates in demonstrating the efficacy of ABA or in drawing young investigators to the field. The first author (Matson) considers this body of research by Azrin as the single most important factor in attracting him to a career in behavior psychology research and practice. Additionally, it should be noted that the range of topics covered was important and it also pointed out the wide array of problems that could be solved with this technology.

JABA, like BRAT, was a success from the start. It continues to be a leader in the publication of papers on ABA. BRAT, on the other hand, has moved more into the cognitive behavior therapy paradigm in recent years. The same can be said for the *Journal of Behavior Therapy and Experimental Psychiatry* founded in 1970. Initially, articles were with one to three participants using single case designs. However, as noted earlier, there are now many journals that publish ABA papers. And, we are of the opinion that BRAT and other journals which have drifted away from content on ABA a bit, underscore yet another important advancement. These trends demonstrate the continuing expansion and influence of learning based methods.

Lovaas

The name most associated with ABA research in ASD in the early years of its application has, to the minds of many, been Ole Ivar Lovaas. A professor of psychology at UCLA, like Eysenck, he has been a controversial figure. And like Skinner, Lovaas was able to capture the general public's attention with some of his research and clinical practice. One of the most influential pieces in his career was an article published in *Life Magazine* in 1965 which would be the equivalent of a major piece on one of the prime time TV newsmagazine programs today. The article was titles *Screams, Slaps and Love: A Surprising Shocking Treatment Helps Far-Gone Mental Cripple*s. And, of course the treatment procedures described in this article were one of the major controversies to embroil Lovaas. Taken in the context of 1965, being able to effectively treat children with ASD was still a relatively new phenomenon. Thus, despite the draconian methods of treatment described in the article, Lovaas and his methods were generally well received. We have described two studies on the topics of ABA research with ASD, but such publications were still a trickle at the time. The *Life Magazine* article describes "enraged bellows" by an adult therapist at an autistic boy, and "slaps to the face." The article describes Lovaas' most drastic innovation of these punishment methods, the contingent shock room, which was used as a last resort. Shocks could be remotely applied to the child's back via small electrodes for engaging in stereotyped and ritualistic behaviors. The article also stresses how patience and tenderness were lavished on the children by staff. Rewards including food and approval were given along with 10 min breaks every hour for "affectionate play." The piece ends on a generally favorable view of the program, describing the improvements in the children as a tremendous accomplishment. Furthermore, in the article, it is reported that parents could not deal with their children's problems on their own, and thus were very happy with the assistance offered. They were very supportive of Lovaas and his program.

Lovaas was distinct from many other researchers in ABA in that his efforts were exclusively with autism, and he continued to work in the area for over four decades. Second, the focus was on comprehensive interventions (treating multiple target behaviors across multiple domains), while most other ABA researchers were emphasizing one or two specific target behaviors or problems in a given study. In this context, the research of Azrin was more consistent with the norm of the time. This philosophy of treatment, employed by Lovaas, led to a second controversy and a popular trend in interventions in the area of ASD, namely 'Early Intensive Behavioral Interventions' (EIBI).

While ABA has now been popular for over four decades, as with any field, there are a few topics which garner the greatest amount of attention. At the time of this writing, two areas are being researched and discussed more than any of the other topics in ABA. These are EIBI and functional assessment. This latter topic will be discussed in more detail later. However, first a brief history of EIBI.

EIBI

The first study we could identify that dealt specifically with EIBI was published by Lovaas, Koegel, Simmons, and Long (1973). The study was essentially a narrative description of several cases. Most importantly however, these authors laid out the fundamental notion of a comprehensive treatment model for young autistic children across a range of target behaviors including stereotypies, echolalia, appropriate verbal behavior, social behaviors, appropriate play, I.Q. and general adaptive behavior measures. The formula was to be repeated by Lovaas and others, and was to take existing ABA methods, put them in a package, and treat a broad range of positive skills the child needed to acquire while decelerating various challenging behaviors all at the same time. Various authors have since published EIBI interventions emphasizing different ABA procedures, using either parents or professionals or both as trainers, employing different settings, for different lengths of time per week (typically 20–40 h). However, the core elements of the Lovaas et al., study can be found in all of these intervention programs.

The best known and most controversial of the EIBI studies, in our view, is Lovaas, 1987. Participants averaged 32 months of age in the experimental group and 35 months of age for controls. The intensive ABA group of 19 children received 40 h of one to one training a week for 2 years or more while the less intensive ABA control group received one to one treatment for 10 h a week also for 2 years or more. In a nutshell, the more intensive intervention produced better effects and Lovaas claimed he has cured autism in the intense treatment group with 47% attaining normal functioning. Needless to say, controversy ensued. Clients were not randomly assigned with the most motivated families being in the intensive group. Similarly, the claims of cure were challenging and on the whole, others have not been able to replicate Lovaas' results (Mudford, Martin, Eikeseth, & Bibby, 2001). Having said this, while Lovaas' claims may have been a bit overenthusiastic, there have been enough gains demonstrated in replication studies to demonstrate benefits. This conclusion is possible despite the fact that most EIBI studies have had substantial methodological shortcomings. The number of papers published to date which have shown effects, although perhaps not cure, lead to the conclusion that EIBI can be very beneficial, at least for a substantial number of young children with ASD (Matson & Smith, 2008). However, one size does not fit all, and that is the (aq)??severity of ASD, the co-occurrence of ID or co morbid psychopathology, age of the child when identified, and resources and family commitment may all dictate various types and intensities of EIBI treatments. So, the final judgment in our view is that EIBI is a powerful, exciting, and important advance in the treatment of ASD. However, the problems with the technology, which at this part are largely a function of major gaps that still exist in our knowledge of the procedures, need to be acknowledged. Furthermore, overhyping any procedure can do it harm in the long run since living up to expectations can be problematic. It is our view that a cautious but optimistic approach will be the most effective for advancing EIBI in the long run.

FA and EFA

The second big issue in ABA in recent years has been the advent of functional assessment (FA). FA was developed to identify and maintain variables in the environment. First established as experimental functional assessment (EFA), rating scales, scatterplots and other methods have also been added to the methodology. Some experts have debated about the authors who employed these methods first. Some of the names that have been mentioned are Montrose Wolfe and Edward

Carr (Matson & Minshawi, 2007). However, it is clear that Brian Iwata, a professor of psychology at the University of Florida, Gainesville is the person who has published the most on the topic, and is associated with its great popularity. He and his associates have been the most responsible for the refinement of EFA methods. The most cited paper on the topics, and the one which helped launch the technology into widespread use was the Iwata, Dorsey, Slifer, Bauman, and Richman (1982) paper. In their study, the authors describe the use of operant methods to establish environmental events that maintain their challenging behaviors such as self-injury and aggression. The Iwata et al. paper utilizes nine adults with developmental disabilities and self-injury. Separate experimental conditions of play materials present or absent, demands to engage in tasks or activities being presented at high vs. low rates, and social attention when it was either absent, non contingent or contingent. The condition that produced the highest rates of self-injury would thus give the clinician clues about what was causing the challenging behavior, and how contingencies could be altered to decelerate these behaviors. With some modifications, most of the Iwata et al. study's components have been employed in the EFA literature. Most of the EFA research papers include two to four participants. As of 2003 (see Hanley, Iwata, & McCord, 2003), 277 research papers had been published on the topic, with 180 of these appearing in JABA.

The EFA is a powerful technology, and some experts argue that it should be used exclusively as the means of identifying and maintaining variables of challenging behaviors. However, in practice, most efforts using EFA has been in research laboratories and university settings The biggest issue with EFA is the amount of time required to implement the technology. This issue has led to the development of FA checklists that can be completed in minutes vs. many hours. The best researched of these FA checklists to date is the Questions About Behavior Function (QABF; Matson & Vollmer, 1995).

Certification

One of the big problems that has confronted ABA in recent years is that the technology has rapidly surpassed the ability of professionals to implement the large need. This issue is no better exemplified than in ASD. ABA has rapidly proven to be the treatment of choice. As we have noted, with ASD you have a high incidence of very serious disorder that requires intensive remediation at a very young age. A major development in helping to meet this need has been the development of the Behavior Analyst Certification Board (BACB). While some masters and doctoral programs in psychology, special education and communication disorder do an excellent job of preparing their students in this area, unfortunately most do not. Thus, it has been noted that severe shortages in professionals who can deliver quality services has developed (Shook & Neisworth, 2005). BACB is a nonprofit corporation established in 1998 to meet certification needs identified by consumers such as state governments. They have continued to update certification tests and standards based on job analysis and input from experts in ABA.

There have been a number of people who have played a n key role in the development of these standards. The most influential of these has been Gerry Shook, a Ph.D. psychologist in Tallahassee, Florida. He has been instrumental in getting this huge effort off the ground. BACB accreditation has gained steadily in popularity to the point that California, Florida, Texas, Pennsylvania, New York, and Oklahoma have transferred their certification responsibilities to the BACB national office, according to their website. The BACB credentialing occurs at over 200 sites nationally and 150 sites internationally. There are approximately 5,300 BACB professionals certified at this time, with a projected increase of about 1,000 additional BACB certified professionals for each year into the foreseeable future.

Overview

The field of ABA has grown from very humble beginnings with the initial influence of German experimental psychology, followed by Witmer, Watson, and Skinner as transition figures. They brought the notions of a science of human behavior to the United States which continues to be the epicenter for ABA research worldwide. Having said that, there have been expansions of the field as it has spread to many countries. A major impetus for grass roots acceptance and the spread of ABA has been enhanced markedly by the phenomenal worldwide interest in ASD. This interest has expanded at an amazing rate with no end in sight. The expansion in interest has been across a wide range of disciplines, which in turn, we predict, will help expand the popularity of ABA. Our crystal ball tells us to look for new developments in the areas of treatment and training of ASD adults, expansions of communication based ABA procedures such as the Picture Exchange Communication Program (PECS), and in the area of Vocal Output Communication Aids (VOCA). Furthermore, federal and state mandates, to provide services to ASD children will dramatically expand ABA practices. As just one example, the Louisiana State Legislature just passed a bill allowing ABA treatments of ASD coverage under health insurance. Developments such as these will lead to dramatic expansion of programs on early identification and early treatment. Along these lines, the authors are involved in the Louisiana Early Steps Initiative which screens all 18–30 month old children statewide who are at risk for ASD and other developmental disabilities. At this writing, over 100 evaluators are involved in the project and over 2,000 children will be screened yearly.

ABA methods, especially FA, behaviorally based reinforcement programs and deceleration methods have proven to be the bread and butter treatments for the challenging behaviors of children with ASD (Matson, Bernavidez, Compton, Paclawskyj, & Baglio, 1996). More emphasis on these effective treatments and the application of these methods to comorbid psychopathology in ASD such as obsessive compulsive disorder are likely to see marked development and expansion in years to come. This book then, which reviews the research on ABA for persons with ASD, would appear to be timely, and hopefully can be another brick in the scientific wall that leads to a better means of assisting the individual child with ASD.

References

Beers, C. (1908). *A mind that found itself*. New York: Longmans, Green.

Boring, E. G. (1950). *History of experimental psychology* (2nd ed.). New York: Appleton – Century-Crofts.

Cover Johnes, M. (1924). A laboratory study of fear: The case of Peter. *Pedogogical Seminary, 31*, 308–315.

Eysenck, H. J. (ed). (1960). *Behaviour therapy and the neurosis*. New York: Pergaman Press.

Eysenck, H. J. (1997). *Rebel with a cause: The autobiography of Hans Eysenck*. Edison, N. J.: Transaction Publications.

Ferster, C. B., & DeMeyer, M. K. (1961). The development of performances in autistic children in an automatically controlled environment. *Journal of Chronic Disease, 13*, 312–345.

Fombonne, E. (1999). The epidemiology of autism. A review. *Psychological Medicine, 29*, 769–786.

Hanley, G. P., Iwata, B. A., & McCord, B. E. (2003). Functional analysis of problem behavior: A review. *Journal of Applied Behavior Analysis, 36*, 147–185.

Hineline, P. N., & Laties, V. G. (2006). Society for the experimental analysis of behavior. *Society for the Experimental Analysis of Behavior Newsletter, 29*, 1–3.

Iwata, B. A., Dorsey, M. F., Slifer, K. J., Bauman, K. E., & Richman, G. S. (1982). Toward a functional assessment of self-injury. *Journal of Applied Behavior Analysis, 27*, 197–209.

Kanner, L. (1943). Autistic disturbances of affective contact. *Nervous Child, 2*, 217–250.

Labrador, F. J. (2004). Skinner and the rise of behavior modification and behavior therapy. *The Spanish Journal of Psychology, 7*, 178–187.

Laties, V. G. (2008). The journal of the experimental analysis of behavior at fifty. *Journal of Experimental Analysis of Behavior, 89*, 89–95.

Lovaas, O. I. (1987). Behavioral treatment and normal educational and intellectual functioning in young autistic children. *Journal of Consulting and Clinical Psychology, 55*, 3–9.

Lovaas, O. I., Koegel, R., Simmons, J. Q., & Long, J. S. (1973). Some generalization and follow-up measures on autistic children in behavior therapy. *Journal of Applied Behavior Analysis, 6*, 131–166.

Magnusson, P., & Saemundsen, E. (2001). Prevalence of autism in Iceland. *Journal of Autism and Developmental Disorders, 31*, 153–163.

Matson, J. L., Benavidez, D. A., Compton, L. S., Paclawskyj, T. R., & Baglio, C. S. (1996). Behavioral treatment of autistic persons: A review of research from 1980 to the present. *Research in Developmental Disabilities, 17*, 433–466.

Matson, J. L., & LoVullo, S. V. (2008). Trends and topics in autism spectrum disorders research. *Research in Autism Spectrum Disorders,* . doi:10.1016/j.rasd.2008.06.005.

Matson, J. L., & Minshawi, N. F. (2007). Functional assessment of challenging behavior: Toward a strategy for applied settings. *Research in Developmental Disabilities, 28*, 353–361.

Matson, J. L., & Smith, K. R. M. (2008). Current status of intensive behavioral interventions for young children with autism and PDDNOS. *Research in Autism Spectrum Disorders, 2*, 60–74.

Matson, J. L., & Vollmer, T. (1995). *Questions about behavior function (QABF)*. Baton Rouge, LA: DisabilityConsultants. org.

Mudford, O. C., Martin, N. T., Eikeseth, S., & Bibby, P. (2001). Parent-management behavioral treatment for pre-school children with autism: Some characteristics of UK programs. *Research in Developmental Disabilities, 22*, 173–182.

Shook, G. L., & Neisworth, J. T. (2005). Ensuring appropriate qualifications for applied behavior analyst professionals: The Behavior Analyst Certification Board. *Exceptionality, 13*, 3–10.

Skinner, B. F. (1948). *Walden two*. New York: Prentice Hall.

Skinner, B. F. (1976). *Walden revisited*. New York: MacMillon.

Watson, J. B. (1919). *Psychology from the standpoint of a behaviorist*. Philadelphia and London: J. B. Lippincott Co.

Watson, J. B., & Rayner, R. (1920). Conditioned emotional reactions. *Journal of Experimental Psychology, 3*, 1–14.

Witmer, L. (1907). Clinical psychology. *Psychological Clinic, 1*, 1–9.

Wolf, M. M., Risley, T. R., & Mees, H. L. (1964). Application of operant conditioning procedures to the behaviour problems of an autistic child. *Behavior Research and Therapy, 1*, 305–312.

Chapter 2
Applied Behavior Analysis and Its Application to Autism and Autism Related Disorders

Joel E. Ringdahl, Todd Kopelman, and Terry S. Falcomata

This chapter will be basic foundations. The theory behind operant conditioning will be the first part of the chapter. Next terms and concepts will be reviewed such as reinforcement, shaping, etc. The presentation of these concepts will include applications to autism. The chapter will conclude with current developments in theory (e.g., functional assessment, positive behavioral supports)

Introduction

Along with the rising prevalence of autism spectrum disorders, there has been a heightened focus on identifying treatments that address the symptoms underlying these disorders in the USA. These symptoms can be grossly categorized into two areas: (1) Behaviors of excess including vocal and motor stereotypies, echoic speech, and rigidity, and (2) behaviors of deficit such as delays in the areas of communication, peer relations, and independent functioning. Many of the behavioral hallmarks of autism have been addressed through strategies based on applied behavior analysis (ABA). This chapter will provide an overview of ABA, including its basic foundations and a discussion of relevant terms and concepts. Several examples from the scientific literature will be described to illustrate how ABA has been used to evaluate and treat the core symptoms associated with autism. At the conclusion of the chapter, we will briefly discuss current developments

and future directions in the application of ABA within the field of autism.

In depth coverage of each of the topics will not be possible given the space limitations of a chapter. Readers are encouraged to independently delve further into the literature, using the cited studies, texts, and chapters referenced in the following pages.

Conceptual Basis and Foundation of Applied Behavior Analysis

Applied behavior analysis (ABA) as a science was established in the early second half of the twentieth century as an approach to the evaluation and selection of change of human behavior based on the operant conditioning principles most famously championed by B. F. Skinner. Operant conditioning can be defined as the process through which the environment and behavior interact to shape the behavioral repertoire of an organism or individual (Skinner, 1953). By 1968, ABA had gained enough of a following in the scientific community that a journal was established (*Journal of Applied Behavior Analysis or JABA*) to publish empirical studies related to the applied behavior analysis of human responding. In the inaugural issue of *JABA*, Baer, Wolf, and Risley (1968) published an article outlining the defining characteristics of ABA. Baer et al. drew a distinction between applied behavior analysis and similar laboratory analysis. Three minimally defining characteristics of ABA were obvious: applied, behavioral, and analytic. Four other defining features were also suggested by Baer et al. Specifically, ABA should be technological, conceptually systematic, effective, and "display some generality" (p. 92).

J.E. Ringdahl (✉)
Department of Pediatrics, Division of Pediatric Psychology, Children's Hospital of Iowa, Center for Disabilities and Development, 100 Hawkins Drive, Iowa City, IA, 5222427011, USA
e-mail: joel-ringdahl@uiowa.edu

J.L. Matson (ed.), *Applied Behavior Analysis for Children with Autism Spectrum Disorders*, DOI 10.1007/978-1-4419-0088-3_2, © Springer Science+Business Media, LLC 2009

In the behavioral context, Baer et al. (1968) established *applied* to mean that the behavior or stimulus addressed was chosen because of its importance to humankind and society, rather than its importance to theory. In addition, the applied nature of the behavior or stimulus of interest should be determined by its context, and should be closely related to the subject being studied. For example, from a laboratory perspective, eating might be a behavior of interest due to its general relationship to metabolism. However, from an applied perspective, eating is a behavior of interest if that behavior is being studied to address individuals who eat too little or too much (Baer et al.). Thus, the range of behavior and stimuli appropriate for applied study can vary widely. Similarly, the range of individuals appropriate for applied study can vary widely.

Behavioral means that the focus should be on what individuals can be brought to do, rather than what they can be brought to say (Baer et al., 1968). Given that behavior is a physical event, its study (or close monitoring) requires precise measurement. Thus, in any ABA program, a method by which the behavior of interest will be measured and that which is reliable and agreed upon by multiple observers must be established. There must be a clear answer to the question regarding whose behavior changed, the observer or the observed. For example, observer drift can result in an apparent change in behavior. However, the change is not due to the behavior of the target individual, but to the measurement behavior of the observer. Calculating interobserver agreement (IOA) is a method by which behavior analysts attempt to demonstrate that the change in behavior is attributable to the individual observed, and not the observers. Several strategies exist to measure IOA. While the exact calculations differ, each strategy requires that multiple, independent observers observe the same situations either simultaneously or via video recordings. For a detailed description of IOA, its benefits, and methods for calculating, the reader is directed to Cooper, Heron, and Heward, Chap. 5.

Analytic refers to the notion that ABA requires a believable demonstration of the events responsible for the behavior. An analysis of behavior has been achieved when an experimenter (scientist, parent, teacher, care provider) can exercise control over the behavior (Baer et al., 1968). Because of this characteristic, demonstrations of ABA are often conducted using some sort of single-subject research design. Baer et al. specifically mentioned two types of designs in their seminal

article: reversal and multiple baseline. Reversal designs consist of measuring a behavior in the absence of the variable of interest until steady state responding is achieved. At that point, the variable of interest is applied and its effect on behavior is again measured. If a change is observed, the variable is discontinued or altered (Baer et al.). When the behavior returns to the previous level, the variable is applied again. Multiple baseline designs are used when behavior is likely to be irreversible (e.g., riding a bicycle) or when a reversal is undesirable (Baer et al.). A multiple baseline evaluation consists of establishing two or more baselines and introducing the independent variable in a sequential manner across the baselines (Kennedy, 2005). Both design strategies allow for a demonstration of prediction and control related to the behavior of interest. (For a comprehensive handling of the various designs employed in ABA, the reader is directed to the text on single-case experimental designs by Kennedy).

ABA's emphasis on *technological* means that the "techniques making up a particular behavioral application are completely identified and described" (p. 95). This characteristic is an attempt to ensure that examples of ABA can be reliably replicated by those reading the account (Baer et al., 1968.).

Conceptually systematic highlights ABA's relevance to principle. This characteristic is meant to tie the technological descriptions to basic principles of behavior analysis. For example, Baer et al. (1968) suggested that describing "exactly how a preschool teacher will attend to jungle-gym climbing in a child frightened by heights is good technological description; but further to call it a social reinforcement procedure relates it to basic concepts of behavioral development" (p. 96).

ABA should also be *effective*. That is, the behavioral techniques should produce large enough effects to be of practical value (Baer et al., 1968). In addition, the behavior change resulting from ABA should be durable over time, across a variety of settings, and/or spread to related behavior. That is, the change should have *generality*.

These characteristics help to define ABA as a methodology that can be used to select change, and evaluate human behavior. It is important to note that, in the context of this chapter, ABA does not refer to a specific package designed to address the challenges of autism spectrum disorders. Rather, ABA refers to the conceptual framework upon which multiple approaches are based.

Concepts and Application

A number of treatments have been identified that address the social, communicative, and behavioral deficits and excesses exhibited by many individuals with an autism spectrum diagnosis. In this section, several of the ABA concepts upon which those treatments are derived will be defined and discussed. These concepts, along with treatment examples from the literature, have been separated into consequence-based and antecedent-based approaches. In addition, combined treatments (e.g., one antecedent and one consequence, or two or more of each), as well as a brief description of some packaged approaches, will be reviewed.

Consequence: Punishment and Punishment-Based Procedures

Punishment procedures are those consequence-based procedures that decrease the future likelihood of the target behavior. There are two broad classes of punishment: positive punishment and negative punishment. Both classes of procedures result in the decreased likelihood of future target behavior. The difference comes in the presentation or removal of a stimulus. In a positive punishment program, an aversive stimulus is presented (positive = presented) contingent on the target behavior and results in a decreased likelihood of future responding. In a negative punishment program, a stimulus is removed (negative = removed) contingent on the target behavior, likewise resulting in a decreased likelihood of future responding.

Positive Punishment

The contingent presentation of aversive stimuli (i.e., positive punishment) has been largely reduced as effective reinforcer assessment technologies have emerged (e.g., functional analysis of problem behavior). Historic examples of positive punishment programs include the use of electric shocks, water mist, aversive tastes, and physical holds. In cases where positive punishment strategies are currently used, their inclusion in a treatment program typically occurs in combination with other, reinforcement-based procedures (e.g., Ringdahl, Christensen, & Boelter, in press).

Risley (1968) examined the impact of positive punishment procedures to decrease dangerous climbing behaviors displayed by a 6-year-old girl diagnosed with autism and an emotional disturbance. Of note, extinction (ignoring the child's climbing), timeout from social interactions, and attention provided contingent on the absence of climbing had been implemented for an extended amount of time without success prior to the introduction of the aversive punishers. Contingent on climbing, an experimenter shouted "No!," ran to the child, and shocked her on the calf or lower thigh. After several sessions, the shock was replaced at home with a spanking by the mother and then by a time-out in a chair. Immediate reductions in climbing were observed in both settings when these punishment procedures were used. The decrease in climbing was maintained when the shocking device was removed from the home. However, the reductions in the child's behavior in the laboratory were found to only occur in the presence of the stimulus conditions associated with the experiment. That is, the child continued to climb if the experimenter was absent, if the experimenter was present but not in the room where the experiment had been conducted, and when the shock device was absent. Some desired and undesired side effects were noted to occur following the use of the punisher.

Foxx and Azrin (1973) implemented an overcorrection procedure to reduce the self-stimulatory behaviors exhibited by four children, one of whom, Mike, had been diagnosed with autism. Overcorrection is a type of positive punishment that requires the individual to repeat an appropriate form of the target, problem behavior (termed positive practice overcorrection) or repair the damage caused by the problem behavior and bring the environment to a condition better than its original state (termed restitutional overcorrection) contingent on each occurrence of that behavior (Cooper et al., 2007). At the beginning of the experiment, Mike engaged in almost continuous hand-clapping. Contingent on hand-clapping, he was required to complete 5 min of Functional Movement Training. During this training, Mike was taught to move his hands in one of five positions (e.g., hands above his head, hands in his pockets, hands behind his back). Compared to baseline, an immediate decrease to near-zero rates of hand-clapping was observed when the Functional Movement Training overcorrection procedure was implemented. Following several days without hand-clapping, a verbal warning procedure was instituted in which Mike was told to stop engaging in the hand-clapping. Overcorrection was only implemented if Mike did not stop clapping. No hand-clapping was observed during this treatment phase.

Negative Punishment

In contrast to positive punishment, procedures based on negative punishment continue to be used and described in the ABA literature. Two types of negative punishment procedures common in the ABA literature are response cost and timeout from reinforcement. Response cost procedures are negative reinforcement procedures that result in the loss of a specified amount of a reinforcer contingent on each occurrence of the target response (Cooper et al., 2007). Timeout from reinforcement consists of the contingent loss of access to positive reinforcers or the loss of opportunities to earn positive reinforcers for a specified time following a target behavior (Cooper et al.).

Hagopian, Bruzek, Bowman, and Jennett (2007) designed treatments to reduce the destructive behavior exhibited by three individuals diagnosed with autism. Initially, reinforcement-based treatments were implemented to treat problem behavior occasioned by interruption of free-operant behavior. Reinforcement-based treatment only (i.e., differential and noncontingent reinforcement) resulted in sustained decreases for one of the three participants. Time out procedures were implemented for the remaining two participants (hands-down time out for one, exclusionary time out for the other) contingent on problem behavior because the reinforcement-based treatment did not reduce problem behavior to acceptable levels. Problem behavior was further reduced when the time out procedures were implemented. The hands-down time out procedure was subsequently dropped from the treatment package for that participant. However, the exclusionary time out procedure remained a component of treatment for the remaining participant.

Athens, Vollmer, Sloman, and St. Peter Pipkin (2008) also examined the relative effects of a response cost procedure for decreasing inappropriate vocalizations exhibited by a child with autism and Down syndrome. The child's vocalizations consisted of loudly and repetitively using words out of context and loudly and repetitively making unintelligible sounds. Results of a functional analysis indicated that the participant's vocalizations were maintained by automatic reinforcement. Two treatments packages, both including a response cost component, were compared. One treatment consisted of noncontingent attention, a contingent demand, and response cost (brief loss of access to a toy). The other treatment consisted only of response cost and the presentation of a contingent demand. Both packages effectively reduced the child's inappropriate vocalizations. The authors noted that the package without non-contingent attention was easier to implement. In both treatments, response cost was rarely implemented. Although not formally evaluated, it is possible that the presentation of the demand served as a positive punisher that contributed to the decreased use of the response cost procedure.

There are several potential concerns and drawbacks in implementing punishment-based procedures. First, such procedures do not explicitly program for the teaching of appropriate behavior. Second, punishment-based procedures do not program for the delivery of reinforcers. Third, punishment-based procedures can result in stimulus-specific treatment gains, where the desired change in behavior is only exhibited in the presence of the punisher (e.g., Risley, 1968). Other concerns include negative emotional side effects, short-lived effectiveness, potential for abuse (Vollmer, 2002), development of escape and avoidance behavior, and undesirable modeling (Cooper et al., 2007). Given these drawbacks, reinforcement-based treatments are typically implemented as a first step in the treatment of behavior problems. And, when punishment-based procedures are implemented, they are often accompanied by reinforcement-based procedures.

Consequence: Reinforcement and Reinforcement-Based Procedures

Like punishment, reinforcement can be defined by its effect on behavior. Reinforcement refers to the response-dependent presentation (positive reinforcement) or removal (negative reinforcement) of a stimulus resulting in an increased likelihood of responding. With the emergence of assessment technologies designed to reliably identify stimulus preferences and reinforcers instrumental in the maintenance of appropriate and inappropriate behavior, reinforcement programs have become the foundation for programs that address the behavioral deficits and excesses exhibited by individuals with autism. There are many and varied reinforcement-based procedures described in the ABA literature including token economies and differential reinforcement. Within these programs, reinforcers can be delivered immediately following a response, intermittently following fixed or varied numbers of responses, or following specific time parameters (e.g., the first response following 60 s). Alternatively, the reinforcers can be delivered in a delayed fashion with a token, or other icon, used to help bridge the time gap (i.e., a token economy). Finally, single responses can be targeted for increase (e.g., exhibiting a particular communicative response), complex responses can be targeted for increase (e.g., reading), or a series of approximations toward a final response goal (i.e., shaping) or a series of interconnected discrete responses (i.e., chaining) can be targeted. Within the context of autism, clinical issues targeted by reinforcement procedures include appropriate communication, social interactions, and other academic, vocational, and independent living skills. The reader is directed to Ferster and Skinner (1957) for a comprehensive description of various reinforcement schedules.

Reinforcement provides the basis for many strategies and is rarely, if ever, the sole component of treatment. For that reason, examples of positive and/or negative reinforcement as singular approaches to treatment will not be provided. Instead, the application of positive and negative reinforcement will be discussed within the context of other reinforcement-based treatments including token economies and differential reinforcement.

Token Economy

Token economies refer to the delivery of a conditioned reinforcer that can later be exchanged for another reinforcer. Typical conditioned reinforcers include tokens (hence, the term), points, and stickers. This type of reinforcement system has several advantages, including some resistance to satiation effects, the ability to implement it with relative ease in large-group settings, and, in such settings, the ability to use uniform reinforcers for several individuals (Rusch, Rose, & Greenwood, 1988). Cooper et al. (2007) defined three components of a token economy: (1) A list of target responses, (2) tokens or points to be earned, and (3) a menu of items for which tokens and/or points can be

exchanged. In typical application, tokens are usually not of any particular value by themselves. Their reinforcing value comes from the opportunity to exchange them for other, more salient reinforcers (Rusch et al.).

Tarbox, Ghezzi, and Wilson (2006) used a token economy system to increase the eye contact exhibited during discrete trial training of a 5-year-old boy with autism. The study was conducted at a day treatment center for children with developmental disabilities. During baseline, the child was given a verbal prompt to attend to the tutor at the start of each instructional trial. The token reinforcement condition was identical to baseline except that the child received a token (star sticker) contingent on meeting the eye contact requirement. Once the child earned a predetermined number of tokens, he could exchange them for a brief break from instruction. A schedule thinning condition was added in which the number of tokens required to gain access to the reinforcer was increased by a factor of five. In addition, a delay to reinforcement component was added in which the child was required to wait before receiving the back-up reinforcer. Compared to baseline sessions, a substantial increase in eye contact was observed when the token economy system was used. This high rate of eye contact was maintained during schedule thinning. Variable rates of eye contact were observed as the delay to the reinforcement was increased.

In addition to targeting sustained attention, token economy systems have also been used to improve the on-task physical activity time of children with autism. Mangus, Henderson, and French (1986) trained a peer tutor to deliver tokens to five children with autism contingent on their meeting a goal for on-task behavior during a physical activity (i.e., walking on a balance beam). The rate of token delivery was individualized for each of the five children based upon their performance during the last 3 days of a baseline phase. After receiving five tokens, the children could exchange the tokens for edible reinforcers selected from a reinforcement menu. On-task physical activity increased for four of the five participants only when the token economy intervention was in place (i.e., lower levels of on-task activity occurred when the token system was removed).

Extinction

Catania (1998) defines operant extinction as, "discontinuing reinforcement of responding" (p. 389). In application, this type of procedure is used as a behavior reduction technique, and requires that the reinforcer maintaining responding is known so that it can be withheld. The procedure is straightforward as it does not require the delivery of reinforcers or punishers. Thus, alternative behavior does not have to be monitored from a procedural standpoint. However, there are other considerations with the procedure that will be discussed later in this section.

While extinction can be an effective behavior-reduction technique, there are a number of considerations to take into account prior to implementation. First, extinction procedures effectively reduce, if not eliminate, individuals' exposure to reinforcing stimuli. Second, extinction procedures do not teach the individual any appropriate methods for recruiting meaningful reinforcers. And, third, extinction procedures can result in an initial increase in target problem behavior (i.e., an extinction burst occurs) and/or can result in variations in response topography, such as the emergence of aggressive behavior (Lerman, Iwata, & Wallace, 1999).

One way to alleviate the drawbacks related to extinction-only procedures is to couple them with some sort of reinforcement-based procedure. This combination of procedures (extinction for problem behavior and reinforcement for some other response) is referred to as differential reinforcement and will be the focus of the following section. Lerman et al. (1999) reported that when extinction was coupled with differential-reinforcement programs, noncontingent reinforcement, or a manipulation of some antecedent variable, the likelihood of extinction bursts (i.e., increases in problem behavior concurrent with the onset of treatment) was reduced as was the emergence of response variations such as aggression.

Differential Reinforcement

Differential reinforcement procedures are consequence-based procedures that include two key components: (1) reinforcement of one response class (i.e., responses maintained by the same reinforcer or reinforcers), and (2) extinction or withholding of reinforcement for a separate response class (Cooper et al., 2007). In application, the response class targeted for reinforcement includes appropriate responses while the response class targeted for extinction includes inappropriate

responses (though exceptions can be found). There are a number of differential reinforcement strategies that have been used to address behavioral challenges exhibited by individuals with autism.

Differential Reinforcement of Alternative Behavior

Perhaps the most frequently applied differential reinforcement strategy is differential reinforcement of alternative behavior (DRA). When applied as a behavior reduction strategy, the procedure includes extinction for the target inappropriate or undesired response and contingent delivery of reinforcers following an appropriate response alternative. Reinforcer selection is often based on a pre-treatment assessment designed to identify the function of the inappropriate or undesired response (e.g., an analogue functional analysis; Iwata, Dorsey, Slifer, Bauman, & Richman, 1982/1994). The selected alternative response can vary and might include responses such as compliance (Reed, Ringdahl, Wacker, Barretto, & Andelman, 2005) or communication (Carr & Durand, 1985). The incorporation of appropriate communicative responding into DRA programs is formally known as functional communication training (FCT). FCT has emerged as one of the most frequently applied treatments to reduce severe problem behavior such as aggression and SIB (Tiger, Hanley, & Bruzek, 2008). In FCT program, the reinforcer maintaining problem behavior is identified. Then, an appropriate communicative alternative is identified. Finally, the individual is exposed to the situations that evoke problem behavior. Appropriate responding is prompted and differentially reinforced, with prompt fading. Appropriate communicative responses can vary and include simple gestures such as reaching (Grow, Kelley, Roane, & Shillingsburg, 2008), the use of augmentative communication devices (Ringdahl et al., 2009), manual sign (Shirley, Iwata, Kahng, Mazaleski, & Lerman, 1997), and spoken or vocal responses (Carr & Durand). While appropriate communication is reinforced, FCT also often includes an extinction component for problem behavior.

Not all examples of FCT in the literature have included the extinction component for problem behavior. However, it has been demonstrated that FCT without the extinction component is minimally effective. For example, Hagopian, Fisher, Sullivan, Acquisto, and LeBlanc (1998) reported that FCT without extinction was somewhat effective for 11 ($N=25$) participants. Though decreases were observed for some of the 11 participants, none achieved a 90% reduction in problem behavior (90% reduction being considered a clinically significant outcome). In addition, three of the 11 participants actually exhibited a 50% or greater increase in problem behavior when the extinction component was not in place. The same study reported a 90% or greater reduction in problem behavior for 44% of the participants (11 of 25) when extinction was included. Thus, the existing literature suggests that when FCT is conducted in accordance with the schedule parameters defined by DRA, it is an effective treatment.

In a series of three experiments, Charlop, Kurtz, and Casey (1990) used a DRA procedure to increase task responding and decrease problem behaviors for children diagnosed with autism. In all of the experiments, the children's stereotyped speech, delayed echolalia, and perseverative behavior were evaluated as potential reinforcers for desired behaviors. In Experiment 1, several sessions were conducted in which four children with autism were required to complete work tasks. In some of the sessions, a preferred food was used as a consequence following accurate responding. In other sessions, the child was able to engage in a stereotypy for accurate responding. In other sessions, the children were allowed to choose either an edible or to engage in the stereotypy contingent on accurate responding. The work tasks that were selected and the stereotypic behavior that served as potential reinforcers varied across the four children. In all sessions, a correction trial was conducted if the child did not produce an accurate response. All children exhibited the highest percentage of correct responding during the condition in which their stereotypy was made available as a contingency. In Experiment 2, similar procedures were used with three children with autism to evaluate the potential effectiveness of delayed echolalia as a reinforcer for correct task performance. A higher percentage of correct responding was observed when delayed echolalia was provided as a consequence than when food was delivered as a consequence. In Experiment 3, a comparison was made for three children with autism between the use of perseverative behavior with specific objects, food, and with stereotypies as potential reinforcers for correct task performance. The highest percentage of correct responding occurred during sessions in which perseverative behavior was available as a consequence. Of note, negative side effects in the form of increases in stereotyped, perseverative, or echolalic behaviors were not observed at the work setting or in the children's homes.

Ringdahl et al. (2002) compared the relative effectiveness of DRA procedures with and without instructional fading for decreasing the destructive, aggressive, and self-injurious behaviors of an 8-year-old girl diagnosed with autism and mental retardation. Results of a functional analysis indicated that the child's disruptive behaviors were maintained by negative reinforcement in the form of escape from instructional demands. DRA without instructional fading consisted of providing the participant with an instruction approximately every other minute. Compliance (i.e., independent completion of the instruction in the absence of disruptive behaviors) resulted in a brief break. Disruptive behaviors during instruction resulted in presentation of another instruction and restoration of the environment. In DRA with instructional fading, no instructions were delivered for three consecutive work sessions. The rate of instruction was then gradually increased (i.e., one instruction delivered every 15 min, followed by adding one instruction every 15 min following each 45-min session with no disruptive behaviors). Initially, high rates of disruptive behavior were observed during the DRA without instructional fading condition. However, the rate of disruptive behaviors decreased across sessions. In the DRA with instructional fading condition, disruptive behaviors occurred at low rates from the outset. The rate of instruction was equivalent in the DRA with and without instructional fading conditions by the end of treatment.

Brithwaite and Richdale (2000) used FCT to target the aggressive and self-injurious behaviors displayed by a 7 year-old boy with autism and an intellectual disability. The evaluation and treatment occurred as part of the child's discrete trial training program at his school. Results of a behavioral interview and an A–B–C observation suggested that the child's disruptive behaviors were maintained by access to preferred items and by escape from difficult tasks. During a training phase, the child was taught a phrase to vocally request a preferred object (e.g., "I want (slinky) please") during tangible sessions and help with a task (e.g., "I need help please") during work sessions. FCT treatment consisted of providing the child with access to the reinforcer (either the toy or help) contingent on an appropriate communicative request. The disruptive behavior was placed on extinction. Substantial reductions in the disruptive behaviors occurred in both the tangible and escape conditions. Specifically, a 99% reduction in disruptive behaviors occurred between baseline and treatment involving FCT for tangible items, and a 90% reduction in disruptive behaviors occurred between baseline and treatment in the FCT escape condition. Corresponding increases in use of the taught phrase were also observed. The inclusion of a delay to reinforcement component did not lead to an increase in disruptive behaviors in either the tangible or escape conditions.

DRA programs can also incorporate negative reinforcement. For example, Reed et al. (2005) used combined fixed-time (i.e., response independent) and contingent schedules of negative reinforcement to treat the destructive behavior exhibited by an 8-year-old boy diagnosed with autism, moderate mental retardation, a seizure disorder, and significant communication deficits. Results of a functional analysis demonstrated that this participant's destructive behavior was maintained by negative reinforcement. During the first treatment phase, a differential negative reinforcement of compliance procedure was implemented in which the child could take a break as soon as he had completed a work task. Compared to baseline, low rates of destruction and high rates of work completion were observed during the differential negative reinforcement treatment. Next, lean and dense schedules of fixed-time escape were added to the differential negative reinforcement treatment. Lower levels of destruction and higher levels of compliance were observed when the fixed-time escape lean schedule was used. This finding suggests that combining a differential negative reinforcement of compliance treatment with a lean schedule for escape can be effective in treating problem behavior maintained by negative reinforcement.

Differential Reinforcement of Incompatible Behavior

Differential reinforcement of incompatible behavior (DRI) can also be considered a type of DRA. However, in this procedure, the alternative response is specified as one incompatible with the target inappropriate response. For example, hands in pockets might be the incompatible response reinforced in the DRI-based treatment of stereotypic hand flapping. By contrast, exhibiting the appropriate vocal response "help" is not physically incompatible with pinching the teacher.

A DRI procedure was used by Smith (1987) to decrease the pica behavior (i.e., ingestion of paper clips, paper, bottle caps, and other nonfood items) of a man diagnosed with autism and profound mental retardation. The study was conducted in a department store where the participant worked. During the baseline phase of the study, the number of incidents of pica was tabulated and attempts at ingestion of metal items were blocked. The DRI treatment consisted of identifying behavior incompatible with pica. Incompatible responses included the participant keeping his hands on his work, staying in his work area, and keeping his mouth clear. Each of these responses was reinforced approximately every 15 min through access to a preferred food, drink, or a preferred activity. Praise was also provided on a 10-min schedule contingent on the participant having a clear mouth, keeping his hands on his work, and remaining in his assigned work location. The experimenter provided verbal redirection if the participant reached for a nonedible item, or the experimenter removed that item before the participant could reach it. An ABAB design was used to evaluate the effectiveness of the treatment. Relative to baseline rates, a substantial reduction in the total number of pica incidents was observed when the DRI treatment was in place. Specifically, mean rates of pica each day was 21 during baseline, 7 during the DRI treatment, 12 during a reversal to baseline, and 5 when the DRI was re-implemented. At a 1-year follow-up, the mean number of instances of pica per day was 0.5.

Differential Reinforcement of Low Rates

Differential reinforcement of low rates of behavior (DRL) is a reductive procedure that has its effect by providing a schedule of reinforcement that is leaner (i.e., reinforcement rate is lower) than what was operating in the pre-treatment environment. The behavior targeted for reduction results in reinforcement following a specified time period that includes the absence of the behavior. The length of that time period is systematically increased to achieve lower rates of the target response. DRL is also referred to as differential reinforcement of diminishing rates, or DRD). One difference with this procedure relative to other DR procedures is that it is not intended to eliminate the target response. Rather, it is intended to reduce the frequency with which the response is exhibited.

Handen, Apolito, and Seltzer (1984) described the use of a DRL procedure to reduce the repetitive verbalizations of an adolescent male diagnosed with autism and mental retardation. The study was conducted in the community residence where the participant resided. The participant had a several year history of repeating statements or asking the same questions hundreds of times each day. During baseline, the investigators tape recorded the participants' verbal responses over a 7-day period and then tabulated the frequency of repetitive verbalizations (i.e., saying any word, phrase, or sentence more than once). No consequences were provided for verbalizations. During the DRL treatment, a 3×5 inch index card was used during each session. The card contained the number of boxes that corresponded to the allowed number of verbalizations within that session. A check was placed through a box each time a verbalization occurred. If the participant met the DRL criterion goal at the end of the session (i.e., having at least one empty box on the card), he received a token. The token could be exchanged immediately following a session for an item from a reinforcement menu or saved. Over the course of the experiment, the criterion level for verbalizations was systematically decreased from a rate of 4.4 to 0.3 repetitions per minute. Relative to baseline, the DRL procedure resulted in a substantial reduction in the participant's rate of verbalizations.

Differential Reinforcement of Other Behavior

Differential reinforcement of other behavior (DRO) can be distinguished from other DR-based procedures in that it does not specify a response following which reinforcers should be delivered. Instead, DRO entails providing the programmed reinforcer following intervals during which no occurrences of the target response were exhibited. DRO programs can incorporate either positive reinforcers (e.g., attention, points, and/or preferred activities) or negative reinforcers (e.g., breaks from non preferred activities). In typical application, the reinforcer provided is determined by the function of the target problem behavior or is one that has been demonstrated as more valuable than the reinforcer(s) maintaining the target problem behavior. Differential reinforcement of the omission of behavior and differential reinforcement of zero rates of behavior are other terms used interchangeably with DRO.

Shabani and Fisher (2006) implemented a DRO and schedule thinning procedure to decrease a fear of needles displayed by an adolescent male with autism, mental retardation, and Type 2 diabetes. The evaluation was conducted in an outpatient clinic. During baseline trials, the participant was given a verbal and physical prompt to place his left hand and arm between an outline of his hand and arm that was drawn on posterboard and attached to the top of the table. The therapist then slowly moved a lancet toward the participant's index finger for a blood draw. Baseline trials were terminated when the participant pulled his arm away or if a draw was successfully completed. During the stimulus fading and DRO treatment, the lancet was positioned a set distance from the participant's hand for 10 s. The initial distance was selected based upon observation that the participant did not exhibit signs of distress of hand withdrawal. If the participant kept his hand and arm between the outline for the entire 10-s interval, he immediately received access to a food item that had been previously identified through a preference assessment. If the participant moved his arm more than 3 cm from the outline in any direction, the trial was terminated and the experimenter turned away for 10 s. The distance between the lancet and the patient's hand was systematically reduced whenever a criterion goal of 100% successful trials for two or three consecutive sessions (i.e., 61, 46, 31, 15, 8, 5, and 1 cm) was obtained. Following distance fading, blood draws were attempted. During the baseline trials, the participant withdrew his hand every time a blood draw was attempted. The DRO and fading intervention was successful in systematically increasing the patient's acceptance of closer proximity between his hand and arm and the lancet. At the completion of fading, blood draws were completed with no refusal behaviors in the clinic room as well and in the nurse's station.

Newman, Tuntigian, Ryan, and Reinecke (1997) used a DRO procedure to decrease the disruptive behaviors of three children who had been diagnosed with autism. The evaluation was conducted in a school setting for two of the participants and at home for the third participant. Disruptive behaviors consisted of out-of-seat behavior for two participants and inappropriate nail-flicking (i.e., repetitive contact between fingertips and the nails of another finger) for other participant. A baseline assessment was conducted in which the participants each received ten noncontingent tokens during 10-min sessions. The tokens were traded for food or a break. During the DRO intervention, the children were given a token at the end of each time interval contingent on not engaging in the targeted behavior. As in baseline, the tokens could be traded in after 10-min. The participant's behavior was compared under prompted and unprompted conditions. In the prompted DRO condition, the participants were provided with verbal prompts to take a token at the end of a time interval if problem behavior did not occur. In the unprompted DRO condition, the participants were not reminded to take a token. Out-of-seat behavior occurred nearly 100% of the time during baseline for both participants who exhibited this behavior. When the DRO procedure was implemented, out-of-seat behavior reduced to below 10% by the end of treatment. Similar results were obtained with nail-flicking. Of note, these reductions in problem behavior occurred during both the prompted and unprompted DRO conditions, suggesting that the children were able to manage their behavior.

Similar to DRA, DRO schedules can incorporate negative reinforcement. For instance, Buckley and Newchok (2006) used a negative reinforcement procedure to decrease the screaming and ear covering behaviors of a 7-year-old boy who had been diagnosed with a pervasive developmental disorder. These behaviors were evoked by his hearing different genres of music. Treatment consisted of the examiner playing music and telling the child that the music would be turned off if he could sit quietly with his hands down until a timer beeped. The timer was reset if the target problem behaviors occurred while the music was playing. The interval of time that the music was played was increased contingent on low rates of disruptive behavior in two consecutive sessions. The mean percentage of disruptive behavior dropped from 52% during baseline to 5% during the negative reinforcement treatment.

Thinning Differential Reinforcement Schedules

DR programs are not without their limitations. One such limitation is that the individual can access reinforcers on a frequent basis, resulting in labor-intensive programs when reinforcement delivery requires the presence of a care giver. In addition, if the individual spends much of the time acquiring and consuming reinforcers, other goals and activities might suffer. For example, if an individual is taught as part of a DRA/FCT program that

every request for break result in a cessation of academic instruction, they could conceivably entirely escape/avoid their school work, thus hindering academic progress. To alleviate this concern, many DR programs will focus on reducing the availability of the reinforcer by increasing the response requirement needed to obtain the reinforcer or implementing a delay to reinforcement.

Roane, Fisher, Sgro, Falcomata, and Pabico (2004) described a schedule thinning procedure for two children with autism who were evaluated for aggressive behavior. Results of a functional analysis indicated that the children's aggressive behavior was maintained by positive reinforcement. For both participants, treatment consisted of access to 20 s of positive reinforcement contingent on appropriate responding. A substantial decrease in aggression was observed for both children in treatment relative to baseline. At the onset of treatment, the participants had continuous access to response cards that gained them access to positive reinforcement. To increase the treatment's feasibility for caregivers, a reinforcement thinning procedure was evaluated in which access to the response cards was restricted for a fixed amount of time. For both of the children, low levels of aggressive behavior were maintained when schedule thinning in the form of card restriction was implemented. The authors noted that, by limiting access to alternative responding, caregivers may be able to reduce their direct involvement in treatment.

Hagopian, Contrucci Kuhn, Long, and Rush (2005) evaluated the effects of schedule thinning following the implementation of FCT for three children diagnosed with an autism spectrum disorder who displayed aggressive, self-injurious, and disruptive behaviors. Treatment consisted of functional communication training targeting the functional analysis condition in which the highest rate of problem behavior was observed. A reduction in the target problem behavior occurred for all participants. A schedule thinning procedure was then implemented. Schedule thinning consisted of instructing the children that they needed to wait after manding for delivery of the reinforcer (either access to attention or to a preferred tangible items). The length of the delay between manding and reinforcer delivery was progressively increased until a terminal schedule goal was obtained (4 min). The criterion for increasing the delay was two consecutive sessions with a rate of problem behavior at or below 0.2

responses per min. If problem behavior occurred at a rate of greater than 0.2 responses per min across two consecutive sessions, the delay was reduced to the previous response schedule where the terminal goal had been achieved. For all three participants, the treatment goal of at least 4 min was achieved.

Shaping and Chaining

While differential reinforcement procedures are usually used to reduce some target inappropriate response(s), other reinforcement-based procedures have been developed to establish responses or repertoires. Two such procedures used with individuals with autism include shaping and chaining. Shaping is the process of differentially reinforcing successive approximations toward a desired response (Cooper et al., 2007). Shaping can be considered a differential reinforcement procedure during which the target response is slightly altered as the individual exhibits responses that are more and more similar to the desired terminal response. Behavioral chains are collections of discrete responses that are performed in rapid and accurate sequences (Rusch et al. 1988). Reinforcement-based acquisition programs sometimes focus on systematically and sequentially reinforcing each of the responses in a chain to establish a particular skill. This process is described as chaining, with two types of chaining (forward and backward) being most often described in the literature. In forward chaining, the responses in a behavioral chain are taught and reinforced in their naturally occurring order (Cooper et al.). Reinforcement might initially be delivered following the completion of Step 1. During the next phase of forward chaining, reinforcement would be delivered following Steps 1 and 2, and so on until all responses are exhibited in the correct order. Backward chaining consists of the teacher or therapist completing all but the last response in a behavior chain, and providing the reinforcer contingent on the individual completing the final response. In the next phase of backward chaining, the reinforcer would be delivered after the individual had completed the next-to-last and final response, and so on until all responses are exhibited in the correct order.

Ricciardi, Luiselli, and Camare (2006) used a shaping procedure to treat specific phobia exhibited by a child with autism. In their study, an 8-year-old boy with autism was differentially provided with reinforcement (access to preferred items) for closer and closer approaches to phobic stimuli. Initially, the child was allowed ongoing access to the preferred items, regardless of proximity to phobic stimuli. Preferred items were then only allowed if the participant successfully approached and stayed within 5 m of the phobic stimuli, then 4, 3, 2 m, and finally 1 m. The use of this shaping procedure successfully resulted in the participant approaching phobic stimuli.

Jerome, Frantino, and Sturmey (2007) used a chaining procedure to help adults with autism acquire internet skills. A 13-step task analysis was generated to develop the skills necessary to access a specific internet site. Initially, the teacher completed the initial 12 steps of the task analysis. An errorless prompting procedure was used to teach step 13 and reinforcement (access to a internet activity along with an edible) was provided contingent on the participants' completing step 13 of the task analysis. Once that behavior was exhibited at criterion, the prompting procedure was applied to the 12th step and reinforcement was delivered after completing steps 12 and 13. Once that combination was exhibited at criterion, the prompting procedure was applied to the 11th step, and reinforcement was delivered following completion of steps 11–13. This process continued until the participants were able to independently exhibit all 13 steps. Both participants were able to acquire all 13 steps, one participant in a single 40-min training session, the other across five 40-min training sessions.

Antecedent Approaches to Treatment

ABA programs have traditionally focused on the response-reinforcement relationship. However, as programs have evolved over the years, the focus has shifted from consequence-based approaches to approaches that focus on manipulating the antecedents relevant to target behavior. In this chapter, we will provide a description of four foci of antecedent-based treatments described in the ABA literature.

Establishing Operations

Establishing operations are those events that alter the reinforcing efficacy, or value, of the reinforcers maintaining a response (Michael, 1982). Establishing operations can be further differentiated by their specific effect on the value of the reinforcer. *Motivating operations (MOs)* are operations that increase the value of the reinforcer. The most basic example of this operation includes deprivation. *Abolishing operations (AOs)* are operations that decrease the value of the reinforcer. The most basic example of this operation includes satiation (Laraway, Snycerski, Michael, & Poling, 2003). MOs result in increased response rates maintained by the reinforcer, whereas AOs result in decreased response rates maintained by the reinforcer.

EOs manipulation has been applied to the treatment of behavior problems exhibited by individuals with autism and other disabilities. Two approaches have been taken in this respect: (1) Providing the reinforcer on a fixed-time, or noncontingent basis (e.g., Reed et al., 2005), and (2) pre-session exposure to the functional reinforcer (i.e., the reinforcer known or hypothesized to maintain the target response).

Taylor et al. (2005) manipulated EOs to increase the frequency of social initiations directed toward peers by three children with autism. The study was conducted in each student's classroom. Prior to intervention, none of the children were observed to initiate requests for preferred items with peers. Preferred snacks for both the participants and peers were identified through free operant preference assessments and were restricted during the school day to increase their desirability. During the MO absent condition, the snack items were presented on separate plates placed in front of the participant and the peer, and the teacher instructed the children to, "have a snack." During the MO present condition, only the peer had access to the snack food. If the participant made an appropriate mand toward the peer for the snack item, the peer handed the participant a small portion of the snack. For all three participants, elevated rates of manding for snacks were observed only in the MO present condition. Participants successfully manded for novel food items or toys when observed during follow-up observations. These results indicated that requesting can be increased through the direct manipulation of establishing operations in the form of the availability of preferred snack items.

Gutierrez et al. (2007) manipulated establishing operations as part of a procedure for teaching children to mand for preferred items in a school setting. Three of the four children included in the study had been diagnosed with autism. The fourth participant displayed behavioral characteristics consistent with an autism spectrum disorder. Each of the participants rarely requested items either vocally or nonvocally and had minimal exposure to picture cards prior to the study. During the initial phases of the study, the participants were taught to exchange picture cards in order to gain brief access to preferred items, activities, and edibles. In the EO manipulation condition, two cards which had been used for training were placed in front of the participant, and the participant had free access to one of the items that he or she had previously manded for in the study. Access to the other preferred item was restricted (e.g., if the child had previously used a picture card to mand for a toy or an edible, during the EO phase he was given access to the edible but not the toy or vice versa). Three of the participants consistently manded for a preferred item when the EO for that item was present and did not typically mand when the EO was absent. These findings suggest that the manipulation of EO's during picture exchange training can help determine whether children are able to accurately discriminate between manding (handing someone a card) and a desired response (gaining access to an outcome that is symbolically represented by that card).

Stimulus Control

Stimulus control is an outcome that emerges after repeated pairings between specific stimuli and consistent consequences. According to Sulzer-Azaroff and Mayer (1991), stimulus control is demonstrated when a particular behavior is predictably occasioned by specific antecedent stimuli. Stimulus control can be systematically achieved only by reinforcing specific responses in the presence of a unique stimulus. Or, stimulus control can emerge naturally as individuals' behavior is exposed to different contexts and their respective reinforcement schedules. For example, a child might learn that requesting bathroom breaks is always reinforced (i.e., the child is allowed to leave the classroom) when Teacher A is asked. However, Teacher B never allows the child to leave following such requests. In this scenario, requests will maintain in the presence of Teacher A and eventually decrease in the presence of Teacher B. Stimulus control can also emerge when punishment is the consistent consequence. For example, if one parent always respond to a problem with an aversive consequence (e.g., spanking), but another parent does not provide any consistent consequence, problem behavior would likely decrease in the presence of the first parent only, because that parent's presence and punishment have been paired.

Anglesea, Hoch, and Taylor (2008) used a stimulus control procedure as part of a treatment to decrease the rapid eating of three teenagers with autism. The total number of seconds of eating time to consume the target food was compared during sessions when a vibrating pager provided the teenagers with prompts to take a bite versus the total number of seconds of eating time when the pager was inactivated. All attempts to take bites before the pager vibrated were blocked. Training sessions were conducted to teach the participants to consume food only when the pager vibrated. When the vibrating pager was used, the participant's eating rate for the target foods decreased and was comparable to the length of time that it took a typical adult to consume the same foods. A reduction in the total number of seconds of eating time for the target foods was not observed when the pager was inactive. All participants ate one bite of food immediately following vibration of the pager on 100% of occasions during probe sessions, suggesting that the pager vibration exerted stimulus control over bite taking.

Transfer of stimulus control is a treatment strategy that can be followed when differentially high levels of problem behavior are correlated with specific stimuli. Ray, Skinner, and Watson (1999) treated problem behavior exhibited by a child with autism using a stimulus control procedure. Prior to treatment, compliance with demands was differentially higher when the participant's parent delivered the instruction compared to when the teacher delivered instruction. The teacher was then paired with the parent during instructional situations. Initially, instructional sessions were composed of 75% (3 of 4) parent-delivered instructions and 25% (1 of 4) teacher-delivered instructions. Compliance was high with both adults. Over time, the teacher-delivered instructions increased as parent-delivered instructions decreased. Compliance continued at high levels. By the end of treatment, the parent-delivered instructions were entirely eliminated and compliance continued to be exhibited at high levels. These results suggested that stimulus control over compliance was successfully transferred from the parent to the teacher.

Prompt Procedures

Prompts have been defined by Cooper et al. (2007) as antecedent stimuli that occasion specific responses and are supplemental to a behavioral treatment. There are at least two broad categories of prompts: response prompts and physical prompts. Response prompts such as physical guidance target behavior. Stimulus prompts target the conditions that exist prior to the occurrence of a target behavior. Stimulus prompts are often used as a means to occasion behavior. Once responding is more frequent and reliable in the presence of naturally occurring stimuli, these auxiliary stimuli can be removed.

DeQuinzio, Townsend, Sturmey, and Poulson (2007) used prompting as part of a treatment plan for teaching three young children with autism to imitate facial models. Prior to treatment, all of the children did not accurately imitate varying facial expressions (e.g., they cried when others smiled at them or laughed when others cried). *Smile, frown, surprise,* and *anger* were the facial expressions targeted for imitation in this study. During baseline, the experimenter modeled one of the facial expressions. During imitation training, a combination of prompting, modeling, differential reinforcement, and error correction procedures was utilized. Specific to this section of the chapter, prompting consisted of a least-to-most hierarchy in which the experimenter started by providing a verbal statement ("do this") if the participant had not imitated a facial model within 5 s of its presentation. If the participant still did not imitate the facial model, the experimenter provided another verbal statement and also modeled two facial motor movements that were topographically related to the target response. If the child still did not imitate the motor movements, the experimenter then manually prompted the correct response (e.g., used two fingers to turn the corners of the participant's mouth up). If the child did not imitate the motor movement following this manual prompt, the experimenter next combined the manual prompt with a verbal statement (e.g., "that's smiling"). All children consistently displayed high rates of imitation of some of the facial models in training relative to baseline.

Prompts have also been used to increase the social initiations of children with autism. Taylor and Levin (1998) used a tactile prompting device (vibrating pager) to teach a student with autism to initiate verbal interactions toward an adult during play activities.

Social initiations were defined as a verbal statement that occurred in the absence of verbal models, when it was related to the context of the activity, was directed towards another person, and that was a complete sentence. Three conditions were compared: a no-prompt condition in which the tactile device was not placed in the child's pocket and verbal models were not provided, a verbal prompt condition in which an adult therapist modeled a social initiation every minute, and a tactile prompt condition in which the pager was placed in the child's pocket and was preset to vibrate every minute. Teaching sessions were conducted in which the child's hand was placed on top of the pager when it vibrated and a verbal initiation was modeled by an adult therapist. A most-to-least hierarchy was used to fade the prompts until the child was able to independently make verbal initiations each time the pager vibrated. During follow-up probes, the child sat at a table with two typically developing children and participated in cooperative learning activities. Neither the participant nor the peers were provided with instructions or consequences for initiating verbal interactions or responding to each other. Frequency of initiations was compared across conditions in which the pager was in the child's pocket and programmed to vibrate every 60 s, when the pager was not activated, and when the pager was not in the child's pocket. Across three different play activities with an adult therapist, the child displayed a substantially higher frequency of verbal initiations with the tactile prompt compared to the no-prompt or verbal prompt conditions. Likewise, the child initiated verbal interactions more frequently with peers when the tactile prompt was activated than when the prompt was not activated or was unavailable. These findings suggest that the pager served as an effective tactile prompt for increasing the child's verbal initiations with adults and peers. Shabani et al. (2002) extended these findings by incorporating a prompt fading program to remove or reduce the reliance on prompts.

Choice

Providing a choice within behavioral treatment programs has been demonstrated to be an effective strategy for reducing problem behavior (e.g., Dibley & Lim, 1999). Within the context of behavioral treatment, choice can be considered an antecedent variable because

it is in operation before the target response occurs and not in response to a behavior. Within a concurrent-operants arrangement, Thompson, Fisher, and Contrucci (1998) evaluated the relative preference for choice making of a 4-year-old boy diagnosed with pervasive developmental disorder. The child had been referred for the evaluation of destructive behavior and, prior to conducting the experiment, had been noted to exhibit problem behaviors when he was not able to make choices. During the initial portion of the assessment, a paired-choice preference assessment was conducted and a most preferred item (cola) was identified. During the concurrent-operants assessment, the child could touch one of three switches. Each switch resulted in a different outcome. The "no-choice" switch resulted in the examiner pouring the child cola into a cup. The "choice" switch resulted in the examiner pouring the identical amount of cola into a cup, but the child was allowed to choose how the cola was delivered (i.e., which cup the cola was poured into, whether a straw was provided, etc). A "control" switch produced no programmed consequence. Findings from the study were that the child consistently pressed the "choice" switch at higher rates than the "no-choice" switch, even when the "choice" option resulted in a substantially lower rate of reinforcement. This result indicates that choice in how the reinforcer was delivered was a potent variable for this child.

Combining Antecedent and Consequence-Based Components

In practice, the treatments described so far throughout this chapter are often combined to form larger treatment packages. Antecedent and consequence-based interventions are oftentimes combined as part of a comprehensive treatment program. For example, the referenced Reed et al. (2005) study included a differential reinforcement component (i.e., breaks contingent on compliance) and a noncontingent reinforcement component (i.e., fixed time delivery of breaks). The noncontingent reinforcement component can be conceptualized as an antecedent approach that would affect the MO for escape-related behavior. Thus, motivation to engage in problem behavior, previously demonstrated to be maintained by escape, should have been reduced because the participants had access to this reinforcer on a fixed-time basis.

ABA-Based Comprehensive Approaches to Autism Treatment: Intervention Programs that Utilize Applied Behavior Analysis Procedures

Over the past four decades, several wide-ranging interventions and treatment programs have been developed to address the difficulties in social interactions, communication, and restricted and repetitive behaviors that are commonly displayed by individuals with an autism spectrum diagnosis. In this section, a brief overview of three widely utilized programs that utilize applied behavior analysis procedures will be provided. References will be provided for each of these programs so that the reader can obtain additional information if desired.

UCLA Young Autism Project

The UCLA Young Autism Project (YAP) is an intensive home-based intervention program for young children with autism developed by Ivaar Lovaas and colleagues (http://www.lovaas.com/). This intervention is sometimes referred to as discrete trial teaching. In the original YAP study, children in the intensive-treatment group received as much as 40 h of intervention weekly for at least 2 years (Lovaas, 1987). The focus of therapy was on increasing language, attending, imitation, social behavior, play, and self-care skills, and decreasing disruptive behaviors. Intensive teaching was provided through a discrete trial format. Please reference Lovaas (1981) and Maurice, Green, & Luce (1996) for specific information on discrete trial teaching procedures and curriculum. Children in the minimal-treatment group received similar services but for only 10 h a week, and a third control group of children received an eclectic mix of interventions. Compared to their baseline performance, children in the intensive-treatment group gained an average of 37 IQ points over the course of the treatment, representing an average difference of 31 points higher in comparison to the control group. In addition, 47% of the children in the intensive group successfully completed first grade in a regular education setting. A follow-up study was conducted with those children who successfully completed first grade without support. At the age of 13, eight of these nine students were continuing to succeed in regular education

settings without support. This group continued to perform significantly higher than the control group on measures of intelligence and adaptive abilities (McEachin, Smith, & Lovaas, 1993). Based upon the results of these studies and others, the UCLA YAP model has been described as one of the most empirically validated interventions (Simpson, 2005). Subsequent to the seminal article by Lovaas, the methodology based on the YAP program has been widely utilized in home and school settings. See Reichow and Wolery (2009) for a listing of articles that have utilized this methodology. Of note, some concerns have been raised about the methodological procedures that were employed by Lovaas (Gresham & MacMillan, 1998). In an analysis of early intensive behavioral intervention programs based on the YAP methodology, Reichow and Wolery noted that the YAP model has produced strong effects for many children. However, not all children responded positively to this intervention, suggesting that additional research is needed to identify modifications in procedures or alternative intervention procedures that would benefit this subgroup.

Pivotal Response Training

Pivotal response training (PRT) is a model that combines applied behavior analytic procedures and developmental approaches to provide opportunities for children with autism spectrum disorders to learn within natural environmental settings (http://psy3.ucsd.edu/~autism/prttraining.html). PRT was developed by Drs. Robert and Lynn Koegel at the University of California Santa Barbara. The model focuses on pivotal areas, defined as those areas that, when targeted, result in meaningful collateral changes in other areas of functioning and responding (Koegel & Koegel, 2006). Pivotal areas that have been identified are: (1) Motivation, (2) Responsivity to multiple cues, (3) Self-management, (4) Self-initiations, and (5) Empathy. Motivational strategies that are applied in PRT include: following the child's lead, using preferred items and activities, teaching within natural contexts, providing clear instructions, providing choices, reinforcement of attempts, varying and interspersing tasks, and using naturally occurring reinforcers (Dunlap, Iovanne, & Kincaid 2008). Instead of a focus on teaching discrete skills through repeated trials, PRT targets developmental skills within natural environments. An emphasis is placed on family involvement in the design and delivery of the intervention, data collection and monitoring, and implementation of interventions in both home and school settings. To date, research on PRT has demonstrated that this model can result in improvements in areas such as language acquisition, play skills and social interactions, and decreases in challenging behaviors. In addition, several studies using PRT have demonstrated generalization of skills and high levels of parent acceptability.

Treatment and Education of Autistic and related Communication-Handicapped Children

The treatment and education of autistic and related communication-handicapped children (TEACCH) program contains several components focused on modifying the environment to meet the individualized needs of individuals with autism (http://www.teacch.com/). This intervention is often referred to as structured teaching (Simpson, 2005). TEACCH was developed by Eric Schopler and colleagues at the University of North Carolina in the early 1970s. Over the past three decades, TEACCH programming has been used in classrooms and in community settings across the world. The four main components of the TEACCH program are: (1) Physical organization and structure, (2) Daily schedules, (3) Work systems, and (4) Task structure. Examples of these four components that are commonly used in classroom, community, and home settings include: establishing clear visual and physical boundaries in rooms to minimize visual and auditory distractions, developing physically separate work and leisure areas in classrooms, the use of schedules (e.g., object, picture, icon, or written word schedules) to increase independence, individualized work systems to increase an individual's understanding of what and how much work needs to be done, and incorporating visual structure within tasks. Please see Mesibov and Howley (2003) and Mesibov, Shea, and Schopler (2004) for details on TEACCH procedures. Through the use of visual and external organization procedures, TEACCH attempts to increase an individual's understanding of situations and expectations, thereby decreasing anxiety and frustration related to compre-

hension and communication difficulties. Because of TEACCH's focus on environmental manipulations aimed to improve learning and limit frustration, the program can be viewed as containing a series of antecedent-based strategies. Although TEACCH is widely used and has been described as a Promising Practice, fewer evaluative studies have been published in peer-reviewed journals relative to studies of early intensive behavioral intervention programs (Simpson) to date.

Future Directions and Summary

A number of areas are ripe for future research and application involving the use of ABA methodology with individuals with autism spectrum disorders. Within the area of early identification, recent research has suggested that autism can be reliably identified in many children as young as 12–18 months of age. Given the demonstrable positive effects of early intervention, it will be important to determine if ABA procedures can be tailored to working with toddlers recently diagnosed or strongly suspected of having an autism spectrum disorder.

Individualizing treatment based upon our knowledge of autism is another area of future focus. As more has been learned about the heterogeneous presentation of autism spectrum disorders, clinicians can increasingly focus on isolating key components that are most likely to lead to successful outcomes for different subgroups. It might be the case, for example, that different cognitive and communicative patterns may preclude or predispose individuals on the spectrum to treatment strategies that rely more heavily on antecedent-based interventions. Research can also increasingly focus on issues related to clinical outcomes. For instance, with respect to generalization and maintenance of skills, what represents the best mode of delivery for treatment: discrete trial training or training in naturally occurring situations?

Finally, outside of the clinical and research realm, the rapid increase in the number of individuals diagnosed with autism will most likely mean that the policies put in place to assist such individuals will require close review. At the time that this chapter was written, eight states have passed legislation requiring private insurance companies to cover autism services, including ABA (www.autismvotes.org). Given the high costs that can be associated with ABA services, these state initiatives may play a key role in determining the accessibility of ABA for children and families impacted by autism.

In the preceding pages, we have attempted to provide an overview of ABA concepts as well as studies that illustrate how these concepts have been used to address the social, communicative, and behavioral concerns exhibited by many individuals diagnosed with autism spectrum disorders. While each of these concepts can be investigated in more depth (and, the reader is invited to do so), what should be apparent is the long-standing empirical nature of evaluation and treatments based upon ABA methodology. It is important to note that, although it did not emerge as an approach specific to autism, ABA has yielded substantial contributions specific to this population.

References

Anglesea, M. M., Hoch, H., & Taylor, B. A. (2008). Reducing rapid eating in teenagers with autism: Use of a pager prompt. *Journal of Applied Behavior Analysis, 41*, 107–111.

Athens, E. S., Vollmer, T. R., Sloman, K. N., & St. Peter Pipkin, C. (2008). An analysis of vocal stereotypy and therapist fading. *Journal of Applied Behavior Analysis, 41*, 291–297.

Baer, D. M., Wolf, M. M., & Risley, T. R. (1968). Some current dimensions of applied behavior analysis. *Journal of Applied Behavior Analysis, 1*, 91–97.

Brithwaite, K. L., & Richdale, A. L. (2000). Functional communication training to replace challenging behaviors across two behavioral outcomes. *Behavioral Interventions, 15*, 21–36.

Buckley, S. D., & Newchok, D. K. (2006). Analysis and treatment of problem behavior evoked by music. *Journal of Applied Behavior Analysis, 39*, 141–144.

Carr, E. G., & Durand, V. M. (1985). Reducing behavior problems through functional communication training. *Journal of Applied Behavior Analysis, 18*, 111–126.

Catania, A. C. (1998). *Learning* (4th ed.). Upper Saddle River, NJ: Prentice Hall.

Charlop, M. H., Kurtz, P. F., & Casey, F. G. (1990). Using aberrant behaviors as reinforcers for autistic children. *Journal of Applied Behavior Analysis, 23*, 163–181.

Cooper, J. O., Heron, T. E., & Heward, W. L. (2007). *Applied behavior analysis* (2nd ed.). Upper Saddle River, NJ: Prentice Hall.

DeQuinzio, J. A., Townsend, D. B., Sturmey, P., & Poulson, C. L. (2007). Generalized imitation of facial models by children with autism. *Journal of Applied Behavior Analysis, 40*, 755–759.

Dibley, S., & Lim, L. (1999). Providing choice making opportunities within and between daily school activities. *Journal of Behavioral Education, 9*, 117–132.

Dunlap, G., Iovannone, R., & Kincaid, D. (2008). Essential components for effective autism educational programs. In J. Luiselli (Ed.), *Effective practices for children with autism*. Oxford: Oxford University Press.

Ferster, C. B., & Skinner, B. F. (1957). *Schedules of reinforcement*. East Norwalk, CT: Appleton-Century-Croft.

Foxx, R. M., & Azrin, N. H. (1973). The elimination of autistic self-stimulatory behavior by overcorrection. *Journal of Applied Behavior Analysis, 6*, 1–14.

Gresham, F. M., & MacMillan, D. L. (1998). Early intervention project: Can its claims be substantiated and its effects replicated? *Journal of Autism and Developmental Disorders, 28*, 5–13.

Grow, L. L., Kelley, M. E., Roane, H. S., & Shillingsburg, A. M. (2008). Utility of extinction-induced response variability for the selection of mands. *Journal of Applied Behavior Analysis, 41*, 15–24.

Gutierrez, A., Vollmer, T. R., Dozier, C. L., Borrero, J. C., Rapp, J. T., Bourret, J. C., et al. (2007). Manipulating establishing operations to verify and establish stimulus control during mand training. *Journal of Applied Behavior Analysis, 40*, 645–658.

Hagopian, L. P., Bruzek, J. L., Bowman, L. G., & Jennett, H. K. (2007). Assessment and treatment of problem behavior occasioned by interruption of free-operant behavior. *Journal of Applied Behavior Analysis, 40*, 89–103.

Hagopian, L. P., Contrucci Kuhn, S. A., Long, E. S., & Rush, K. S. (2005). Schedule thinning following communication training: Using competing stimuli to enhance tolerance to decrements in reinforcer density. *Journal of Applied Behavior Analysis, 38*, 177–193.

Hagopian, L. P., Fisher, W. W., Sullivan, M. T., Acquisto, J., & LeBlanc, L. A. (1998). Effectiveness of functional communication training with and without extinction and punishment: A summary of 21 inpatient cases. *Journal of Applied Behavior Analysis, 31*, 211–235.

Handen, B. L., Apolito, P. M., & Seltzer, G. B. (1984). Use of differential reinforcement of low rates of behavior to decrease repetitive speech in an autistic adolescent. *Journal of Behavioral Therapy and Experimental Psychiatry, 15*, 359–364.

Iwata, B. A., Dorsey, M. F., Slifer, K. J., Bauman, K. E., & Richman, G. S. (1994). Toward a functional analysis of self-injury. *Journal of Applied Behavior Analysis, 27*, 197–209. (Reprinted from Analysis and Intervention in Developmental Disabilities, 2, 3–20, 1982).

Jerome, J., Frantino, E. P., & Sturmey, P. (2007). The effects of errorless learning and backward chaining on the acquisition of internet skills in adults with developmental disabilities. *Journal of Applied Behavior Analysis, 40*, 185–189.

Kennedy, C. H. (2005). *Single-case design for educational research*. Boston, MA: Allyn & Bacon.

Koegel, R. L., & Koegel, L. K. (2006). *Pivotal response treatments for autism: communication, social, and academic development*. Baltimore, MD: Brookes Press.

Laraway, S., Snycerski, S., Michael, J., & Poling, A. (2003). Motivating operations and terms to describe them: Some further refinements. *Journal of Applied Behavior Analysis, 36*, 407–414.

Lerman, D. C., Iwata, B. A., & Wallace, M. D. (1999). Side effects of extinction: Prevalence of bursting and aggression during the treatment of self-injurious behavior. *Journal of Applied Behavior Analysis, 32,* 1–8.

Lovaas, O. I. (1981). *Teaching developmentally disabled children: The me book.* Baltimore, MD: University Park.

Lovaas, O. I. (1987). Behavioral treatment and normal educational and intellectual functioning in young autistic children. *Journal of Consulting and Clinical Psychology, 55,* 3–9.

Mangus, B., Henderson, H., & French, R. (1986). Implementation of a token economy by peer tutors to increase on-task physical activity time of autistic children. *Perceptual and Motor Skills, 1,* 97–98.

Maurice, C., Green, G., & Luce, S. C. (1996). *Behavioral intervention for young children with autism.* Austin, TX: Pro-Ed.

McEachin, J. J., Smith, T., & Lovaas, O. I. (1993). Long-term outcome for children with autism who received early intensive behavioral treatment. *American Journal on Mental Retardation, 97,* 359–372.

Mesibov, G., & Howley, M. (2003). *Accessing the curriculum for pupils with autistic spectrum disorders: Using the TEACCH programme to help inclusion.* London: David Fulton Publishers.

Mesibov, G. B., Shea, V., & Schopler, E. (2004). *The TEACCH approach to autism spectrum disorders.* New York, NY: Springer.

Michael, J. (1982). Distinguishing between discriminative and motivational functions of stimuli. *Journal of the Experimental Analysis of Behavior, 1,* 149–155.

Newman, B., Tuntigian, L., Ryan, C., & Reinecke, D. (1997). Self-management of a DRO procedure by three students with autism. *Behavioral Interventions, 12,* 149–156.

Ray, K. P., Skinner, C. H., & Watson, T. S. (1999). Transferring stimulus control via momentum to increase compliance in a student with autism: A demonstration of collaborative consultation. *School Psychology Review, 28,* 622–628.

Reed, G. K., Ringdahl, J. E., Wacker, D. P., Barretto, A., & Andelman, M. S. (2005). The effects of fixed-time and contingent schedules of negative reinforcement on compliance and aberrant behavior. *Research in Developmental Disabilities, 3,* 281–295.

Reichow, B., & Wolery, M. (2009). Comprehensive synthesis of early intensive behavioral interventions for young children with autism based on the UCLA young autism project model. *Journal of Autism and Developmental Disorders, 39*(1), 23–41.

Ricciardi, J. N., Luiselli, J. K., & Camare, M. (2006). Shaping approach responses as intervention for specific phobia in a child with autism. *Journal of Applied Behavior Analysis, 39,* 445–448.

Ringdahl, J. E., Christensen, T. J., & Boelter, E. W. (2009). Further evaluation of idiosyncratic functions for severe problem behavior: Aggression maintained by access to walks. *Behavioral Interventions* doi:10.1002/bin.289

Ringdahl, J. E., Falcomata, T. S., Christensen, T. J., Bass-Ringdahl, S. M., Lentz, A., Dutt, A., et al. (2009). Evaluation of a pre-treatment assessment to select mand topographies for functional communication training. *Research in Developmental Disabilities, 30*(2), 330–341.

Ringdahl, J. E., Kitsukawa, K., Andelman, M. S., Call, N., Winborn, L., Barretto, A., et al. (2002). Differential reinforcement with

and without instructional fading. *Journal of Applied Behavior Analysis, 35,* 291–294.

Risley, T. R. (1968). The effects and side effects of punishing the autistic behaviors of a deviant child. *Journal of Applied Behavior Analysis, 1,* 21–34.

Roane, H. S., Fisher, W. W., Sgro, G. M., Falcomata, T. S., & Pabico, R. R. (2004). An alternative method of thinning reinforcer delivery during differential reinforcement. *Journal of Applied Behavior Analysis, 37,* 213–218.

Rusch, F. R., Rose, T., & Greenwood, C. R. (1988). *Introduction to behavior analysis in special education.* Prentice Hall: Englewood Cliffs, NJ.

Shabani, D. B., & Fisher, W. W. (2006). Stimulus fading and differential reinforcement for the treatment of needle phobia in a youth with autism. *Journal of Applied Behavior Analysis, 39,* 449–452.

Shabani, D. B., Katz, R. C., Wilder, D. A., Beauchamp, K., Taylor, C. R., & Fischer, K. J. (2002). Increasing social initiations in children with autism: Effects of a tactile prompt. *Journal of Applied Behavior Analysis, 35,* 79–83.

Shirley, M. J., Iwata, B. A., Kahng, S., Mazaleski, J. L., & Lerman, D. C. (1997). Does functional communication training compete with ongoing contingencies of reinforcement? An analysis during response acquisition and maintenance. *Journal of Applied Behavior Analysis, 30,* 93–104.

Simpson, R. L. (2005). *Autism spectrum disorders: Interventions and treatments for children and youth.* Thousand Oaks, CA: Corwin Press.

Skinner, B. F. (1953). *Science and human behavior.* New York, NY: The Free Press.

Smith, M. D. (1987). Treatment of pica in an adult disabled by autism by differential reinforcement of incompatible behavior. *Journal of Behavioral Therapy and Experimental Psychiatry, 18,* 285–288.

Sulzer-Azaroff, B., & Mayer, G. R. (1991). *Behavior analysis for lasting change.* New York, NY: Harcourt Brace College Publishers.

Tarbox, R. F., Ghezzi, P. M., & Wilson, G. (2006). The effects of token reinforcement on attending in a young child with autism. *Behavioral Interventions, 21,* 155–164.

Taylor, B. A., & Levin, L. (1998). Teaching a student with autism to make verbal initiations: Effects of a tactile prompt. *Journal of Applied Behavior Analysis, 31,* 651–654.

Taylor, B. A., Hoch, H., Potter, B., Rodriguez, A., Spinnato, D., & Kalaigan, M. (2005). Manipulating establishing operations to promote initiations toward peers in children with autism. *Research in Developmental Disabilities, 26,* 385–392.

Thompson, R. H., Fisher, W. W., & Contrucci, S. A. (1998). Evaluating the reinforcing effects of choice in comparison to reinforcement rate. *Research in Developmental Disabilities, 18,* 181–187.

Tiger, J. H., Hanley, G. P., & Bruzek, J. (2008). Functional communication training: A review and practical guide. *Behavior Analysis in Practice, 1,* 16–23.

Vollmer, T. R. (2002). Punishment happens: Some comments on Lerman and Vorndran's review. *Journal of Applied Behavior Analysis, 35,* 469–473.

Chapter 3
Assessment Methods

Frederick Furniss

Functional assessment, experimental functional analysis, operationally defining target behaviors, interval recording, and single case research designs will be the focus here. The unique aspects of operant evaluation and assessment methods, and how they can be applied to the evaluation of autism will be stressed.

Phases of Behavioural Assessment

The goal of applied behaviour analysis is to enable clients to make improvements in socially important behaviours which thereby produce significant improvements in the quality of life of the client and socially significant others. Assessment is an essential first step in this process, which enables the behaviour analyst and the client to (1) define the key behaviours to be changed, (2) identify environmental conditions which will support the changes to be made and (3) define any environmental conditions which are currently impeding the desired changes.

The assessment process itself may be conceptualized as comprising five stages:

1. Preassessment: gaining an overview of the client's situation and defining possible important areas for intervention.
2. Identification of priority targets for behaviour change, including behaviours to be strengthened and behaviours to be replaced/reduced.
3. Definition and measurement of baseline (preintervention) levels of target behaviours.
4. Evaluating functional relationships between environmental conditions and target behaviours and developing hypotheses regarding interventions which will produce desired behaviour change.
5. Testing the behaviour change hypotheses thus developed.

This chapter describes some key questions to be addressed at each stage of the process and some of the methods and tools available to the behaviour analyst in seeking to answer these questions.

Preassessment

When working with children with autism spectrum disorders (ASD), initial acquaintance with the child will often suggest that there are many areas in which behaviour change might benefit the child and her/his significant others. The child may have many obvious problems with social, communication, or play skills, and may engage in stereotyped, self-injurious, or aggressive behaviours which discourage other people from engaging with him/her and limit his/her participation in educational and recreational activities. An important initial task is therefore to identify from a potentially large number of possible targets for intervention a realistic number of key targets for initial attention.

One approach to this problem is to use standardized descriptive assessments of adaptive and problematic behaviours. Such scales can be distinguished into two categories by their scope. Generalised behaviour rating scales assess a range of domains of adaptive or

F. Furniss (✉)
The Hesley Group, Hesley Hall, Stripe Road, Doncaster, DN11 9HH, U.K.
e-mail: fred.furniss@hesleygroup.co.uk

J.L. Matson (ed.), *Applied Behavior Analysis for Children with Autism Spectrum Disorders*,
DOI 10.1007/978-1-4419-0088-3_3, © Springer Science+Business Media, LLC 2009

potentially problematic behaviour, each of which in turn may consist of a number of sub-domains. Assessments such as the Vineland Adaptive Behavior Scales (de Bildt, Kraijer, Sytema, & Minderaa, 2005), and the AAIDD Adaptive Behavior Scale – School: Second Edition (ABS-S:2) (Lambert, Nihira, & Leland, 1993) can provide the behaviour analyst with a broad overview of the child's abilities and by providing developmental norms, enable the clinician to evaluate the child's abilities in various domains in comparison with those of children without developmental disabilities. The AAIDD ABS-S:2 and other instruments such as the Developmental Behavior Checklist (Einfeld & Tonge, 1995) similarly provide a broad overview of potential problematic behaviours. Although such assessments can provide indications concerning priority areas for intervention, they typically include only a few items assessing each domain and sub-domain and therefore provide limited assistance in selecting target behaviours for intervention. More specialized assessments focussing on single domains or sub-domains such as language (Luyster, Kadlec, Carter & Tager-Flusberg, 2008), stereotyped behaviours (Rojahn, Matlock, & Tassé, 2000; Rojahn, Tassé, & Sturmey, 1997) or mealtime behaviours (Lukens & Linscheid, 2008) may provide more specific indications of potential target behaviours. Final selection of target behaviours will however almost certainly require further attention in the second stage of the assessment process.

Although identification of areas of adaptive and problem behaviour for intervention is a key goal of the preassessment process, the behaviour analyst should also at this stage gather further basic information regarding potential target behaviours. Estimates of approximate frequency of occurrence of problem behaviours, for example, may well be of value in deciding how to structure more detailed assessment. Efficient assessment of a behaviour estimated to occur many times per hour will require a different approach than that required for a major problem which however occurs less than once per month (Ball, Bush, & Emerson, 2004). It is also important at the preassessment phase to identify any behaviours which pose sufficiently severe risks to the child and/or other people that it may be necessary to devise and implement an emergency crisis management plan (Willis & LaVigna, 1985) in advance of a comprehensive assessment being completed (Ball et al.).

Identification of Priority Targets for Behaviour Change

The use of developmental assessments as described above may suggest general foci for intervention. Developmental appropriateness is however only one consideration in selecting target behaviours for intervention. For adaptive behaviours, children with ASD will often show deficits in many areas relative to peers without disabilities, and so determination of priorities for intervention must involve selection among many possible relevant targets. For potentially problematic behaviours, children with ASD may show behaviours which are developmentally common, such as stereotyped behaviours, which in children without disabilities may resolve without intervention but which in children with ASD will often require intervention if they are not to become chronic. The behaviour analyst will therefore often need, in consultation with the child and his/her significant others, to determine priority behaviours for intervention from a large number of possibilities. Cooper, Heron, and Heward (2007) and others suggest a number of questions which may usefully be asked in making this choice:

1. Will the behaviour elicit reinforcement in the client's natural environment and hence be likely to be maintained without artificial programming of contingencies (Ayllon & Azrin, 1968)?
2. Is the behaviour a necessary prerequisite for learning a useful skill?
3. Will the behaviour increase the client's access to environments in which other important behaviours can be learned and used?
4. Will changing this behaviour predispose others to interact with the client in a way which will enhance quality of life and promote further development? If a child frequently spits on to his/her hands and plays with the spittle, this behaviour may merit intervention, not only because of the direct harm which it may cause to the child, which may be mild, but because it may discourage other children and adults from engaging with the child.
5. Is the behaviour a "behavioural cusp" or "pivotal behaviour"? Acquisition of some behaviours may facilitate further development, not simply because they are components of a more complex skill, but because the acquisition of the behaviour enables

the child to engage with a range of previously inaccessible learning opportunities. Rosales-Ruiz and Baer (1997) describe "behavioural cusps" as behaviours which bring the learner's repertoire into contact with new environments and contingencies of reinforcement and punishment, and suggest crawling, generalized imitation, and reading as possible examples. Koegel, Koegel, and McNerney (2001) describe "pivotal behaviours" as behaviours the acquisition of which results in corresponding changes in other adaptive behaviours.

6. Is a behaviour proposed as a developmental target chronologically age-appropriate?

7. What degree of risk to the child or others does the behaviour pose? In some cases problem behaviours (e.g. self-injury, aggression or dangerous climbing) or lack of adaptive skills (e.g. failure to inhibit ongoing behaviour in response to "no" from carers) may put the child or others at sufficient risk that the behaviour must be a priority for intervention (Ball et al., 2004).

8. If the target behaviour is to be reduced, what adaptive behaviour will be taught or strengthened to enable the child to meet the need previously fulfilled by the problem behaviour (Goldiamond, 1974)?

9. Are necessary resources in place to achieve change in the proposed target behaviour? The experience, knowledge and skill of the behaviour analyst herself and of the child's carers will influence the probability that specific target behaviours can be changed (Ball et al., 2004; Cooper et al., 2007).

10. What is the history of previous change attempts? The behaviour analyst should carefully review records relating to previous attempts to change potential target behaviours. Records indicating previous successes with related target behaviours or a history of limited impact on a behaviour despite well-planned and faithfully implemented change programmes may be useful in selecting change targets which can be achieved within meaningful timescales.

Even after consideration of all these questions, a substantial number of potential target behaviours for change may well be identified, and final selection of target behaviours for intervention will probably involve a process of discussion and negotiation between the child, his/her parents, other involved professionals such as teachers and speech and language therapists, and the behaviour analyst. Legal frameworks and associated codes of practice (e.g. the UK Mental Capacity Act) may well prescribe, depending on the age of the young person and his/her capacity to evaluate the proposed intervention, who has ultimate responsibility for deciding on whether a particular intervention should proceed, who that person should consult before reaching their decision, and how any serious irreconcilable disagreement between key interested parties may be resolved. In most cases however a systematic joint approach to the issue, perhaps involving structured ratings of proposed targets by interested parties according to the above criteria (Cooper et al., 2007) will achieve consensus. Where this proves impossible, a joint commitment to objective evaluation of the degree to which intervention is producing expected benefits to the child, and to regular review of the appropriateness of the intervention target, may reassure those with unresolved doubts and allow intervention to begin.

Definition and Measurement of Baseline Levels of Target Behaviours

The history of interventions used in attempts to produce change in the behaviours of people with developmental disabilities includes many examples of interventions which have been widely used and often assumed to be effective, but were found to be ineffective when carefully evaluated in controlled research (e.g. Tyrer et al. 2008). In the case of children with ASD, behaviour analytic interventions have both been subject to more scientific scrutiny than many other widely used interventions and have a stronger evidence base for their efficacy (Eikeseth, 2009). The practising behaviour analyst should however remember that (1) much of the evidence supporting the efficacy of behavioural interventions for problems such as self-injury comes from studies using single-subject experimental designs, which may be particularly susceptible to bias in publication of studies with positive rather than negative outcomes (Kahng, Iwata, & Lewin, 2002), and (2) although complex interventions can be successfully implemented by service staff such as teachers (e.g. Sigafoos & Meikle, 1996), some of the evidence for treatment effectiveness comes from data collected during defined time periods with interventions implemented by highly skilled staff, with only a minority of studies reporting data on generalization of treatment effects (DeLeon, Rodriguez-Catter & Cataldo, 2002; Kahng et al., 2002). The measurement of change in the individual case is therefore not just central to the ethos of behaviour analysis; it is also required by the current state of the science, which despite its undoubted strengths is continuing to work towards effective technological (Baer, Wolf, & Risley, 1968) solutions to many serious problems of childhood development.

Defining Target Behaviours

Measurement of baseline levels of the target behaviours requires that they first be operationally defined. Definitions may be based on function or topography (Cooper et al., 2007). Function-based definitions identify the target behaviour as any behaviour which produces a specific effect on the environment (including the child's own body). Topographically-based definitions identify the target behaviour by describing its form or (often) by providing a general description of a class of behaviours together with specific descriptions of behaviours which are to be recorded as members of the class. Examples of both are given in Table 3.1.

In general, functional definitions are to be preferred over topographical descriptions as they provide a comprehensive definition of all possible relevant behaviours. Definition in terms of topography may however be necessary in cases where either a behaviour does not necessarily result in a functional outcome (e.g. a child may say "hello" to a peer who does not respond), or when the outcome may be produced by other events (e.g. a peer may respond positively if a child hits them as well as if the child says "hello"). In some cases it may be useful to define the target behaviour in terms of both topography and function, e.g. where it is necessary to define a behaviour in terms of qualitative features as well as outcome (e.g. it may be necessary to define self-injury as any forceful contact between the child's hand and head). An example of such a mixed definition is also given in Table 3.1.

Whether the target behaviour is defined functionally or topographically, the definition should be phrased in terms of observable aspects of the behaviour (and where relevant its environmental consequences), should be sufficiently clear so that experienced observers can agree as to whether a particular behavioural episode does or does not constitute an example of the target behaviour, and should be exhaustive in the sense that so far as possible it should include all possible exemplars of the target behaviour class. An adequate behavioural definition should enable an observer to classify any segment of the child's stream of behaviour as including or not including the target behaviour.

Measuring Baseline Levels of the Target Behaviour

General Considerations

Measuring baseline levels of the target behaviour will generally require direct or indirect observation of the child's behaviour. Again, depending on the local legal framework and the age of the child/young person, the consent of the child, the consent of parents, or, in the case where the young person in terms of age would normally have the right to decline assessment but is judged to lack capacity to make an informed decision, a decision as to whether observation is in the best interests of the young person, will be required.

Table 3.1 Examples of function-based, topographically based, and mixed definitions of target behaviours

Type of definition	Behaviour label	Behaviour definition	Source
Function-based	Hand mouthing	Insertion of the hand or fingers past the plane of the upper and lower lips, or protrusion of the tongue out of the mouth onto the hand or fingers	Goh et al., 1995, pp. 271–272
Topographically based	Social initiation	Approaching the experimenter, emitting any verbal (e.g. "Let's play", "Let's move the table", or "Let's sit down") or gestural (e.g. taking him by the hand) behaviour and leading him toward the activity previously viewed on the video	Nikopoulos and Keenan, 2007, p. 680.
Mixed	Spitting	Wiping with her hand, licking or projecting from her mouth saliva onto herself, any other person, or any object or surface	Garbutt and Furniss, 2007, p. 128.

An appropriate observation period will also need to be identified (Miltenberger, 2001). The preassessment process should enable the behaviour analyst to select a time period, location, and observation period appropriate to gain a representative estimate of the baseline level of the behaviour. For high-frequency behaviours, a relatively brief observation period may suffice, whereas for lower-frequency behaviours, especially those reported to occur throughout the whole day, a procedure which allows for continuous observation and recording may be necessary. In all cases, the behaviour analyst should balance the need for reliable and representative information with the principle of using the least intrusive method. If, for example, the target behaviour is believed to occur to the same extent in school or preschool as in the child's home, observation in the school may be preferred if this is a commonplace occurrence, but observation in the home may be preferred if observation in the school would draw peers' attention to the fact that the child is receiving unusual professional intervention. If observation can be reliably undertaken by persons normally present in the child's environment, (the child him/herself, parents, or teachers), this option is preferable to the intrusive introduction of specialist observers. If, however, use of specialist observers is the only option for gaining reliable observations, the benefit in terms of improved intervention design may warrant the increased intrusion. In all cases, however, the behaviour analyst before beginning any potentially intrusive observation should (1) define circumstances or areas in which observations will be suspended to maintain the child's dignity and privacy and (2) ensure that the child is able to end an observation session if he/she so desires. In the case of children with limited communication skills, this may require definition of an area accessible to the child where observations are not pursued.

Measures of Behaviour

Assuming that the target behaviour has a discrete beginning and end, its occurrences can be counted. To enable meaningful comparison of counts across observation periods, counts are generally used together with the duration of the observation period to derive the rate or frequency of the target behaviour, defined as the number of occurrences of the behaviour per unit time. Meaningful comparison of rates of target behaviours may itself, however, require reference to the length of the observation period, measurement (in the case of skill development) of rates of both correct and incorrect responding, and consideration of possible changes in complexity of the behaviour being counted. Cooper et al. (2007) provide more detailed discussion of these subtleties of rate measures and how they may be addressed.

For some target behaviours, duration rather than rate will be a more appropriate measure. This may be because (1) single episodes of a behaviour (e.g. screaming) may occur for very variable durations, (2) a target behaviour (e.g. cooperative play), although composed of discrete behaviours, is functionally defined by the reciprocation of the peer and hence is more usefully defined as extended in time or (3) the target behaviour (e.g. head-hitting), although occurring as a discrete behaviour which could be counted, typically occurs in "bursts" of variable duration and it is suspected that the "burst", rather than the individual blow to the head, may be the functional unit of behaviour (Hall & Oliver, 1992). In each case, either the total time (or percentage of the total observation time) for which the behaviour occurred, or the mean duration of individual episodes, may be the most relevant measure of the target behaviour.

Depending on the specific target behaviour and the goals and possible methods of intervention being considered, other measures of behaviour may be relevant. Intensity of behaviour may be relevant if the goal of intervention is to modify the audibility of speech or severity of tissue damage resulting from self-injurious behaviours, and measurement of mean interresponse time (mean length of time between successive occurrences of the target behaviour) may be useful in planning initial parameters for differential reinforcement interventions (Cooper et al., 2007).

Other measures may be appropriate depending on the specific aims of intervention. For example, where the goal of intervention is to strengthen a behaviour under specified contextual conditions (e.g. to pass an object when requested to do so by a peer), the relevant measure may be the proportion of appropriate opportunities on which the target behaviour is performed. Where the goal is for the child to learn a new skill which comprises an organised chain of behaviours, a useful measure of progress may be the number or proportion of task analysis steps which the child performs correctly.

Evaluation of interventions by measuring change in the level of the target behaviour(s) is central to the ethos of behaviour analysis and should always be addressed in behavioural interventions. It will often be the case however, that the intervention is intended to produce change not only in a target behaviour (e.g. spontaneously approaching peers to engage in play, or screaming) but also in other behaviours of the child, peers or caregivers (e.g. engaging in social play, positive comments from peers, taking the child on visits to friends or family). Such putative collateral benefits can be operationally defined and measured in similar fashion to target behaviours, providing a partial basis for the behaviour analyst to objectively evaluate the social validity (Wolf, 1978) of the subsequent intervention.

Observation and Recording Methods

Continuous Recording Methods

In continuous recording, the observer takes data from every occurrence of the target behaviour during the observation period. In *event recording*, the observer keeps a tally of each occurrence of the target behaviour(s). The tally may be simply kept using paper and pencil, with the advantage that the count can be made within defined time segments of the observation period (i.e. *frequency-within-interval recording*, Miltenberger, 2001), providing additional information as to the clustering of behaviours. However, if use of paper and pencil is inappropriate or difficult (for example, if it would draw undue peer attention to the fact that the child is being observed, or if the observer has to observe while also undertaking other tasks) wrist- or hand-held counters of the kind used to tally golf strokes, numbers of passengers present on aeroplanes, stock held in grocery stores, etc. may be used. Event recording can often be accurately conducted by observers with minimal training and can be used to measure frequency/rate of behaviour. Event recording is useful if rate is a useful measure of the behaviour, if the beginning and end of an episode of behaviour are clearly defined, and if the behaviour occurs at a rate which the observer's responses can match. If the client's self-injury, therefore, typically comprises single blows of the head against hard surfaces at a rate of approximately one per minute, event recording may be suitable. If however the self-injury presents as sequences of very

rapid hand-head blows, with "bursts" of self-injury varying widely in duration, and in conditions where it is difficult to discern whether a blow is an isolated event or the initiation of a "burst", event recording probably is not an appropriate observation method.

In the latter case, the observer may wish to continuously record the *duration* of the behaviour, either by measuring the total time occupied by the behaviour, or or by measuring the duration of each episode and the duration of each inter-episode interval. The first may be readily accomplished using a digital stopwatch, while episode length and inter-episode interval length may be recorded using a stopwatch plus paper and pencil. The first method will enable calculation of the overall percentage of time occupied by the behaviour, the second will in addition enable calculation of mean and range of episode lengths, and the final option would additionally enable the observer to calculate inter-response times. In the latter two cases, as with event recording, the observer will need to decide how to deal with brief interruptions in the behaviour. If a child interacting with a peer suspends the interaction for 2 s to look towards an adult entering the room and then resumes the interaction, is this to be recorded as a single episode of social interaction or as two shorter episodes with an inter-response time of 2 s? Such questions should be addressed by the operational definition of the target behaviour, but the observer may well need to "field-test" the definition in preliminary observations in order to refine the definition to deal with all such circumstances.

In *real-time* recording methods, the exact second of onset and offset of each episode of target behaviours within the observation period is recorded. Such methods can be used to calculate all of the measures derived from event or duration records (frequency/rate, total duration, total duration as a percentage of the observation period, mean and range of episode lengths, etc.). A number of systems for real-time observation running on handheld computers are now available (Emerson, Reeves, & Felce, 2000; Kahng & Iwata, 2000). Such systems have the advantage of allowing the observer to readily record multiple target behaviours both of the child and of significant others in the environment together with other environmental events. The potential advantages of such systems are discussed further in the next section of this chapter.

In *product recording*, the observer does not directly record the child's behaviour, but instead records a measure related to the product of the child's behaviour, e.g. number of arithmetic problems successfully completed during the observation period. Product recording may be useful where it is difficult or socially inappropriate to directly observe the behaviour.

To evaluate the impact of a toilet training programme Lancioni, Van Bergen, and Furniss (2002), for example, used direct event recording of one target behaviour (self-initiated toileting). Inappropriate urinations were however not recorded directly; instead, "small accidents" and "large accidents" were measured by observing the impact on the learner's clothing. The value of product recording of course depends on the extent to which the product measured is reliably and exclusively produced only by the target behaviour of the client (Cooper et al., 2007; Miltenberger, 2001).

Sampling Methods

If the behaviour analyst does not have access to real-time recording methods, it may be difficult to use continuous recording methods in situations where multiple target behaviours (or a single target behaviour of more than one client) are to be measured. This difficulty will be compounded if the analyst additionally wishes to record target behaviours of other people directed towards the client, or other environmental events, as will frequently be required for purposes of functional assessment (see further below). It may also be difficult to use continuous recording methods if the target behaviour occurs at very high rate, or if it is difficult to operationally define the onset and offset of episodes of behaviour. In such circumstances one of a number of sampling methods may be helpful. All are based on the principle that the recording procedure is not structured by the episodes of the behaviour. Rather, the observations are made at a series of predetermined time periods (which are either momentary or typically of 5–20 s duration), and the presence or absence of the behaviour in that time period is recorded.

In *whole-interval* recording, the observation period is divided into a series of brief time intervals (typically 5–20 s in duration). For each interval, the observer records at the end of the interval whether or not the target behaviour was observed throughout the whole of that interval. Data are typically summarized in terms of the percentage of total intervals in which the behaviour was recorded, a measure which may be taken as an estimate of the percentage of observation time for which the behaviour occurred and used to derive an estimate of its total duration during the observation period. It will be obvious that whole-interval recording may be expected to produce conservative estimates in this regard, since if a behaviour (e.g. social interaction) is observed to occur for 9 s in a 10 s recording interval, the presence of the behaviour will not be recorded in that interval. It will also be apparent that whole-interval records may be used to estimate mean episode length and inter-response interval for the target behaviour, but that the precision of these estimates will vary inversely with the length of the recording interval.

Partial-interval recording uses a similar procedure, but the observer records the behaviour as present within an interval if it was observed at any time during the interval. Thus, the child is recorded as engaged in social interaction during a 10 s interval even if such interaction is observed for only 1 s of that interval. The data is again typically summarized in terms of the percentage of intervals during which the behaviour was present, and this measure is again often taken as an estimate of the percentage of the observation time in which the behaviour is occurring. It will this time be apparent that the method would be expected to provide an inflated estimate of the actual presence of the behaviour, and that this inflation will be greater with greater interval lengths.

Both whole- and partial-interval methods require the observer to accurately measure the passage of time during the recording period. Wristwatches, stopwatches, taped audio cues, or paging devices may be used to indicate the transitions between intervals. Observers should always actively record the presence or absence of each observed behaviour during each interval, as if intervals are left unmarked it is easy to become confused as to which of the sequence of intervals is currently underway (Cooper et al., 2007). The necessity to observe and record simultaneously can be avoided by dividing the observation period into observation and recording periods, e.g. 10 s for observation, 5 s for recording.

In *momentary time sampling*, observations are made momentarily at predetermined time intervals. Thus, the observer using momentary time sampling with a 20 s interval, records only if the behaviour is occurring at the time of momentary observations (typically with a nominal 1 s or sometimes 2 s duration) at 20, 40, 60 s (etc.) following the beginning of the observation period. Data is again usually summarized in terms of the percentage of intervals during which the behaviour was present, and this measure is again often taken as an estimate of the percentage of the observation time for which the behaviour occurs. Momentary time sampling is particularly useful if the behaviour analyst wishes to simultaneously record the behaviour of many clients (e.g. on-task behaviour of a whole class of students). However, it can only be used if the behaviour can be defined independently of its temporally extended social context (e.g. it can be used to record social interaction, but not social interaction reciprocal to a peer's initiation), and is not generally useful for measuring low-frequency or typically very brief behaviours (Saudargas & Zanolli, 1990).

Figure 3.1 illustrates a general-purpose recording form which may be adapted for frequency-within-interval, whole- or partial-interval, or momentary time sample, recording, while Fig. 3.2 illustrates how such a form would be completed for each method given the stream of behaviour illustrated.

Comparison of Sampling Methods

A limited amount of empirical work has compared continuous duration recording measures of the percentage of observation time occupied by a target behaviour with estimates derived from sampling methods and/or has investigated whether use of different methods leads to different conclusions on questions such as the relative levels of a behaviour under two or more conditions. Recent work on the first issue has confirmed findings from earlier studies (e.g. Murphy & Goodall, 1980) showing that partial interval recording, as would be expected, over-estimates the percentage of time for which the target behaviour is present. Gardenier, MacDonald, and Green (2004, Experiment 1) showed that in comparison with results from continuous duration recording, 10 s partial-interval recording yielded substantial over-estimates of the percentages of time during which 15 children with ASD engaged in stereotyped behaviours, with the mean figure from partial interval recording exceeding that of continuous recording by a factor greater than 1.5. Gardenier et al. (Experiment 2) then demonstrated that the 10 s partial-interval method substantially over-estimated the duration of stereotypy even for samples in which continuous recording showed stereotypy occurring for 40% of observation time or more. Momentary time sampling with intervals of 10,

20 or 30 s generated both under- and over-estimates of the percentage of time occupied by stereotypy across different observation samples, but this method reliably yielded more accurate estimates than the partial interval record. Rapp et al. (2007) considered the extent to which continuous duration recording, 10 s partial-interval recording, and 10- and 20-s momentary time sampling might impact on conclusions regarding functional relationships between environmental contexts (e.g. treatment conditions) and a target behaviour and regarding functional relationships between two target behaviours. Comparisons were considered using both reversal and alternating treatment approaches (Cooper et al., 2007) to examine functional relationships. Momentary time sampling with 10 s intervals reliably, and with 20 s intervals generally, led to conclusions regarding functional relationships that were identical to those reached using continuous recording. With some data distributions however, the partial interval method led to different conclusions regarding functional relationships than those derived from the continuous recording data.

Meany-Daboul, Roscoe, Bourret, and Ahearn (2007), examining three datasets from reversal designs, also found slightly higher agreement on functional relationships between continuous duration recording and momentary time sampling than between continuous duration recording and partial-interval recording when judgements concerning functional relationships were based on visual inspection of the data by experienced behaviour analysts. However, when agreement between two analysts applying criteria proposed by Fisher, Kelley, and Lomas (2003) was evaluated, momentary time sampling and partial interval data yielded equal numbers of agreements with continuous duration recording. Meany-Daboul et al., noting that partial-interval sampling is also used in situations where frequency data would be the continuous recording method of choice, also compared agreements for two datasets between frequency records and momentary time sampling and partial interval data. In these cases, both expert visual analysis and application of structured criteria to judgements on functional relationships produced slightly higher levels of agreement between judgements based on continuous frequency recording and partial interval data than between continuous frequency recording and data from momentary time sampling.

More research is needed on the extent to which differing data distributions affect the extent to which sampling methods produce estimates agreeing with

Behaviour Monitoring Chart

Client's Name: [   ]   Date/time of observation: [   ]

Behaviours/Events to be Recorded:

Behaviour A = [   ]

Behaviour B = [   ]

Behaviour C = [   ]

Behaviour D = [   ]

Type of Recording (circle method used)

Frequency Count: Tick once each time the behaviour occurs; enter 0 if it does not occur in that interval

Partial Interval: Tick if the behaviour occurs at any time during that interval or write 0 if it does not

Whole Interval: Tick if the behaviour occurs throughout the whole of the interval, write 0 if it does not

Momentary Time Sample   Tick if the behaviour was occurring in the final second of the interval, write 0 if it was not.

Interval Length: [   ]

Interval Number	Time Period	Behaviour A	Behaviour B	Behaviour C	Behaviour D
1					
2					
3					
4					
5					
6					
7					
8					
9					
10					
11					
12					
13					
14					
15					
16					
17					
18					
19					
20					
TOTAL NO. OF OCCURRENCES/INTERVALS					
FOR SAMPLING METHODS: PERCENTAGE INTERVALS WITH BEHAVIOUR RECORDED					

Fig. 3.1 General purpose observation form for frequency-within interval, partial-interval, whole-interval or momentary time sample recording

Behaviour Monitoring Chart

Client's Name: | Anthony Nigel OTHER | Date/time of observation: | 1st. September 2008, 13.30 |

Behaviours/Events to be Recorded:

Behaviour A = | Hand-to-head hits |

Type of Recording (circle method used)

Frequency Count: Tick once each time the behaviour occurs within an interval; enter 0 if it does not occur in that interval

Partial Interval: Tick if the behaviour occurs at any time during that interval or write 0 if it does not

Whole Interval: Tick if the behaviour occurs throughout the whole of the interval, write 0 if it does not

Momentary Time Sample: Tick if the behaviour was occurring in the <u>final second</u> of the interval, write 0 if it was not.

Interval Length: | 5 Seconds |

Behaviour per second of observation (X = occurrence, 0 = non-occurrence)	Interval Number	Time Period	Observation/recording method			
			Frequency within interval	Partial interval	Whole interval	Momentary time sample
X X X X 0	1	0-5s	√√√√	√	0	0
0 0 0 0 0	2	6-10s	0	0	0	0
0 X X X X	3	11-15s	√√√√	√	0	√
X X X X X	4	16-20s	√√√√√	√	√	√
X 0 0 0 0	5	21-25s	√	√	0	0
TOTAL NO. OF OCCURRENCES/INTERVALS			14 occurrences	4 intervals	1 interval	2 intervals
FOR SAMPLING METHODS: PERCENTAGE INTERVALS WITH BEHAVIOUR RECORDED				4/5 x 100% = 80%	1/5 x 100% = 20%	2/5 x 100% = 40%

Fig. 3.2 Comparison of records completed by frequency-within interval, partial-interval, whole-interval and momentary time sample recording

continuous records. If duration is the dimension of behaviour of primary interest, if the aim of recording is to produce an accurate estimate of the percentage of observation time occupied by the behaviour, and if a sampling method is to be used, momentary time sampling, with an interval of 10 s if possible, should be the method of choice. If comparison of levels of behaviour under different conditions, as in evaluating the impact of intervention, is of greater concern than estimating the actual level of the behaviour, then momentary time sampling is generally to be preferred for behaviour where duration is of primary interest and partial-interval recording for data is to be preferred where frequency is of primary interest.

Evaluating the Accuracy and Reliability of Data Collected by Direct Observation

The accuracy of any measure of the frequency or duration of a behaviour refers to the extent to which the data collected match the "true" frequency or duration value (Johnston & Pennypacker, 1993). The accuracy of behavioural data will be affected by a number of factors including the comprehensiveness and clarity of definition of the target behaviour, the extent of training and practice which observers undertake prior to collecting clinical data, observer fatigue, the number of different behaviours/events being recorded, and so on. In principle, the accuracy of any specific system for observation could be evaluated by using the system to collect data from videorecorded sequences of relevant social interactions with known properties. In clinical practice, however, the "true" values of levels of behaviour will generally not be known. In these circumstances, unable to determine the accuracy of the data collected, the behaviour analyst will nevertheless at least wish to evaluate its reliability. Reliability refers to the extent to which repeated application of the observation system to a specific segment of behaviour results in identical measures. A high degree of reliability does not guarantee the accuracy of the data, but inadequate reliability is a strong indicator of likely inaccuracy. Reliability may be evaluated by having a single observer repeat observation and recording of videorecorded events. A high degree of reliability thus measured however leaves open the possibility that the degree of reliability achieved, is dependent on unknown factors as well as on the observation system employed.

For this reason, the measure of reliability most often employed in behaviour analysis is interobserver agreement, namely, the extent to which two observers, using the same definitions of behaviour, appropriately trained in the use of a specific observation and recording technique, and independently observing the same events, agree on the level of behaviour observed. Cooper et al. (2007) review a range of approaches applicable to measure interobserver agreement, dependent on the dimension of behaviour which is of interest and the observation system used. Where interval recording or time sampling is used, the simplest method of evaluating interobserver agreement is to directly compare whether the two observers agree or disagree on the presence or absence of a behaviour at each interval of the observation system. The extent of interobserver agreement may then be evaluated by counting the number of intervals at which the two observers agree, dividing this figure by the number of agreements plus the number of intervals at which the two observers disagree, and expressing the resulting figure as a percentage (see Fig. 3.3). If a behaviour occurs infrequently, however, the fact that this method measures agreement regarding both the occurrence and nonoccurrence of a behaviour means that it may yield high levels of agreement in cases where the two observers rarely agree on the occurrence of a behaviour. This difficulty may be addressed by calculating occurrence interobserver agreement in which the above calculation is performed using only those intervals at which at least one observer has recorded the behaviour as present (Fig. 3.3, shaded rows). An alternative approach is to evaluate the extent of agreement using Cohen's kappa, a statistic which indicates the extent of agreement while taking into account the extent to which the proportion of intervals at which a behaviour is recorded as present will affect the probability of "agreement" occurring by chance.

A long tradition in applied behaviour analysis holds that when interobserver agreement is measured by interval-by-interval percentage agreement, a minimum mean level of agreement of 80% is desirable (Cooper et al., 2007). Conventions for use of kappa with observational data are less well established, but a minimum mean kappa value of 0.6 is often cited as necessary for data to be worth analyzing. Applied researchers will generally aim to assess interobserver reliability in approximately one third of observational sessions, distributed over the course of a study. If the practitioner applied behaviour analyst has the time and resources (e.g. to videorecord sessions) necessary, such standards

Behaviour Monitoring Chart

Client's Name: | Anthony Nigel OTHER | Date/time of observation: | 1st. September 2008, 14.10

Behaviours/Events to be Recorded:

Behaviour A = | Appropriate interaction with peers

Type of Recording (circle method used)

Partial Interval: Tick if the behaviour occurs at any time during that interval or write 0 if it does not

Interval Length: | 20s

Interval Number	Time Period	Record of first observer	Record of second observer	Agree (A) or disagree (D)?
1	0min 1s - 0min 20s	√	√	A
2	0min 21s - 0min 40s	√	√	A
3	0min 41s - 1min 0s	√	√	A
4	1min 1s - 1min 20s	0	√	D
5	1min 21s - 1min 40s	√	√	A
6	1min 41s - 2min 0s	0	√	D
7	2min 1s - 2min 20s	0	0	A
8	2min 21s - 2min 40s	0	0	A
9	2min 41s - 3min 0s	0	0	A
10	3min 1s - 3min 20s	√	√	A
11	3min 21s - 3min 40s	√	√	A
12	3min 41s - 4min 0s	0	√	D
13	4min 1s - 4min 20s	√	√	A
14	4min 21s - 4min 40s	0	0	A
15	4min 41s - 5min 0s	0	0	A
16	5min 1s - 5min 20s	√	0	D
17	5min 21s - 5min 40s	√	√	A
18	5min 41s - 6min 0s	√	√	A
19	6min 1s - 6min 20s	√	0	D
20	6min 21s - 6min 40s	0	0	A
21	6min 41s - 7min 0s	0	0	A
22	7min 1s - 7min 20s	0	0	A
23	7min 21s - 7min 40s	0	0	A
24	7min 41s - 8min 0s	0	0	A
25	8min 1s - 8min 20s	√	0	D
TOTAL NO. OF OCCURRENCES/INTERVALS		12	12	
FOR SAMPLING METHODS: PERCENTAGE INTERVALS WITH BEHAVIOUR RECORDED		12/25 X 100% = **48%**	12/25 X 100% = **48%**	

Interobserver agreement =   Number of intervals with agreement   X 100%
(interval-by-interval)   Number of intervals with agreement plus number with disagreement

= 19/25 X 100% = 76%

Interobserver agreement = Number of intervals with agreement with one observer scoring presence X 100%
(occurrence)   Number of intervals with agreement plus number with disagreement

= 9/15 X 100% = 60%

Fig. 3.3 Calculation of inter-observer agreement using interval-by interval and occurrence only approaches

are equally applicable in clinical practice. In other situations, e.g. when data is being collected by a teacher or by parents, evaluating interobserver agreement may be difficult. Nevertheless, the applied behaviour analyst should, wherever possible, attempt such evaluation. If the teacher is collecting data using a scatterplot (see below) with hourly intervals, for example, and the behaviour analyst is collecting observational data using a 10 s partial-interval record for 2 h per week, simply ensuring that observations are conducted within a time-frame aligned with that of the teacher's scatterplot will enable the behaviour analyst to evaluate interobserver agreement between her data (when collapsed across the hour) and the scatterplot data.

Evaluating Functional Relationships Between environmental Conditions and Target Behaviours

Goals of Functional Assessment

The penultimate stage of assessment in behaviour analysis is to investigate relationships between the target behaviour(s) and environmental conditions and to generate hypotheses regarding the relationships which are inhibiting the acquisition or use of adaptive behaviours and/or supporting the use of problem behaviours. In behaviour analysis this process, referred to in its broadest sense as functional assessment, analyses such relationships in terms of the concepts employed in the experimental analysis of behaviour. The first question therefore, is to attempt to define the operants (functional classes) of which the target behaviour is a member, since other processes (e.g. reinforcement) act upon operants (Skinner, 1938) rather than the individual topographically defined behaviours which are members of operant classes. An operant is a class of behaviour defined by functional identity; that is, any behaviour which produces the same effect on the environment is a member of the operant. The importance of striving to conduct functional assessments based on operant classes can be readily appreciated by considering a practical example. Assume that a child's self-injury is presumed to be reinforced by escape from task demands. An intervention of teaching the child to use a symbol to request a break from activities may be proposed, and the child may be taught to obtain a break by using the symbol. If however, self-injury also continues to result in escape from demands, then escape symbol use and self-injury comprise topographically dissimilar members of the same operant class, and reinforcing symbol use will strengthen all members of the operant class including self-injury. Although this strengthening may not be immediately apparent if the prosocial communicative response requires less effort than self-injury, the entire functional class including self-injury may be strengthened in terms of rate of occurrence and resistance to extinction (Derby, Fisher, Piazza, Wilke, & Johnson, 1998). Successful intervention will therefore probably require extinction or time-out contingencies to be in effect for problem behaviour in addition to reinforcement of the communicative response (Shirley, Iwata, Kahng, Mazaleski, & Lerman, 1997; Wacker et al., 1990).

An initial hypothesis regarding topographically dissimilar behaviours which may be members of a single operant class, can increase the efficiency of the assessment process, since investigation of relevant antecedents and consequences can then be conducted for the hypothesized operant class rather than for each individual topographically defined behaviour. Frequent co-occurrence of target behaviours, or consistent occurrence in a particular sequence, are initial indicators of possible common functional class membership. Such co-occurrence is however only a limited indicator of functional identity, and the behaviour analyst will often prefer the more laborious path of evaluating the function of topographically defined individual behaviours, and deriving hypotheses about operant class membership from the results of these assessments.

Having developed a working hypothesis regarding operant class membership or having reached a decision to assess individual behaviours, the behaviour analyst will next wish to identify possible positive or negative reinforcement processes maintaining those behaviours. In doing so, the behaviour analyst will remain aware that reinforcement processes are only one possible set of processes maintaining behaviours, which may also be directly elicited by processes such as aversive stimulation (Azrin, Rubin, & Hutchinson, 1968), reinforcement schedules (Emerson, 1996) or shifts in reinforcement schedules (including shifts into extinction) (Hutchinson, Azrin, & Hunt, 1968; Kelly & Hake, 1970), and may also come to be elicited by previously neutral stimuli through Pavlovian conditioning (Lyon & Ozolins, 1970). The behaviour analyst working with children with ASD will also be mindful that in addition to the processes of positive social reinforcement, escape from task demands, and automatic reinforcement which are frequently identified as maintaining problem behaviours in children with developmental disabilities (Iwata et al., 1994; Kurtz et al. 2003), problem behaviours may also be maintained by escape from idiosyncratically aversive sensory stimulation (Reese, Richman, Belmont, and Morse, 2005). Further, effective tangible reinforcers for children with ASD, in addition to those often identified for children with other (or no) disabilities, may include items used in specific repetitive behaviours (Reese et al.).

Almost by definition, behaviours regarded as problematic will evoke a response from carers. Therefore, even where a reliable relationship between a problem behaviour and a hypothesized reinforcer (e.g. interaction with carers) has been identified, if this relationship has been identified by a purely descriptive assessment, there will always be grounds to doubt whether it represents a functional reinforcement relationship. Confidence in the existence of a functional relationship will be substantially increased if it is found that the problem behaviour is more likely to occur in the presence of the relevant establishing operation (EO) (Cooper et al., 2007), such as relative deprivation of interaction with carers.

The establishment (where possible) of hypothetical operant classes and the identification of relationships between hypothesized operants and possible reinforcement processes and EOs will therefore be central to the functional assessment process, irrespective of the specific assessment methods used. Where possible, the assessment will also attempt to identify relevant discriminative stimuli which may control the production of the target behaviour, and potential functionally equivalent replacement behaviours which might be strengthened to replace the target behaviour. Functional assessment will also endeavour to assess the relative efficiency of the target behaviour and potential replacement behaviours in terms of relative response effort and the reinforcer magnitude, latency, and schedule of the reinforcement processes currently maintaining target and potential replacement behaviours. Finally, particularly if only a descriptive assessment is to be conducted, the behaviour analyst will seek information on any previous intervention programmes and their effect on the target behaviour. Such information may be especially useful in determining the status of hypothesized response-reinforcer rela-

tionships. If a behaviour hypothesized to be maintained by contingent carer attention has not been reduced by a previous well-implemented intervention to increase levels of noncontingent carer attention, for example, the behaviour analyst may doubt whether the behaviour-attention relationship is functional in nature.

Approaches to Functional Assessment

All methods of functional assessment are designed to gather information relevant to identifying operant classes, reinforcement processes, EOs, and the other information outlined above. Methods of functional analysis may be categorised along two principal dimensions: firstly whether information is gained directly by observation of the behaviour of the child and others or indirectly by questioning carers, and secondly whether information is gained by observing naturally occurring sequences of events in the child's natural environment or whether the behaviour analyst investigates functional relationships by manipulating environmental conditions and observing the effects on the child's behaviour. Combination of categorisation along these dimensions results in three widely recognised approaches to functional assessment. *Indirect* methods use interviews or questionnaires to gather the above information from informants who spend considerable time with the child, such as parents or teachers, generally asking informants to provide generic descriptions of events which (for example) typically follow occurrences of the target behaviour. *Direct observation* or *descriptive* methods gather information by observing sequences of events (including the target behaviour) in the child's natural environment. *Experimental* methods (often referred to as functional analyses or sometimes as analogue assessments) use manipulation of levels of potential relevant antecedents and/or response-event contingencies and observation of effects on levels of the target behaviour to identify EO-behaviour-reinforcer relationships.

Methods of Indirect Functional Assessment

Methods of indirect functional assessment fall into two broad groups. Semi-structured interview schedules such as the Functional Assessment Interview

(O'Neill et al., 1997) provide a format for the clinician to gather a wide range of descriptions of the form, interrelationships, context, consequences and history relating to a problem behaviour, together with information on the client's communicative abilities and possible socially appropriate behaviours which might be reinforced as functional alternatives to problem behaviour. Rating scales such as the Motivation Assessment Scale (Durand & Crimmins, 1988) and the Questions About Behavioural Function scale (Vollmer & Matson, 1995) can typically be completed much more rapidly by asking questions intended to evaluate in broad terms, a limited number of predetermined hypotheses regarding behavioural function. The manuals for such scales often indicate that they may be completed directly by the third-party informant, but in much of the research evaluating the reliability and validity of such scales, they have in fact been completed by the alternative method of a professional completing the scale by interviewing an informant.

Semi-structured Interviews

The Functional Assessment Interview (FAI) (O'Neill et al., 1997) is the most widely researched of the semi-structured interview schedules. The FAI includes questions on topography, frequency, duration and intensity of problem behaviours, co-occurrence (as an indicator of potential operant class co-membership), a range of potential distal motivating operations, temporally proximal antecedents, possible maintaining consequences, and the relative efficiency of the problem behaviour in terms of response effort and schedule and immediacy of hypothesised reinforcers. It also includes questions on prosocial behaviours hypothesised to be functionally equivalent to the problem behaviour, the client's usual methods of communicating a range of needs and desires, possible general reinforcers, and the history of change attempts. The Functional Assessment Interview provides a schematic diagram for summarizing information as an aid to identifying possible functional relationships, but no criteria or decision rules for this purpose.

Hartwig, Heathfield, and Jenson (2004) describe a computerized functional behavioural assessment "expert system", the Functional Assessment and Intervention Program (FAIP). Users answer questions on identifying information about the client and setting, and respond

to questions on antecedents and consequences related to an identified target behaviour. The user is then asked to confirm (or reject) antecedents and consequences which the program identifies on the basis of the user's earlier responses. The program then formulates hypotheses regarding possible functions of the target behaviour (obtain attention, obtain tangible items, gain sensory stimulation, or escape/avoid task demands). After prompting the user to support (or reject) each hypothesis proposed, the program then generates a list of evidence-based interventions relevant to the selected behavioural functions and student characteristics.

A number of other semi-structured instruments have recently been published, many in the course of efforts to extend applications of positive behavioural supports to regular school settings, intended to broaden the range of contextual variables investigated and/or reduce the time taken to complete the assessment and/or to provide versions suitable for use with students as well as teachers. An example is the Teacher Functional Behavioural Assessment Checklist (Stage, Cheney, Walker, & LaRoque, 2002).

Reliability of Questionnaire Methods of Functional Assessment

Because most questionnaire assessments do not provide decision rules for developing hypotheses regarding the functions of target behaviours, leaving the user to develop hypotheses regarding functional relationships, there has been little research on the psychometric properties of such measures. Reese et al. (2005) however, using the FAI in a comparison of functions of problem behaviour in children with and without autism, conducted the FAI with the parents of 46 children presenting problem behaviours. The functions of the problem behaviours were categorized into six categories, three "standard" functions (gain attention, escape demand, or gain tangible item), and three hypothesised "autism-specific" functions (e.g. escape sensory stimulation). For 27 cases, a second trained rater independently repeated the categorisation on the basis of the recorded interviews. Occurrence reliability was 81% for the "gain attention" function, 84% for "escape demand" and 93% for "gain item". The FAIP, in contrast, does incorporate a heuristic process for identification of function. Hartwig et al.

(2004) had 19 pairs of raters familiar with individual clients complete the FAIP within 2 days of each other, focussing on the same problem behaviour, and then asked the primary rater to re-complete the FAIP approximately 30 days later. Overall inter-observer agreement on function was 71%, and overall test-retest agreement on function was 81%.

Rating Scales

The Motivation Assessment Scale (MAS) developed by Durand and Crimmins (1988) is a 16-item questionnaire with the likelihood of problem behaviour occurring in various situations rated on a seven-point Likert-type scale. Originally designed to assess the influence of social attention, tangible, escape and sensory consequences on self-injury, the questionnaire has since been used with other topographies of problem behaviour (Duker & Sigafoos, 1998).

The Questions About Behavioral Function (QABF) scale, (Vollmer & Matson, 1995) is a 25-item questionnaire designed to identify the function of any challenging behaviour in people with intellectual disabilities. The five subscales of the assessment relate to five possible functions; attention, escape, non-social, physical (i.e. behaviour associated with pain or physical discomfort) and tangible. Each function has five corresponding items on the scale, which informants rate on a Likert-type scale, with respect to how often the behaviour occurs in particular contexts.

Where problem behaviours are multifunctional, assessment using the MAS or QABF may provide limited information regarding the relative importance of alternative functions. To address this problem, the Functional Assessment for Multiple Causality (FACT) developed by Matson et al. (2003) uses a forced-choice question procedure aimed at clarifying the relative importance of alternative functions of multifunctional problem behaviour.

As with semi-structured interviews, a number of other functional analysis checklists are available, e.g. the Problem Behaviour Questionnaire (Lewis, Scott, & Sugai, 1994). More recently, attempts have also been made to develop questionnaires such as the Contextual Assessment Inventory (McAtee, Carr, & Schulte, 2004), designed to assess the extent to which a broad range of contextual variables may be functionally related to problem behaviour.

Reliability and Subscale Internal Consistency of Rating Scales for Functional Assessment

Early evaluations of the psychometric properties of the MAS suggested that it had acceptable internal consistency, construct validity, test-retest and inter-rater reliability, and predictive validity (Bihm, Kienlen, Ness, & Poindexter, 1991; Durand & Crimmins, 1988). However, subsequent research on the MAS has found indices of inter-rater reliability substantially lower than those found by Durand and Crimmins (Duker & Sigafoos, 1998; Newton & Sturmey, 1991; Shogren & Rojahn, 2003; Sigafoos, Kerr, & Roberts, 1994; Spreat & Connelly, 1996; Zarcone, Rodgers, Iwata, Rourke, & Dorsey, 1991), although findings on test-retest reliability continue to suggest that this is acceptable (Barton-Arwood, Wehby, Gunter, & Lane, 2003; Shogren & Rojahn, 2003). Mixed results have also been reported for internal consistency of the subscales of the MAS, with acceptable values of Cronbach's alpha reported by Duker and Sigafoos (1998), Freeman, Walker, and Kaufman (2007), and Shogren and Rojahn (2003), but with Newton and Sturmey (1991) finding high levels of internal consistency not only for the subscales of the MAS but also for the entire scale, suggesting the possibility that the high levels of consistency for the subscales may be an artefact resulting from a factor such as perceived problem severity affecting ratings given for items throughout the scale.

Similarly, early research on the reliability of the QABF suggested that it demonstrated very satisfactory levels of inter-rater and test-retest reliability and subscale internal consistency (Paclawskyj et al. 2000). As with the MAS, subsequent research however has generally supported findings of acceptable test-retest reliability but found lower levels of inter-rater reliability than those reported by Paclawskyj et al. It has not only (but not consistently for the Physical subscale) confirmed findings of acceptable subscale internal consistency but also sometimes found a high level of internal consistency for the whole scale (Freeman et al., 2007; Nicholson, Konstantinidi, & Furniss, 2006; Shogren & Rojahn, 2003).

Initial evaluations have shown the FACT to have high levels of subscale internal consistency (Matson et al., 2003), but research into other aspects of reliability and validity of the FACT have yet to be published.

It has often been suggested that the psychometric properties of methods of indirect functional assessment may be affected by variables such as the frequency of occurrence of the behaviour being assessed, the topography of behaviour assessed, whether the behaviour is unifunctional or multifunctional, and the level of sophistication of interviewer and interviewee regarding behavioural concepts (Nicholson et al., 2006). To date however little research has examined these questions directly. Duker and Sigafoos (1998) found lower MAS subscale interrater reliability scores for destructive rather than for maladaptive or disruptive behaviours. Nicholson et al. found that QABF interrater reliability was lower for maladaptive versus disruptive and destructive behaviours and higher for behaviours estimated by carers to occur at least once per day versus those said to occur less frequently. Matson and Boisjoli (2007) found that although inter-rater reliability of the QABF was comparable when the scale was used to assess unifunctional behaviours and the primary function of multifunctional behaviours, agreement between raters was considerably lower with regard to the additional functions of the multifunctional behaviours.

Direct Observation (Descriptive) Methods

Direct observation and recording may be conducted by the behaviour analyst herself, by trained assistants, or by people normally present in the child's environment (e.g. parents, teachers, or the child him/herself). The latter option will most often be used when the target behaviour occurs relatively infrequently and when the behaviour analyst herself would have to devote substantial time for observation in order to see sufficient examples of the target behaviour to make analysis possible. If the behaviour analyst decides that she or a trained assistant will undertake the observations, it if often useful to develop some indication as to when the target behaviour is most likely to be observed. An initial indirect questionnaire assessment may provide some indication as to times of day when the behaviour is most likely to occur. If no such assessment has been completed, or if the analyst wishes to further verify the information obtained through a questionnaire assessment, useful information may be obtained by asking carers (or the child him/herself) to complete a *scatterplot* record (Touchette, MacDonald, & Langer, 1985) for a number of days. The scatterplot (see example at Fig. 3.4) is essentially a variant of a partial-interval record using a very long

interval (typically 30 or 60 min). The child's waking day is divided into a series of intervals, and for each period the person keeping the record notes either whether the target behaviour occurred during that period or not, or whether the behaviour occurred extensively, to a limited extent, or not at all.

Scatterplots can be useful in indicating times of day at which subsequent direct observation is most likely to effectively capture occurrences of the target behaviour. Additionally, the results of scatterplots may themselves suggest hypotheses regarding functions of target behaviours. If a behaviour occurs most frequently during periods of scheduled academic instruction, for example, a hypothesis of reinforcement by escape from academic demands may be suggested for further evaluation. There is however little evidence regarding the reliability, validity and utility of scatterplot records. Kahng et al. (1998) collecting scatterplot data on problem behaviours of 20 children and adults with developmental disabilities living in residential facilities, found poor interobserver reliability in five cases and were unable (without statistical analysis) to discern reliable temporal patterns of responding in all the other cases. It might be expected that scatterplot analysis would be most useful where clients participate in tightly timetabled schedules such as may be found in schools, but factors influencing the utility of scatterplots remain to be investigated.

Antecedent-behaviour-consequence (ABC) recording was one of the first functional assessment methods developed for use in applied settings (Bijou, Peterson, & Ault, 1968). In the approach described as *descriptive* (Miltenberger, 2001) or *narrative* (Cooper et al., 2007) ABC recording, the observer records a description (including time of occurrence) of each occurrence of the target behaviour together with events occurring immediately before and after the behaviour. A four-column recording sheet such as that shown in Fig. 3.5 is generally used.

Although it is generally recommended that ABC recording be conducted by trained observers (e.g. Miltenberger, 2001), the primary advantage of descriptive ABC recording is its economy of effort insofar as a record is made only when the target behaviour occurs. In clinical practice therefore, descriptive ABC records will often be used when the observer is a teacher or carer with other responsibilities but perhaps with limited training in behavioural observation or recording, and a potential problem with descriptive ABC records

Client: Anthony Nigel OTHER   Start date: September 1st. 2008

Behaviour to be recorded: Aggression to others

☐ No Aggression   ◨ 1 incident of aggression   ■ 2 or more incidents of aggression

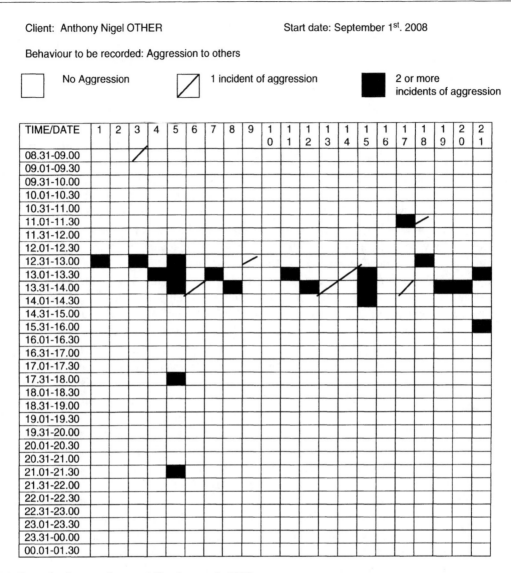

Fig. 3.4 Example of scatter plot record (Touchette et al., 1985)

in such circumstances is that observers may well record inferred mental states or vague descriptions of behavioural states ("got annoyed", "became agitated"), rather than environmental events, as antecedents to the target behaviour. One approach to this problem is to use *checklist* ABC records (Miltenberger) in which antecedents, behaviours and consequences of interest are pre-specified. The ABC recording chart has a column for each event of interest and the observer checks the columns specifying which behaviours, antecedents and consequences were observed at each occurrence of the target behaviour. Such charts may include a wide range of antecedents, behaviours and consequences and be used for exploratory data collection and analysis

(e.g. Fig. 3.6), and carers may be encouraged to carry copies of such charts reduced on to 1,500 mm × 1,000 mm cards and record details of episodes of target behaviours as they occur (Matson, personal communication, 2001). Alternatively, charts may be used (e.g. Fig. 3.7) which list specific antecedents, behaviours and consequences hypothesized to be of interest as a result of a prior indirect assessment (O'Neill et al., 1997).

The use of ABC records enables the behaviour analyst to determine how frequently topographically distinct target behaviours co-occur, facilitating identification of possible operant classes, and also makes it possible to tally the frequency with which particular antecedents and consequences precede and follow target behaviours.

ABC recording sheet

Client's name: A.N. Other

Date and time	Antecedents. Describe what happened just *before* the behaviour. What *was* Anthony doing? Who else was present? What were they doing? What else was happening, etc.?	Behaviour. What exactly did Anthony do? Be as specific as possible.	Consequences. What happened immediately *following* the behaviour. What did you do? What did Anthony do? What did other people do? What else happened?
01/09/08, 12.34 p.m.	Anthony had just gone into the school dining room, accompanied by teacher support assistant N.G. Anthony waited in the queue at the serving counter. When he reached the counter, catering assistant SB asked him if he wanted sausages and mash or salad and baked potato, showing him a plate of each as she asked. Anthony reached out to take both plates. SB said "Anthony, tell me what you want" while keeping hold of the plates.	Anthony shouted loudly, pulled the plates out of SB's hands, and threw the plate with sausages across the dining room. He took the plate with salad and potato, ran to one corner of the room, and started to eat the salad.	NG followed Anthony and asked him to sit down and eat his lunch. Anthony did so. Student PD started crying when Anthony threw the plate.

Fig. 3.5 Example of a completed narrative ABC recording sheet

Exploratory ABC Chart

Client's Name: [   ]   Staff Initials: [   ]   Date: [   ]   Time: [   ]

What happened just before the behaviour?	Behaviour	What happened immediately after?
Particular individual present/entered the room	Self-injury	Given food/drink
Physical discomfort/pain	Aggression towards another person	Received more social contact/attention
Seizure	Property destruction	Received less social contact/attention
Noisy/disruptive environment	Shouting/screaming	Went to quieter and/or less crowded area
No social contact/attention for over one minute	Threatening	Given a task/activity
No involvement in task/activity for over one minute	Swearing	Redirected to current activity
Waiting	Food/drink refusal	Redirected to a different activity
Changing activities/location	Pica	Gained new sensory stimulation
Shift change	Rumination/vomiting	Demands or requests withdrawn/reduced
Food or drink present or being prepared	Repeated non-compliance	Given more help to complete task/activity
Was asked to do something	Teasing/provoking others	Taken out for walk
Task/activity had just begun	Inappropriate sexual behaviour	'Counselled'/spoken to about behaviour
Task/activity had just ended	Running away	Sensory input reduced
Asked to stop activity	Spitting	Other students removed from area
Told that he/she couldn't have or do something	Incontinent of urine	Moved away from others within area
Inappropriate behaviour interrupted	Incontinent of faeces	Physical intervention
Could not get desired item	Smearing faeces	**Complete incident report form as well**
Received corrective feedback	Smearing mucus	**Other (specify):**
Target of teasing or verbal abuse	Sitting down/refusing to move	
Involved in an argument	Socially inappropriate behaviour	
Other (specify):	Other (specify):	

Fig. 3.6 Example of checklist-type ABC chart used for exploratory recording/analysis

Investigatory ABC chart

Client's name:

Please record date and time, initial, and tick all boxes which apply every time a behaviour is noted

Date	Time	Staff Initials	Antecedents (what happened shortly before the behaviour)							Behaviour						Consequences (what happened immediately after the behaviour)				
			Alone, unoccupied	Alone, occupied	Task demand	Noise from other client	Noise from other source	Transition between activities	Other (please specify)	Screaming	Spitting at others	Self-injury	Dropping to floor	Other (Please specify)	Behaviour ignored	Redirected to same activity	Redirected to another activity	Redirected to quieter area	Other (please specify)

Fig. 3.7 Example of checklist-type ABC chart used for hypothesis-testing recording/analysis

In developing hypotheses regarding behavioural function on the basis of such descriptive data, it is important to apply the criterion of internal coherence of the hypothesis outlined earlier. That is, even if increased carer attention reliably follows occurrence of the target behaviour, extreme caution should be exercised in hypothesising a reinforcement function unless the target behaviour is also reliably preceded by reduction in level of carer attention. Further, care is needed where the consequence necessarily implies presence of an antecedent; escape from task demand, for example, can only occur when antecedent occurrence of task demand is given, and both narrative and checklist ABC recording may therefore give an impression of a coherent EO-target behaviour-reinforcement sequence in situations where the behaviour is not functionally related to the antecedents and behaviours recorded.

The fundamental limitation of all forms of ABC records is that a record is made only if the target behaviour occurs and no account is taken of the overall level of occurrence of the relevant antecedents and consequences. For a child with ASD participating in an intensive educational programme, it is likely that task demand will occur prior to problem behaviour irrespective of whether there is a functional relationship between the two events. The only solution to this problem is to observe continuously, using a checklist-style recording form, and recording all occurrences of antecedents and consequences of interest irrespective of whether the target behaviour has occurred, such as in *ABC continuous recording* (Cooper et al., 2007). Use of ABC recording in this way, however, itself faces difficulties if the antecedents of interest are typically extended in time (e.g. reduced levels of social interaction). One solution to this problem is to use one of the time-sampling approaches described earlier. Figure 3.8, based on an example from Oliver (personal communication) shows data from such an observation session. The advantage of such an approach, as illustrated in Fig. 3.8, is that the conditional probability of a behaviour given the occurrence of an antecedent, can be compared with the unconditional probability of the behaviour.

In the example given, the conditional probability of face-slapping when the child is on his/her own playing with toys, and to a lesser extent when he/she is alone and unoccupied, is elevated with respect to the unconditional (overall) probability of the behaviour. Task demand, by contrast, is associated with a conditional probability of face-slapping lower than its unconditional probability. Although such conditional probabilities of one event occurring together with another do not indicate the direction of causality (if any) between the two, their calculation can suggest specific relationships for further investigation. Similarly, the conditional probability of a consequence following a behaviour can be compared with the unconditional probability of the consequence.

As Fig. 3.8 illustrates, simple conditional probability calculations can be applied to paper-and pencil time sampling records. Such calculations can however readily become onerous; for example, the behaviour analyst may well wish to consider not only whether the target behaviour shows elevated probability of occurrence in the same sampling interval as task demand, but also whether its probability is also elevated in several immediately succeeding sampling intervals. Computerized real-time observation and recording can considerably facilitate such analyses. The OBSWIN system (Martin, Oliver, & Hall, 2003), for example, enables the behaviour analyst to readily plot the conditional probability of an event of interest at a range of intervals before, during, and following the occurrence of a target behaviour, and to compare conditional with unconditional probabilities of the event both visually and statistically. Figure 3.9, for example, shows a plot of the conditional probability of task engagement ("engagement") for a child with developmental disabilities, plotted prior to, during, and following episodes of verbal or gestural prompting ("demand") from carers to engage in such activities, produced by the OBSWIN (Martin et al.) "burst analysis" programme.

The horizontal dashed line shows that the overall mean (unconditional) probability of the child being actively engaged was just over 0.4. The burst analysis programme plots the conditional probability of the child being engaged on tasks prior to, during and following 89 separate episodes of demand. The episodes of demand, and the periods between them, will vary in absolute length, and so data are plotted using a "normalise and pool" method in which time (plotted on the horizontal axis) is measured in terms of percentiles of the duration of individual episodes of demand (and the first and second halves of each inter-episode interval) (Hall & Oliver, 2000), allowing data to be pooled across episodes of varying duration. It can be seen that prior to episodes of carer prompting, the conditional probability of the child being engaged is approximately

Behaviour Monitoring Chart

Client's Name: | Anthony Nigel OTHER | Date/time of observation: | 3rd. September 2008

Behaviours/Events to be Recorded:

Behaviour/event A = | Face-slapping

Behaviour/event B = | Unoccupied, on own

Behaviour/event C = | Playing with toys, on own

Behaviour/event D= | Task demand

Type of Recording (circle method used)

Momentary Time Sample | Tick if the behaviour was occurring in the <u>final second</u> of the interval, write 0 if it was not.

Interval Length: | 10s

Interval Number	Time Period	Behaviour A	Behaviour B	Behaviour C	Behaviour D
1	0-10s	√	√	0	0
2	11-20s	0	√	0	0
3	21-30s	√	√	0	0
4	31-40s	√	0	√	0
5	41-50s	√	0	0	0
6	51-60s	√	0	√	0
7	61-70s	0	0	√	0
8	71-80s	0	0	0	0
9	81-90s	√	0	√	0
10	91-100s	0	0	0	√
11	101-110s	0	0	0	√
12	111-120s	0	0	0	√
TOTAL NO. OF OCCURRENCES/INTERVALS		6	3	4	3
FOR SAMPLING METHODS: PERCENTAGE INTERVALS WITH BEHAVIOUR RECORDED		6/12x100%= 50%	3/12x100%= 25%	4/12x100%= 33%	3/12x100%= 25%

UP (face-slapping): (6/12 intervals) = 0.5

CP (face-slapping when unoccupied on own) (2/3 intervals) = 0.67

CP (face-slapping with toys on own) (3/4 intervals) = 0.75

CP (face-slapping with task demand) (0/3 intervals) = 0

UP: unconditional probability
CP: conditional probability of behaviour A given behaviour X

Fig. 3.8 Use of sampling observation to compare unconditional and conditional probabilities of a behaviour

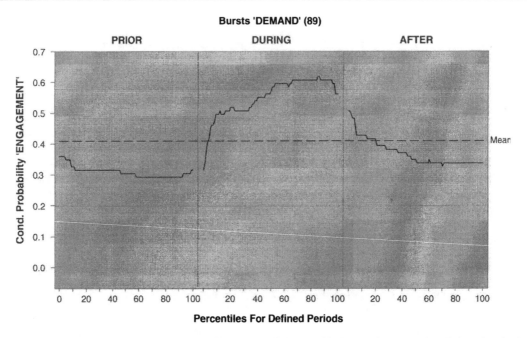

Fig. 3.9 Conditional probability of task engagement ("engagement") for a child with developmental disabilities, plotted prior to, during, and following episodes of verbal or gestural prompting ("demand") from carers to engage in such activities: data from 89 separate episodes of demand plotted using the "normalise and pool" method

0.3–0.35. The initiation of episodes of prompting by carers is accompanied by an initial rapid increase in the conditional probability of the child being engaged, which is followed by a further, more gradual increase in the conditional probability of engagement up to a maximum level of around 0.6. When carers cease prompting, the conditional probability of engagement by the child initially rapidly decreases to its overall mean and then declines further.

However sophisticated the analytic methods applied, purely descriptive approaches to functional assessment are fundamentally limited by their inability to determine whether observed relationships are functional in nature. The difficulty is particularly acute in the case of behaviours maintained by thin schedules of reinforcement, in which even the most exacting descriptive analysis may not identify the relationship. Such problems have inspired the development of descriptive methods incorporating either antecedent manipulations or deliberate sampling of various naturally occurring antecedent conditions. Since, such approaches have been derived from experimental (functional analysis) methodology, they will be covered following discussion of experimental methods.

Experimental Functional Assessment (Functional Analysis)

The functional analysis methodology initially described by Iwata, Dorsey, Slifer, Bauman, and Richman (1982) involves briefly exposing the child to a systematically arranged (analogue) social environment in which certain antecedent conditions are reliably present, and the target behaviour is reliably followed by a specified consequence. A fundamental assumption of the approach is that the target behaviour will be differentially sensitive to contingencies similar to those which maintain that behaviour in the child's natural environment, i.e. that observation of high levels of the target behaviour under a certain set of analogue contingencies implies that similar contingencies maintain the behaviour in the child's natural environment.

The classic paper of Iwata et al. (1982) described four conditions, outlined in Table 3.2, one (Unstructured play) being a control condition and the others ("social disapproval", i.e. contingent attention, "task demand", i.e. contingent escape from task demands, and alone) designed to test hypotheses regarding functions of

Table 3.2 Outline of functional analysis conditions used by Iwata et al. (1982)

Condition label	Hypothesis regarding function of behaviour to be tested	Antecedent condition (motivating operation)	Consequences delivered contingent on problem behaviour
"Social disapproval"	Behaviour maintained by contingent carer attention	Toys available to child. Carer present but does not interact with child, busies him/herself with an activity	Adult verbally expresses concern and/or disapproval of the behaviour paired with brief, nonpunitive physical contact (e.g. puts hand on child's shoulder)
"Academic demand"	Behaviour maintained by contingent escape from task demands	Adult uses 3-step (verbal, modelling, physical guidance) least-to-most prompting to engage the child in difficult educational activities	Adult terminates current task demand and turns away from child for 30 s, with additional 30 s suspension of demands for repeated behaviours
"Alone"	Behaviour maintained by automatic reinforcement (e.g. sensory stimulation)	Child is left alone in room with no toys/activities available and observed from outside room	None
"Unstructured play"	Control condition	Variety of toys available. Adult remains close to child, does not block/restrict any child behaviour, periodically offers toys to child while making no demands, gives social praise and brief physical contact at least once every 30 s provided child is not engaged in problem behaviour	None

self-injury based on Carr's (1977) review of previous studies of this question.

Analogue conditions are typically presented briefly (for 5 or 10 min each) with breaks between conditions and in alternating order, and levels of the target behaviour are recorded (as frequency or duration as most appropriate) in each session. In Iwata et al.'s initial demonstration of the method, sessions were repeated until higher levels of the target behaviour were consistently observed in one condition than in the others. The results of experimental analyses by convention are typically plotted as for an alternating treatments design. As illustrated by hypothetical data in Fig. 3.10, a consistently higher level of the target behaviour in the "social disapproval" (contingent attention) condition is interpreted as supporting a hypothesis that the target behaviour is maintained by positive social reinforcement in the child's natural environment. A consistently higher level of the behaviour in the "task demand" (contingent escape from task demand) condition is taken to indicate a corresponding function for the behaviour in the natural environment, while a higher level of the behaviour in the "alone" condition is generally interpreted as suggesting that the behaviour is maintained by automatic reinforcement. An undifferentiated pattern of responding (similar levels of the target behaviour in all conditions)

may indicate that the behaviour is genuinely multifunctional, that it is maintained by automatic reinforcement, or that it is maintained by some other process not modelled by the analogue conditions.

The method of experimental functional analysis necessarily tests only specified hypotheses regarding the function of problem behaviour. The behaviour analyst may therefore need to design additional conditions to those originally described by Iwata et al. (1982) in order to test hypotheses relevant to a client's behaviour. A hypothesis that problem behaviour is reinforced by contingent access to tangible reinforcers such as toys or snacks, for example, may be tested by a condition in which the tangible is present and visible to the child but access to the reinforcer is given only contingent on occurrence of the problem behaviour. Also, if there is no suggestion from preliminary assessment that the problem behaviour is maintained by a particular reinforcement process (e.g. positive social reinforcement), the corresponding condition ("social disapproval") may be omitted from the experimental analysis.

Use of experimental analysis, particularly for assessment of potentially seriously harmful target behaviours such as aggression or self-injury, poses a number of technical and ethical challenges. At least two skilled persons, one to observe and one to reliably implement

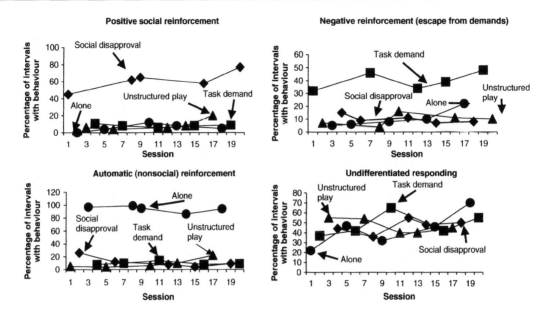

Fig. 3.10 Patterns of responding consistent with alternative functional hypotheses in experimental functional analyses

the assessment conditions, are needed. Experimental analysis intentionally seeks to evoke high rates of problem behaviour. In the case of potentially seriously harmful behaviour, therefore, either a priori decision rules governing conditions in which a condition will be terminated, or the presence of an independent appropriately qualified judge to call a halt if unacceptable harm is occurring, or both, must be arranged (Iwata et al., 1982). Data must be subject to careful review to ensure that artefacts of the assessment process such as sequencing of conditions and the intervals between them do not confuse the interpretation of data. Finally, in the case of extended functional analyses, caution must be exercised with regard to the possibility that repeated exposure to systematic analogue conditions may establish a new function for the target behaviour not previously learned in the child's natural environment (Neef & Peterson, 2007). Developments such as application of experimental analysis to reliable precursor behaviours rather than harmful problem behaviours (e.g. Borrero & Borrero, 2008) may address some of these concerns, which to date however have led several commentators (e.g. Sturmey, 1995) to question whether experimental methods can be routinely applied in everyday clinical practice.

Several researchers have attempted to adapt experimental analysis methodologies to the time and resource constraints typical of clinical settings. Wacker et al. (1994) have developed brief functional analysis procedures typically comprising a single session using the methods of Iwata et al. (1982) followed by a brief evaluation of hypotheses derived from that analysis in a mini-reversal or multielement design. Results from such methods correspond with those from extended functional analyses in over 60% of cases (Kahng & Iwata, 1999). However, these brief analyses fail to identify the functions of challenging behaviours in over 30% of cases, most commonly because the client shows no challenging behaviour during the assessment (Derby et al., 1992). Analyses conducted in settings and by personnel other than those of the client's everyday environment may yield undifferentiated results because specific establishing operations, discriminative stimuli, and reinforcers occasioning or maintaining the problem behaviour in the natural environment are not replicated in the analogue environment (see, e.g., Carr, Yarbrough, & Langdon, 1997; Richman & Hagopian, 1999; Ringdahl & Sellers, 2000). Carr et al. (1997) and Vollmer and Smith (1996) have recommended use of descriptive analyses to identify relevant stimuli for incorporation into experimental analyses. Alternatively, experimental analysis may be implemented in the course of the client's everyday routines by regular carers (Sigafoos & Saggers, 1995).

Structured Descriptive and Context Sampling Approaches

Although the classic methodology of Iwata et al. involves systematic manipulation of both antecedents and consequences, other researchers have conducted functional analyses in which only antecedents are manipulated. Carr and Durand (1985), for example, measured problem behaviours under conditions of reduced carer attention and increased task difficulty and inferred that high levels of problem behaviour in the former condition suggested that the behaviour was maintained by positive social reinforcement, whereas high levels of problem behaviour in the latter condition suggested maintenance by escape from task demands. If the corresponding consequences are not actually delivered during analysis conditions, it would of course be expected that the target behaviour would extinguish over the course of assessment sessions, but levels of behaviour early in sessions may provide a useful indicator of behavioural function.

Anderson and her colleagues (Anderson & Long, 2002; Freeman, Anderson, & Scotti, 2000) have developed this approach into a *structured descriptive assessment (SDA)* strategy in which antecedent variables are systematically manipulated during observation of the client's behaviour in his/her natural environment, while leaving consequences for the client's behaviours un programmed. Anderson and Long, working with four children with severe intellectual disabilities and/or autism, found that the functions of problem behaviours identified by the SDA and analogue experimental analysis were similar in three cases, and that in the two children treated, interventions to address the function identified led to reductions in the behaviour. In the fourth case, a combination of interventions based on the two different functions identified by the SDA and experimental analysis proved necessary to produce and maintain a reduction in problem behaviour.

The SDA methodology requires carers to systematically vary antecedent conditions. An alternative which would further reduce the need for carers to change normal patterns of care, would be to identify naturally occurring contexts systematically associated with different patterns of antecedent conditions. Hodge, Hall, and Oliver (2001) proposed that antecedent conditions prevailing in certain naturally occurring contexts such as individual instruction, group instruction and unstructured time

may parallel those used in analogue assessments in that they reliably involve particular combinations of establishing operations and discriminative stimuli (e.g. task demands, reduced attention but with carers remaining present, withdrawal of attention together with withdrawal of carers) which may differentially impact on behaviours maintained by different consequences. Hodge et al. used sequential analysis of observational data to establish possible functions of the challenging, stereotyped, engaged and disengaged behaviour of three children with intellectual disabilities and then examined levels of those behaviours in four school situations hypothesized to involve antecedent conditions related to the academic demand, reduced attention, alone, and control conditions often used in experimental analyses. For some behaviours, the pattern of probabilities of the behaviour across situations was congruent with that expected from the function suggested by the sequential analysis. This *context sampling descriptive assessment (CSDA)* method (Garbutt & Furniss, 2007) may represent a clinically feasible method for using descriptive assessment to produce some of the information which has traditionally been sought through experimental methods. Demonstration of the utility and validity of the CSDA approach will however require further research which clearly establishes behavioural function through experimental methods and demonstrates variation in levels of problem behaviour across different CSDA contexts consistent with previously identified function.

Convergent and Predictive (Treatment) Validity of Functional Assessment Methods

The fact that experimental analyses directly demonstrate functional relationships may lead to assumptions that such methods have inherently high reliability and validity and that the only justification for using indirect assessments is that they require less time and expertise to implement. All of these assumptions are questionable (Hanley, Iwata, & McCord, 2003; Martin, Gaffan, & Williams, 1999; Matson & Minshawi, 2007). The behaviour analyst considering her choice of functional assessment methodologies for an individual case will wish to refer to empirical research on two questions. Firstly, to what extent do different functional assessment methods lead to identical hypotheses regarding behavioural function? Secondly, in what proportion of cases do the functional hypotheses derived by different methods lead to effective interventions?

Results from systematic studies involving people with severe developmental disabilities suggest (1) a moderate degree of agreement on function between questionnaire assessments and rating scales (Toogood & Timlin, 1996), (2) variable findings with regard to agreement between the MAS and QABF (Freeman et al., 2007; Paclawskyj, Matson, Rush, Smalls, & Vollmer, 2001) and (3) a moderate to high level of agreement between the QABF and experimental assessments (Hall, 2005; Paclawskyj et al. 2001). Of particular note is the fact that agreement between indirect methods and experimental analyses may be higher than that between hypotheses about function based on direct observation and experimental analyses (Hall, 2005; Toogood & Timlin, 1996)

There has been rather little direct research on the issue of the predictive (treatment) validity of indirect functional assessment methods where these have been used as the sole method of functional assessment. Matson, Bamburg, Cherry, and Paclawskyj (1999) examined the predictive validity of the QABF by comparing behavioural change over a period of 6 months in 90 persons with severe and profound intellectual disabilities whose treatment plans for challenging behaviours (self-injury, aggression and stereotypies) were individualized on the basis of QABF assessments (e.g. communication training in cases where the QABF results suggested behaviour reinforced by attention) with the progress of 90 similar residents of the same centre with standardized treatment protocols based on blocking and redirecting in response to problem behaviours. For each topography of challenging behaviour, participants receiving QABF-based treatment plans showed overall percentage reductions in problem behaviour frequency three times greater than for those receiving standard treatments.

The literature employing experimental functional analyses clearly illustrates many cases in which effective interventions have been based on the results of the assessment. Given the predominance of single-case experimental designs in such research however, evidence on the relative predictive validity of different assessment approaches comes mainly from meta-analytic studies. Didden, Duker, and Korzilius (1997) reviewed 482 studies of treatment of problem behaviour in people with intellectual disabilities published from 1968 to 1994, using the "percentage of nonoverlapping data" (PND) approach. Use of a pretreatment functional assessment was associated with better treatment outcome, and studies using experimental functional analyses showed better outcomes than those using "informal assessment". Campbell (2003) reviewed studies of behavioural treatments of problem behaviours in people with autism published between 1966 and 1998. Meta-analysis using the "percentage of zero data" (PZD), but not the "mean baseline reduction" (MBLR) or "percentage of nonoverlapping data" (PND) approaches, suggested both that conducting a pretreatment functional assessment resulted in a better treatment outcome and that within the group of studies employing functional assessments, use of experimental analysis resulted in better treatment outcome than use of other functional assessment methods. Herzinger and Campbell (2007) replicated and extended these findings in a review of studies using functional assessment with people with autistic disorder published between 1998 and 2003. Again, the PZD but not the MBLR or PND approaches showed better treatment outcome for studies using experimental analyses than for those using other methods, of which "informal assessment" was the most commonly reported approach. Didden, Korzilius, van Oorsouw, and Sturmey (2006) reviewed treatment studies involving people with mild intellectual disabilities published between 1980 and 2005. Analysis using PND showed better outcome for studies using experimental than for those using descriptive functional assessment, but no overall advantage for use of functional assessment, whereas the PZD method showed better outcome for studies using pretreatment functional assessment, but no difference in outcome for experimental versus other methods. Didden et al. further note that ABC analysis was the most common nonexperimental method reported in the studies they reviewed, with rating scales such as the MAS and QABF never used.

To date therefore, meta-analytic studies have not specifically examined the relationship between use of indirect methods of functional assessment and treatment outcome. Use of functional assessment in general is associated with better treatment outcome, and there is some evidence that use of experimental methods result in better outcomes than descriptive (direct and indirect) methods when comparisons are made using the PZD method, i.e. the extent to which treatment maintains zero occurrence of target behaviours.

Functional Assessment: A Clinical Approach

Given the current state of our knowledge base regarding the reliability and validity of different methods of functional assessment, it remains appropriate for the behaviour analyst to use a combination of several methods in assessing behavioural function. Given further that decisions regarding the feasibility of different methods of direct observation and experimental approaches require some preliminary estimate of the frequency of the behaviour, and that such methods always require the behaviour analyst (explicitly or implicitly) to identify behaviours, antecedents and consequences likely to be relevant to the analysis, some form of initial indirect assessment using a questionnaire such as the Functional Assessment Interview, with a parent, teacher, carer or the child him/herself as the informant, will often be an essential first step. Where it is essential to gain multiple viewpoints (e.g. if it is important to assess whether a problem behaviour serves identical functions at home and at school), but time is limited, the behaviour analyst may conduct an extended indirect assessment by interview of one key informant while asking others to complete behaviour function rating scales such as the QABF or FACT. Concordance between the functions identified on the basis of these assessments will strengthen confidence in the conclusions reached; disagreement should prompt supplementary questioning of the original informant for the FAI and/or a detailed interview of the informants completing the rating scales to investigate whether the disagreement results from provision of partial or inaccurate information from one or more sources or whether the function of the target behaviour does indeed vary across settings.

If the target behaviour is reported to vary substantially in frequency within or across days, asking carers or the child to complete a scatterplot record for several days may help to more precisely define the frequency of occurrence of the behaviour and time periods when the behaviour is likely to occur. If information from the indirect assessment and scatterplot suggests that the behaviour occurs only once per day or less, then unless the behaviour occurs at highly predictable times or the behaviour analyst has ample time to conduct extensive observations, asking carers to complete checklist ABC records with antecedents, behaviours and consequences

specified on the basis of the previous indirect assessment will probably be the most useful next step in assessment. If for some reason, it has not been possible to conduct an initial indirect assessment, use of exploratory checklist ABC records may be helpful.

If on the other hand, indirect assessment and/or scatterplot records suggest that the behaviour typically happens with relatively high frequency (several times per day or more) and/or regularly occurs at specific times, then direct observation using either time-sampling or real-time measures is probably the preferred next step in assessment. Such approaches enable the behaviour analyst to distinguish antecedents and consequences differentially associated with the target behaviour from those which simply occur with high overall frequency. Again, antecedents, behaviours and consequences of interest can be derived from the previous indirect assessment. If however such approaches do not result in robust hypotheses regarding behavioural function, or if the behaviour occurs with such high frequency that recording of discrete antecedents and consequences is difficult, then assessment methods such as experimental analyses, structured descriptive assessment, or context sampling descriptive assessment may be used. These approaches rely on comparison of rates (or durations) of behaviour across conditions rather than identification of individual antecedent-behaviour-consequence sequences and hence can be used with even very high frequency behaviours.

Functional Assessment: Concluding Comments

The goal in analysing the results of any functional assessment is to develop a working hypothesis regarding the function of a behaviour. The analysis therefore needs to go beyond tabulation of antecedents and consequences co-occurring with or functionally related to the target behaviour, to provide a hypothesis of the processes involved using the conceptual framework of behaviour analysis. The analysis should identify relevant establishing operations, discriminative stimuli, and reinforcement processes, together with potential or actual more adaptive functionally equivalent behaviours. This analysis of the processes currently maintaining the target behaviour should then be used to develop a range of options for intervention which should simultaneously weaken targeted problem behaviours and strengthen functionally equivalent adaptive behaviours. Such interventions may include modifying establishing operations, neutralising the effects of establishing operations, increasing tolerance of establishing operations, avoiding discriminative stimuli, teaching adaptive behaviours functionally equivalent to a problem behaviour, and modifying contingencies to increase the efficiency of adaptive behaviours by comparison with problem behaviours. The final step in the initial assessment, should therefore be to develop from hypotheses concerning processes maintaining the target behaviour, a comprehensive set of hypotheses regarding interventions, which should produce beneficial change in the target behaviour and functional alternatives.

Assessing Stimulus Preferences and Effectiveness of Potential Reinforcers

The goal of functional assessment is to identify events currently reinforcing problem behaviours with a view to modifying the client's repertoire and/or environmental contingencies in ways such that these events will differentially reinforce prosocial behaviours. When the goal of intervention is to teach new behaviours however, the behaviour analyst may also need to identify ecologically "arbitrary" reinforcers which can be used to establish the novel behaviour. For children with ASD in particular, systematic efforts may be necessary to identify effective reinforcers.

This assessment is typically undertaken in two stages. In the first stage, a pool of relatively preferred stimuli is identified and, possibly, ranked in order of preference. One approach to such preference assessment is to ask the child him/herself, or significant others, to identify preferred stimuli using open-ended questions or survey schedules (e.g. Fisher, Piazza, Bowman, & Amari, 1996). However, preferences expressed in such assessments may show only limited correspondence with those suggested by direct observation of the child's behaviour towards those stimuli. In *free operant* assessment of preferences, the child is allowed free access to the items and activities to be assessed and the duration of engagement with each is recorded. Where necessary, the child is encouraged to "sample" each item/activity before the assessment

period. In *trial-based* preference assessments, the child's preferences from a range of sources of stimulation are assessed by systematically observing either choices when items are presented simultaneously (e.g. in pairs; Fisher et al., 1992) or the child's behaviour towards items presented individually (DeLeon, Iwata, Conners, & Wallace, 1999) or simultaneously (Roane, Vollmer, Ringdahl, & Marcus, 1998). In each case, the behaviours observed may be "approach" responses (e.g. looking towards the item), physical contact with the item, or active engagement with/use of the item.

Stimulus preferences change over time and are dependent on contextual factors, and it will often be necessary to frequently re-assess preferences, perhaps even before each individual teaching session. Even stimuli identified as highly preferred in choice-based assessments will not however, necessarily act as effective reinforcers for target behaviours, since the response effort of the target behaviour, and the latency to reinforcement in the teaching situation, may differ from that in the preference assessment (Shore, Iwata, DeLeon, Kahng, & Smith, 1997). In some situations, the behaviour analyst may wish to evaluate the effectiveness of a preferred stimulus as a reinforcer with various response requirements before using it in an intervention programme (DeLeon, Iwata, Goh, & Worsdell, 1997). In clinical practice however, the effectiveness as reinforcers of stimuli/activities identified by preference assessments will often be evaluated directly in the course of the clinical intervention.

Testing the Behaviour Change Hypotheses Developed

The completion of the assessment process will be followed by implementation of one or more of the interventions which are expected to reduce levels of problematic behaviour and strengthen adaptive alternatives. However comprehensive the functional assessment which has been undertaken, it is important to attempt to evaluate whether the interventions implemented are producing the changes expected. The process of testing the change hypotheses is important for four reasons. Firstly, however thorough the functional assessment, the possibility always remains that the processes maintaining the problem behaviour have been incompletely or imperfectly understood. A behaviour believed to be reinforced by escape from task demands may, for example, be reinforced only by escape from task demands phrased in a particular way. Secondly, even if a problem behaviour improves following intervention, the improvement may not be systematically related to the intervention but may be produced by collateral unspecified changes in the social environment (i.e. a "placebo effect"). In this case testing of the change hypothesis is necessary to avoid the client and carers expending effort on a possibly ineffective intervention. The third possibility is that improvement in the target behaviour is functionally related to the intervention, but that significant others attribute the improvement to other, nonspecific factors, e.g. the child "settling in" to a new situation. In this case testing of the change hypothesis may be necessary to persuade significant others not to abandon an ongoing effective intervention. Finally, particularly in the case of severe problem behaviours, in contrast to the analytic method of changing one variable at a time recommended in experimental work, a broadside approach to intervention in which several changes are introduced simultaneously may have been adopted. In such cases, a component analysis may identify which elements of the intervention are responsible for behaviour change.

Testing treatment hypotheses requires ongoing measurement of levels of target and replacement behaviours using the measurement methods described earlier in this chapter in combination with use of elements of single-subject experimental designs such as reversal, alternating treatments, and multiple probe/multiple baseline designs (Cooper et al., 2007).

Assessment Methods: Concluding Comments

The assessment process is a critical component of effective behaviour analytic intervention to assist children with ASD to strengthen adaptive behaviours and replace problem behaviours with more adaptive and effective alternatives. Although many applied psychological approaches to helping children with ASD emphasize the importance of assessment, the foundations of applied behaviour analysis in the experimental analysis of behaviour lead to a particular emphasis on the intervention process itself as an analytic exercise. This emphasis is of particular value when, despite thorough assessment, careful planning, and faithful implementation, a behavioural intervention does not result in the expected positive changes for the client. Such an outcome may be an indication of the current limits of our knowledge. It may also however be an indication that one or more specific parameters critical to the effectiveness of the intervention (e.g. schedule of reinforcement) have been inadequately assessed. Viewing the intervention process as a process of extended assessment of the dynamics of the clinical problem, enables the behaviour analyst to both improve the success rate of clinical interventions and to contribute to the knowledge base of the field by identifying factors affecting intervention effectiveness in the complex environments typically encountered in applied work.

References

Anderson, C. M., & Long, E. S. (2002). Use of a structured descriptive assessment methodology to identify variables affecting problem behavior. *Journal of Applied Behavior Analysis, 35*(2), 137–154.

Ayllon, T., & Azrin, N. H. (1968). *The token economy: A motivational system for therapy and rehabilitation.* New York, NY: Appleton-Century-Crofts.

Azrin, N. H., Rubin, H. B., & Hutchinson, R. R. (1968). Biting attack by rats in response to aversive shock. *Journal of the Experimental Analysis of Behavior, 11*(5), 633–639.

Baer, D. M., Wolf, M. M., & Risley, T. R. (1968). Some current dimensions of applied behavior analysis. *Journal of Applied Behavior Analysis, 1*(1), 91–97.

Ball, T., Bush, A., & Emerson, E. (2004). *Psychological interventions for severely challenging behaviours shown by people with learning disabilities: Clinical practice guidelines.* Leicester: British Psychological Society.

Barton-Arwood, S. M., Wehby, J. H., Gunter, P. L., & Lane, K. L. (2003). Functional behavior assessment rating scales: Intrarater reliability with students with emotional or behavioral disorders. *Behavioral Disorders, 28*(4), 386–400.

Bihm, E. M., Kienlen, T. L., Ness, M. E., & Poindexter, A. R. (1991). Factor structure of the motivation assessment scale for persons with mental retardation. *Psychological Reports, 68*(3 Pt 2), 1235–1238.

Bijou, S. W., Peterson, R. F., & Ault, M. H. (1968). A method to integrate descriptive and experimental field studies at the level of data and empirical concepts. *Journal of Applied Behavior Analysis, 1*(2), 175–191.

Borrero, C. S. W., & Borrero, J. C. (2008). Descriptive and experimental analyses of potential precursors to problem behavior. *Journal of Applied Behavior Analysis, 41*(1), 83–96.

Campbell, J. M. (2003). Efficacy of behavioral interventions for reducing problem behavior in persons with autism: A quantitative synthesis of single-subject research. *Research in Developmental Disabilities, 24*(2), 120–138.

Carr, E. G. (1977). The motivation of self-injurious behavior: A review of some hypotheses. *Psychological Bulletin, 84*(4), 800–816.

Carr, E. G., & Durand, V. M. (1985). Reducing behavior problems through functional communication training. *Journal of Applied Behavior Analysis, 18*(2), 111–126.

Carr, E. G., Yarbrough, S. C., & Langdon, N. A. (1997). Effects of idiosyncratic stimulus variables on functional analysis outcomes. *Journal of Applied Behavior Analysis, 30*(4), 673–686.

Cooper, J. O., Heron, T. E., & Heward, W. L. (2007). *Applied behavior analysis* (3rd ed.). Upper Saddle River, N.J.: Pearson.

de Bildt, A., Kraijer, D., Sytema, S., & Minderaa, R. (2005). The psychometric properties of the Vineland adaptive behavior scales in children and adolescents with mental retardation. *Journal of Autism and Developmental Disorders, 35*(1), 53–62.

DeLeon, I. G., Iwata, B. A., Conners, J., & Wallace, M. D. (1999). Examination of ambiguous stimulus preferences with duration-based measures. *Journal of Applied Behavior Analysis, 32*(1), 111–114.

DeLeon, I. G., Iwata, B. A., Goh, H. L., & Worsdell, A. S. (1997). Emergence of reinforcer preference as a function of schedule requirements and stimulus similarity. *Journal of Applied Behavior Analysis, 30*(3), 439–449.

DeLeon, I. G., Rodriguez-Catter, V., & Cataldo, M. F. (2002). Treatment: Current standards of care and their research implications. In S. R. Schroeder, M. L. Oster-Granite & T. Thompson (Eds.), *Self-injurious behavior: Gene-brain-behavior relationships* (pp. 81–91). Washington, DC: American Psychological Association.

Derby, K. M., Fisher, W. W., Piazza, C. C., Wilke, A. E., & Johnson, W. (1998). The effects of noncontingent and contingent attention for self-injury, manding, and collateral responses. *Behavior Modification, 22*(4), 474–484.

Derby, K. M., Wacker, D. P., Sasso, G., Steege, M., Northup, J., Cigrand, K., et al. (1992). Brief functional assessment techniques to evaluate aberrant behavior in an outpatient setting: A summary of 79 cases. *Journal of Applied Behavior Analysis, 25*(3), 713–721.

Didden, R., Duker, P. C., & Korzilius, H. (1997). Meta-analytic study on treatment effectiveness for problem behaviors with individuals who have mental retardation. *American Journal on Mental Retardation, 101*(4), 387–399.

Didden, R., Korzilius, H., Van Oorsouw, W., & Sturmey, P. (2006). Behavioral treatment of challenging behaviors in individuals with mild mental retardation: Meta-analysis of single-subject research. *American Journal on Mental Retardation, 111*(4), 290–298.

Duker, P. C., & Sigafoos, J. (1998). The motivation assessment scale: Reliability and construct validity across three topographies of behavior. *Research in Developmental Disabilities, 19*(2), 131–141.

Durand, V. M., & Crimmins, D. B. (1988). Identifying the variables maintaining self-injurious behavior. *Journal of Autism and Developmental Disorders, 18*(1), 99–117.

Eikeseth, S. (2009). Outcome of comprehensive psycho-educational interventions for young children with autism. *Research in Developmental Disabilities, 30*(1), 158–178.

Einfeld, S. L., & Tonge, B. J. (1995). The developmental behavior checklist: The development and validation of an instrument to assess behavioral and emotional disturbance in children and adolescents with mental retardation. *Journal of Autism and Developmental Disorders, 25*(2), 81–104.

Emerson, E. (1996). Schedule-induced challenging behavior. *Journal of Developmental and Physical Disabilities, 82*(2), 89–103.

Emerson, E., Reeves, D. J., & Felce, D. (2000). Palmtop computer technologies for behavioral observation research. In T. Thompson, D. Felce & F. J. Symons (Eds.), *Behavioral observation: Technology and applications in developmental disabilities* (pp. 47–59). Baltimore, MD: Paul H. Brookes.

Fisher, W. W., Kelley, M. E., & Lomas, J. E. (2003). Visual aids and structured criteria for improving visual inspection and interpretation of single-case designs. *Journal of Applied Behavior Analysis, 36*(3), 387–406.

Fisher, W. W., Piazza, C. C., Bowman, L. G., & Amari, A. (1996). Integrating caregiver report with systematic choice assessment to enhance reinforcer identification. *American Journal on Mental Retardation, 101*(1), 15–25.

Fisher, W., Piazza, C. C., Bowman, L. G., Hagopian, L. P., Owens, J. C., & Slevin, I. (1992). A comparison of two approaches for identifying reinforcers for persons with severe and profound disabilities. *Journal of Applied Behavior Analysis, 25*(2), 491–498.

Freeman, K. A., Anderson, C. M., & Scotti, J. R. (2000). A structured descriptive methodology: Increasing agreement between descriptive and experimental analyses. *Education and Training in Mental Retardation and Developmental Disabilities, 35*(1), 55–66.

Freeman, K. A., Walker, M., & Kaufman, J. (2007). Psychometric properties of the questions about behavioral function scale in a child sample. *American Journal on Mental Retardation, 112*(2), 122–129.

Garbutt, N., & Furniss, F. (2007). Context sampling descriptive assessment: A pilot study of a further approach to functional assessment. *Journal of Applied Research in Intellectual Disabilities, 20*(2), 127–130.

Gardenier, N. C., MacDonald, R., & Green, G. (2004). Comparison of direct observational methods for measuring stereotypic behavior in children with autism spectrum disorders. *Research in Developmental Disabilities, 25*(2), 99–118.

Goh, H. L., Iwata, B. A., Shore, B. A., DeLeon, I. G., Lerman, D. C., Ulrich, S. M., et al. (1995). An analysis of the reinforcing properties of hand mouthing. *Journal of Applied Behavior Analysis, 28*(3), 269–283.

Goldiamond, I. (1974). Toward a constructional approach to social problems: Ethical and constitutional issues raised by applied behavior analysis. *Behaviorism, 2*(1), 1–84.

Hall, S. S. (2005). Comparing descriptive, experimental and informant-based assessments of problem behaviors. *Research in Developmental Disabilities, 26*(6), 514–526.

Hall, S., & Oliver, C. (1992). Differential effects of severe self-injurious behaviour on the behaviour of others. *Behavioural Psychotherapy, 20*(4), 355–365.

Hall, S., & Oliver, C. (2000). An alternative approach to the sequential analysis of behavioral interactions. In T. Thompson, D. Felce & F. J. Symons (Eds.), *Behavioral observation: Technology and applications in developmental disabilities* (pp. 335–348). Baltimore, MD: Paul H. Brookes.

Hanley, G. P., Iwata, B. A., & McCord, B. E. (2003). Functional analysis of problem behavior: A review. *Journal of Applied Behavior Analysis, 36*(2), 147–185.

Hartwig, L., Heathfield, L. T., & Jenson, W. R. (2004). Standardization of the functional assessment and intervention program (FAIP) with children who have externalizing behaviors. *School Psychology Quarterly, 19*(3), 272–287.

Herzinger, C. V., & Campbell, J. M. (2007). Comparing functional assessment methodologies: A quantitative synthesis. *Journal of Autism and Developmental Disorders, 37*(8), 1430–1445.

Hodge, K., Hall, S., & Oliver, C. (2001). *Distinguishing between social positive and automatic reinforcement in descriptive analyses of problem behaviour.* Paper presented at the first International ABA Conference, Venice.

Hutchinson, R. R., Azrin, N. H., & Hunt, G. M. (1968). Attack produced by intermittent reinforcement of a concurrent operant response. *Journal of the Experimental Analysis of Behavior, 11*(4), 489–495.

Iwata, B. A., Dorsey, M. F., Slifer, K. J., Bauman, K. E., & Richman, G. S. (1982). Toward a functional analysis of self-injury. *Analysis and Intervention in Developmental Disabilities, 2*, 3–20.

Iwata, B. A., Pace, G. M., Dorsey, M. F., Zarcone, J. R., Vollmer, T. R., Smith, R. G., et al. (1994). The functions of self-injurious behavior: An experimental-epidemiological analysis. *Journal of Applied Behavior Analysis, 27*(2), 215–240.

Johnston, J. M., & Pennypacker, H. S. (1993). *Strategies and tactics for human behavioral research* (3rd ed.). Hillsdale, NJ: Erlbaum.

Kahng, S., & Iwata, B. A. (1999). Correspondence between outcomes of brief and extended functional analyses. *Journal of Applied Behavior Analysis, 32*(2), 149–159.

Kahng, S., & Iwata, B. A. (2000). Computer systems for collecting real-time observational data. In T. Thompson, D. Felce & F. J. Symons (Eds.), *Behavioral observation: Technology and applications in developmental disabilities* (pp. 35–45). Baltimore, MD: Paul H. Brookes.

Kahng, S., Iwata, B. A., Fischer, S. M., Page, T. J., Treadwell, K. R., Williams, D. E., et al. (1998). Temporal distributions of problem behavior based on scatter plot analysis. *Journal of Applied Behavior Analysis, 31*(4), 593–604.

Kahng, S., Iwata, B. A., & Lewin, A. B. (2002). Behavioral treatment of self-injury, 1964 to 2000. *American Journal on Mental Retardation, 107*(3), 212–221+234.

Kelly, J. F., & Hake, D. F. (1970). An extinction-induced increase in an aggressive response with humans. *Journal of the Experimental Analysis of Behavior, 14*(2), 153–164.

Koegel, R. L., Koegel, L. K., & McNerney, E. K. (2001). Pivotal areas in intervention for autism. *Journal of Clinical Child Psychology, 30*(1), 19–32.

Kurtz, P. F., Chin, M. D., Huete, J. M., Tarbox, R. S. F., O'Connor, J. T., Paclawskyj, T. R., et al. (2003). Functional analysis and treatment of self-injurious behavior in young children: A summary of 30 cases. *Journal of applied behavior analysis, 36*(2), 205–219.

Lambert, N., Nihira, K., & Leland, H. (1993). *Adaptive behavior scale-school* (2nd ed.). Austin, TX: Pro-Ed.

Lancioni, G. E., Van Bergen, I., & Furniss, F. (2002). Urine alarms and prompts for fostering daytime urinary continence in a student with multiple disabilities: A replication study. *Perceptual and Motor Skills, 94*(3 Pt 1), 867–870.

Lewis, T. J., Scott, T. M., & Sugai, G. (1994). The problem behavior questionnaire: A teacher-based instrument to develop functional hypotheses of problem behavior in gen-eral education classrooms. *Diagnostique, 19*(2–3), 103–115.

Lukens, C. T., & Linscheid, T. R. (2008). Development and validation of an inventory to assess mealtime behavior problems in children with autism. *Journal of Autism and Developmental Disorders, 38*(2), 342–352.

Luyster, R. J., Kadlec, M. B., Carter, A., & Tager-Flusberg, H. (2008). Language assessment and development in toddlers with autism spectrum disorders. *Journal of Autism and Developmental Disorders, 38*(8), 1426–1438.

Lyon, D. O., & Ozolins, D. (1970). Pavlovian conditioning of shock-elicited aggression: A discrimination procedure. *Journal of the Experimental Analysis of Behavior, 13*(3), 325–331.

Martin, N. T., Gaffan, E. A., & Williams, T. (1999). Experimental functional analyses for challenging behavior: A study of validity and reliability. *Research in Developmental Disabilities, 20*(2), 125–146.

Martin, N., Oliver, C., & Hall, S. (2003). *Observational data collection and analysis, version 3.2.* London: Antam Ltd.

Matson, J. L., Bamburg, J. W., Cherry, K. E., & Paclawskyj, T. R. (1999). A validity study on the questions about behavioral function (QABF) scale: Predicting treatment success for self-injury, aggression, and stereotypies. *Research in Developmental Disabilities, 20*(2), 163–176.

Matson, J. L., & Boisjoli, J. A. (2007). Multiple versus single maintaining factors of challenging behaviours as assessed by the QABF for adults with intellectual disabilities. *Journal of Intellectual and Developmental Disability, 32*(1), 39–44.

Matson, J. L., Kuhn, D. E., Dixon, D. R., Mayville, S. B., Laud, R. B., Cooper, C. L., et al. (2003). The development and factor structure of the functional assessment for multiple causality (FACT). *Research in Developmental Disabilities, 24*(6), 485–495.

Matson, J. L., & Minshawi, N. F. (2007). Functional assessment of challenging behavior: Toward a strategy for applied settings. *Research in Developmental Disabilities, 28*(4), 353–361.

McAtee, M., Carr, E. G., & Schulte, C. (2004). A contextual assessment inventory for problem behavior: Initial development. *Journal of Positive Behavior Interventions, 6*(3), 148–165.

Meany-Daboul, M. G., Roscoe, E. M., Bourret, J. C., & Ahearn, W. H. (2007). A comparison of momentary time sampling and partial-interval recording for evaluating functional relations. *Journal of Applied Behavior Analysis, 40*(3), 501–514.

Miltenberger, R. G. (2001). *Behavior modification: Principles and procedures* (2nd ed.). Belmont, CA: Wadsworth/Thomson Learning.

Murphy, G., & Goodall, E. (1980). Measurement error in direct observations: A comparison of common recording methods. *Behaviour Research and Therapy, 18*(2), 147–150.

Neef, N. A., & Peterson, S. M. (2007). Functional behavior assessment. In J. O. Cooper, T. E. Heron & W. L. Heward (Eds.), *Applied behavior analysis* (2nd ed., pp. 500–524). Upper Saddle River, NJ: Pearson.

Newton, J. T., & Sturmey, P. (1991). The motivation assessment scale: Inter-rater reliability and internal consistency in a British sample. *Journal of Mental Deficiency Research, 35*(5), 472–474.

Nicholson, J., Konstantinidi, E., & Furniss, F. (2006). On some psychometric properties of the questions about behavioral function (QABF) scale. *Research in Developmental Disabilities, 27*(3), 337–352.

Nikopoulos, C. K., & Keenan, M. (2007). Using video modeling to teach complex social sequences to children with autism. *Journal of Autism and Developmental Disorders, 37*, 678–693.

O'Neill, R. E., Horner, R. H., Albin, R. W., Sprague, J. R., Storey, K., & Newton, J. S. (1997). *Functional assessment and program development for problem behavior: a practical handbook* (2nd ed.). Pacific Grove, CA: Brooks/Cole.

Paclawskyj, T. R., Matson, J. L., Rush, K. S., Smalls, Y., & Vollmer, T. R. (2000). Questions about behavioral function (QABF): A behavioral checklist for functional assessment of aberrant behavior. *Research in Developmental Disabilities, 21*(3), 223–229.

Paclawskyj, T. R., Matson, J. L., Rush, K. S., Smalls, Y., & Vollmer, T. R. (2001). Assessment of the convergent validity of the questions about behavioral function scale with analogue functional analysis and the motivation assessment scale. *Journal of Intellectual Disability Research, 45*(6), 484–494.

Rapp, J. T., Colby, A. M., Vollmer, T. R., Roane, H. S., Lomas, J., & Britton, L. N. (2007). Interval recording for duration events: A re-evaluation. *Behavioral Interventions, 22*, 319–345.

Reese, R. M., Richman, D. M., Belmont, J. M., & Morse, P. (2005). Functional characteristics of disruptive behavior in developmentally disabled children with and without autism. *Journal of Autism and Developmental Disorders, 35*(4), 419–428.

Richman, D. M., & Hagopian, L. P. (1999). On the effects of "quality" of attention in the functional analysis of destructive behavior. *Research in Developmental Disabilities, 20*(1), 51–62.

Ringdahl, J. E., & Sellers, J. A. (2000). The effects of different adults as therapists during functional analyses. *Journal of Applied Behavior Analysis, 33*(2), 247–250.

Roane, H. S., Vollmer, T. R., Ringdahl, J. E., & Marcus, B. A. (1998). Evaluation of a brief stimulus preference assessment. *Journal of Applied Behavior Analysis, 31*(4), 605–620.

Rojahn, J., Matlock, S. T., & Tassé, M. J. (2000). The stereotyped behavior scale: Psychometric properties and norms. *Research in Developmental Disabilities, 21*(6), 437–454.

Rojahn, J., Tassé, M. J., & Sturmey, P. (1997). The stereotyped behavior scale for adolescents and adults with mental retardation. *American Journal on Mental Retardation, 102*(2), 137–146.

Rosales-Ruiz, J., & Baer, D. M. (1997). Behavioral cusps: A developmental and pragmatic concept for behavior analysis. *Journal of Applied Behavior Analysis, 30*(3), 533–544.

Saudargas, R. A., & Zanolli, K. (1990). Momentary time sampling as an estimate of percentage time: A field validation. *Journal of Applied Behavior Analysis, 23*, 533–537.

Shirley, M. J., Iwata, B. A., Kahng, S. W., Mazaleski, J. L., & Lerman, D. C. (1997). Does functional communication training compete with ongoing contingencies of reinforcement? An analysis during response acquisition and maintenance. *Journal of Applied Behavior Analysis, 30*(1), 93–104.

Shogren, K. A., & Rojahn, J. (2003). Convergent reliability and validity of the questions about behavioral function and the motivation assessment scale: A replication study. *Journal of Developmental and Physical Disabilities, 15*(4), 367–375.

Shore, B. A., Iwata, B. A., DeLeon, I. G., Kahng, S., & Smith, R. G. (1997). An analysis of reinforcer substitutability using object manipulation and self-injury as competing responses. *Journal of Applied Behavior Analysis, 30*(1), 21–41.

Sigafoos, J., Kerr, M., & Roberts, D. (1994). Interrater reliability of the motivation assessment scale: Failure to replicate with aggressive behavior. *Research in Developmental Disabilities, 15*(5), 333–342.

Sigafoos, J., & Meikle, B. (1996). Functional communication training for the treatment of multiply determined challenging behavior in two boys with autism. *Behavior Modification, 20*(1), 60–84.

Sigafoos, J., & Saggers, E. (1995). A discrete-trial approach to the functional analysis of aggressive behaviour in two boys with autism. *Australia and New Zealand Journal of Developmental Disabilities, 20*, 287–297.

Skinner, B. F. (1938). *The behavior of organisms*. New York, NY: Appleton-Century-Crofts.

Spreat, S., & Connelly, L. (1996). Reliability analysis of the motivation assessment scale. *American Journal on Mental Retardation, 100*(5), 528–532.

Stage, S. A., Cheney, D., Walker, B., & LaRocque, M. (2002). A preliminary discriminant and convergent validity study of the teacher functional behavioral assessment checklist. *School Psychology Review, 31*(1), 71–93.

Sturmey, P. (1995). Analog baselines: A critical review of the methodology. *Research in Developmental Disabilities, 16*(4), 269–284.

Toogood, S., & Timlin, K. (1996). The functional assessment of challenging behaviour: A comparison of informant-based, experimental and descriptive methods. *Journal of Applied Research in Intellectual Disabilities, 9*(3), 206–222.

Touchette, P. E., MacDonald, R. F., & Langer, S. N. (1985). A scatter plot for identifying stimulus control of problem behavior. *Journal of Applied Behavior Analysis, 18*(4), 343–351.

Tyrer, P., Oliver-Africano, P. C., Ahmed, Z., Bouras, N., Cooray, S., Deb, S., et al. (2008). Risperidone, haloperidol, and placebo in the treatment of aggressive challenging behaviour in patients with intellectual disability: A randomised controlled trial. *Lancet, 371*(9606), 57–63.

Vollmer, T. R., & Matson, J. L. (1995). *User's guide: Questions about behavioral function (QABF)*. Baton Rouge, LA: Scientific Publishers, Inc.

Vollmer, T. R., & Smith, R. G. (1996). Some current themes in functional analysis research. *Research in Developmental Disabilities, 17*(3), 229–249.

Wacker, D. P., Berg, W. K., Cooper, L. J., Derby, K. M., Steege, M. W., Northup, J., et al. (1994). The impact of functional analysis methodology on outpatient clinic services. *Journal of Applied Behavior Analysis, 27*, 405–407.

Wacker, D. P., Steege, M. W., Northup, J., Sasso, G., Berg, W., Reimers, T., et al. (1990). A component analysis of functional communication training across three topographies of severe behavior problems. *Journal of Applied Behavior Analysis, 23*(4), 417–429.

Willis, T. J., & LaVigna, G. W. (1985). *Emergency management guidelines*. Los Angeles, CA: Institute for Applied Behavior Analysis.

Wolf, M. M. (1978). Social validity: The case for subjective measurement or how applied behavior analysis is finding its heart. *Journal of Applied Behavior Analysis, 11*(2), 203–214.

Zarcone, J. R., Rodgers, T. A., Iwata, B. A., Rourke, D. A., & Dorsey, M. F. (1991). Reliability analysis of the motivation assessment scale: A failure to replicate. *Research in Developmental Disabilities, 12*(4), 349–360.

Chapter 4
Intervention and Treatment Methods for Children with Autism Spectrum Disorders

Nozomi Naoi

Reinforcement, training replacement behaviors, discrete trail training, pivotal response training, behavioral cusps, and related training strategies will be emphasized. Research on these and related methods as they apply to autism will be covered.

Introduction

The aim of this chapter is to provide an overview of the approaches to the treatment of children with Autism Spectrum Disorders (ASD) and to consider the differences across the approaches in terms of theoretical positions, strategies, and targeted skills. Common elements that they share will also be highlighted.

ASD are pervasive developmental disorders characterized by impairments in social interaction, communication, and restricted, repetitive, and stereotyped behaviors (DSM-IV, American Psychiatric Association, 1994). Symptoms of individuals with ASD can range over a wide variety of combinations of these three core behavioral deficits with severities ranging from mild to severe. In addition, individuals with ASD are likely to exhibit a variety of comorbid disorders, including mental retardation, phobias and depression (Matson & Nebel-Schwalm, 2007). Therefore, each person with ASD has a unique combination of symptoms, symptom severities, and comorbid disorders. Furthermore, these symptoms and characteristics of children with ASD change with age and development.

Recently, a variety of intervention strategies have been touted as uniquely effective in promoting language and social development, decreasing maladaptive behaviors, and generally improving autistic symptoms. However, to date many of these strategies have not been supported by scientific evidence obtained from randomized controlled studies. Although some of these nonsupported treatments or intervention approaches may in fact have some positive effects on the development of children with ASD, evidence-based practice is critical for helping parents, professionals, and others to select suitable interventions that fit their children's needs and family resources, which will lead to better outcomes at less cost. In addition, scientific evidence is needed not only for the parents and educators of a child with ASD but also for intervention service providers, who must evaluate the effectiveness of intervention programs in order to improve them.

In this chapter, we review intervention methods with published empirical scientific research to support their findings. Most of the interventions reviewed here are based on the principles of Applied Behavioral Analysis (ABA), but other highly regarded programs are derived from structured teaching, as embodied by the TEACCH programs. These interventions are also discussed.

Applied Behavioral Analysis (ABA)

ABA is based on experimentally derived principles of behavior, such as operant conditioning (Skinner, 1938). In B.F. Skinner's (1938, 1953) analysis of behavior; human behaviors can be analyzed within the

N. Naoi (✉)
Japan Agency of Science and Technology, Department of Psychology, Keio University, 2-15-45 Mita, Minato-Ku, Tokyo, 108-8345, Japan
e-mail: nnaoi@psy.flet.keio.ac.jp

framework of a three-term contingency of operant conditioning, which includes the events that precede behavior (antecedents), the behavior itself, and the stimuli that follow the behavior (consequences). When the presentation or removal of a stimulus following a behavior increases the likelihood that the behavior will be repeated in the future, that consequence is considered to be a reinforcement. On the other hand, when a consequence following a behavior decreases the probability that the behavior will be repeated in the future, the consequence is referred to as a punishment. Reinforcement occurs when the probability of a certain behavior increases due to the presentation of a stimulus (positive reinforcement) or the removal of a stimulus (negative reinforcement) as a behavioral consequence. When the stimulus following the behavior increases the frequency of the behavior, the stimulus is called as positive reinforcer. When removing the stimulus following the behavior increases the frequency of the behavior, the stimulus is called a negative reinforcer. This type of reinforcement is also known as avoidance. Likewise, punishment decreases the probability of a behavior through presentation of a stimulus (positive punishment) or the removal of a stimulus (negative punishment) as a behavioral consequence. Similarly, a stimulus added following the behavior that decreases the probability that the behavior will be repeated in the future is called positive punisher, whereas a negative punisher decreases the probability of a behavior when it is removed. In addition, when a behavior that was positively reinforced in the past is no longer reinforced the probability that the behavior will occur in the future also decreases (e.g., Ayllon & Haughton, 1964; Ducharme & Van Houten, 1994). This procedure is known as extinction. In operant conditioning, when the antecedent stimulus does not elicit or cause the behavior directly but instead influences the likelihood that the behavior will occur, the antecedent stimulus is called a discriminative stimulus.

It is important that a reinforcer or a punisher be functionally defined, and only if a consequential stimulus increases or decreases the likelihood of the recurrence of the behavior can the consequential stimulus be defined as a reinforcer or a punisher. For example, candy or praise is not a positive reinforcer until the possibility of the preceding behaviors increases. Similarly, scolding a child cannot be called a punishment unless the frequency of the preceding behavior has been shown to decline.

Method

ABA is the application of the principles of operant conditioning to increase socially appropriate behaviors using reinforcement and decrease maladaptive behaviors using extinction or punishment.

Behavioral interventions based on ABA frequently involve conducting a functional analysis to determine antecedents and consequences of the child's behavior, selecting "a target behavior" based on the child's individual skills and difficulties, measuring the current levels of the child's behavior as a baseline, and finally implementing a behavioral intervention to increase socially appropriate behavior and/or reduce maladaptive behavior. During intervention, the behavior is continuously measured in order to determine the effectiveness of the intervention and, in general, the generalizations of acquired skills across settings, people, and materials are assessed following the completion of intervention. In addition, follow-up data are frequently collected to evaluate the generalization and maintenance of the behavior (i.e., the success of the intervention).

Functional Analysis

Functional analysis of a child's environment is typically conducted to identify the antecedents and consequences associated with the child's behavior by interviewing, making direct observations, and/or systematically manipulating environmental events (Hanley, Iwata, & McCord, 2003; Hanley, Piazza, & Fisher, 1997; Kennedy, Meyer, Knowles, & Shukla, 2000; Potoczak, Carr, & Michael, 2007). For example, to reduce maladaptive behaviors such as tantrums, a functional analysis of the child's environment is conducted to identify the variables that probably maintain the behavior. The behavioral functions that have been hypothesized to maintain the child's inappropriate behaviors include adult attention, escape from an undesired situation or difficult instruction, access to tangible items and preferred activities, and generation of sensory reinforcement (Carr, 1977; Carr & Durand, 1985; Derby et al., 1992; Durand & Carr, 1987; Hanley et al., 2003; Iwata, Dorsey, Slifer, Bauman, & Richman, 1994; Mace & Belfiore, 1990). When the function of the behavior has been determined to be attention seeking or escape from demands, these conditions are manipulated to reduce the behavior via extinction or punishment and/or to replace the behavior with a more appropriate alternative response that delivers the same results as the inappropriate behavior. For example, if it appears that a child is seeking attention from adults by screaming, the child's screaming is ignored (via extinction) and the child is taught more appropriate replacement behavior to gain attention, such as verbal response "look!" Recently nonaversive procedures that focus on both teaching positive alternative skills and manipulating the environment to prevent the occurrence of inappropriate behavior are increasingly used to treat maladaptive behaviors rather than punishment procedures involving aversive consequences (Carr et al., 2002; Horner, 2000; Horner et al., 1990; Koegel, Koegel, & Dunlap, 1996). Punishment procedures should be used only when positive procedures alone are not effective to reduce maladaptive behaviors and then careful attention should be given to the severity of maladaptive behaviors including potential harm to a child or others and benefits of the procedures to reduce the maladaptive behavior (Davies, Howlin, Bernal, & Warren, 1998; Fisher et al., 1993; Hagopian, Fisher, Sullivan, Acquisto, & LeBlanc, 1998; Matson & LoVullo, 2008; Matson & Taras, 1989; Wacker et al., 1990).

Selecting Target Behaviors

The selection of target behaviors is one of the most important aspects of successful interventions for children with ASD. A variety of child behaviors could be targeted in any intervention based on ABA. However, selecting a target behavior based on the impact on other behavioral domains appears to be important, if the intervention effect is to be optimized.

"A Behavioral Cusp," as defined by Rosales-Ruiz and Baer (1997), is "a behavior change that has consequences for the organism beyond the change itself" (p. 534). In other words, behavioral cusps are considered as behaviors in which changes have more far-reaching consequences when compared to other behaviors, and should therefore be targeted by priority. Bosch and Fuqua (2001) provide guidelines for selecting potentially important target behaviors such as behavioral cusps. The first criterion for a behavioral cusp is changes in the behavior leading to "access to new reinforcers, contingencies, or environments"

not previously encountered (p. 123). Second, the behavioral changes must meet "the demands of the social community of which the learner is a member" (p. 125). Third, the behavioral changes must facilitate "subsequent learning by being either a prerequisite or a component of more complex responses" (p. 124). Fourth, changes in the behavior must interfere with or replace inappropriate behaviors. Last, the changes in response must benefit others such as parents, siblings, or the teachers of the child.

When a behavior is targeted, it must be clearly defined in objective, observable and quantifiable terms. For example, "being nice to friends" is not an objective and observable definition, while "saying good morning to friends in the morning" is a more specific definition. Objective and observable definitions of the target behaviors are necessary to measure behavior, implement intervention strategies, and enhance accountability, which promote communication and collaboration among parents, teachers, and other professionals.

Teaching Procedures

To increase socially appropriate behaviors, ABA focuses on teaching small, measurable units of behavior systematically. Targeted skills are broken down into small steps using task analysis and each step is taught using behavioral techniques such as shaping, prompting, and chaining.

Shaping is a method of conditioning a new behavior by gradually reinforcing successive approximations of the desired target behavior (i.e., what the child already does is reinforced by a positive reinforcer such as an edible item or praise). For example, in teaching a child to write, the child is first reinforced for picking up the pencil. When the child could reliably pick up the pencil, the child is then reinforced for scribbling. Finally, the child is reinforced for drawing a vertical line on a piece of paper.

Prompting is a method used to ensure the child's production of the target behavior by providing various types of assistance, including such approaches as verbal instruction, modeling, gestures, and physical guidance. For example, when a child is taught to discriminate between two items, a physical prompt is used to guide his/her hand to select the correct item.

Prompts gradually fade out or are delayed as the child progresses to avoid prompt-dependency.

In addition, chaining is often used to teach the child to produce a sequence of behaviors. For example, using task analysis, "putting on trousers" can be broken down in to smaller steps such as holding trousers, opening the waistband, putting the right leg into the right trouser leg, putting the left leg into the left trouser leg, pulling trousers up, and fastening the button. In forward chaining, the child is taught holding trousers first (i.e., the initial step). Once the initial step is mastered, the child is taught the second step; opening the waistband. In backward chaining, the child is taught the final step such as fastening the button first. Once the final step in the chain is mastered, the second to last step (pulling trousers up) is taught.

Intervention Strategies Based on Applied Behavior Analysis

Discrete Trial Training (DTT)

DTT and ABA are not synonymous, with DTT being the application of ABA principles within a structured environment in order to teach specific skills. The "discrete trial" refers to a small unit in which an adult (such as the child's teacher) provides a discriminate stimulus, which is then followed by the child response and the reinforcement of the response immediately following the child's response. In general, the discriminate stimulus is delivered verbally in a brief and clear manner (e.g., "Do this"), and the target behavior is broken down into small segments. Only one particular skill is taught at a time in DTT. When the child responds appropriately to the discriminate stimulus, the teacher immediately provides a positive reinforcer such as an edible item, praise, or access to toys or preferred activities. If the child does not give the correct response, the teacher provides prompting to assist the child in responding correctly. As the child progresses, the prompt is gradually faded out so that the child learns to respond to the discriminative stimulus by itself. It is essential that teachers carefully select reinforcers, and reinforce immediately following the child's appropriate responses. Discrete trials are heavily repeated in order to ensure acquisition of a particular target behavior.

Evidence Base

A number of studies have indicated that DTT is useful in the teaching of a wide variety of skills, such as motor, vocal, and verbal imitation (e.g., Baer, Peterson, & Sherman, 1967; Lovaas, Berberich, Perloff, & Schaeffer, 1966; Metz, 1965; Schroeder & Baer, 1972; Young, Krantz, McClannahan, & Poulson, 1994), verbal behaviors including receptive and expressive language skills and alternative communication systems (Carr, Kologinsky, Leff-Simon, 1987; Howlin, 1981; Hung, 1977, 1980; Krantz & McClannahan, 1993; Yoder & Layton, 1988), play skills (Coe, Matson, Fee, Manikam, & Linarello, 1990), and the management of maladaptive behaviors (Piazza, Moes, & Fisher, 1996; Sigafoos & Saggers, 1995) in children with ASD. It is suggested that DTT is useful in teaching new skills and new discriminations between events due to the provision of many learning opportunities within a teaching session (Smith, 2001).

Many comprehensive early intervention programs for children with ASD include the provision of intensive DTT, and these intervention programs have documented effectiveness across a wide range of settings including home, school, and center, and across various levels of symptom severity (Anderson, Avery, DiPietro, Edwards, & Christian, 1987; Fenske, Zalenski, Krantz, & McClannahan, 1985; Harris, Handleman, Gordon, Kristoff, & Fuentes, 1991; Harris, Handleman, Kristoff, Bass, & Gordon, 1990; Lovaas, 1987; McEachin, Smith, & Lovaas, 1993; Sheinkopf & Siegel, 1998; Smith, Buch, & Gamby, 2000).

An early intervention study by Lovaas of the UCLA Young Autism Project is the most frequently cited study demonstrating the effectiveness of DTT for young children with ASD under 4 years of age. Lovaas's program involves an average of 40 h per week of one-to-one instruction administered by trained graduate students and parents at both home and school settings. Nine out of 19 children (about 47%) in the experimental group who received intensive DTT treatment were reported to have average or above scores on IQ tests and less restrictive school placements, compared with only 1 of 40 children of the comparison group (about 2%) who received less intensive interventions over 2 to 3 years (Lovaas, 1987). McEachin et al. (1993) conducted follow-up assessments of the children who participated in the initial Lovaas study (1987), and reported that 8 out of 19 children (42%) in the experimental group had maintained IQ and behavioral gains at a mean age of 11.5 years.

A number of studies have replicated the UCLA Young Autism Project results across a variety of settings, including home and school. Although there were differences between the study of Lovaas (1987) and other replication studies in intensity and duration of treatment, characteristics of children at intake, training curriculum, treatment administrators, and degree of gains shown by the children in the intensive treatment group, these studies have generally reported significant gains in the treated children's intellectual functioning, adaptive skills, and language, as well as less restrictive school placements compared to the comparison group (Anderson et al., 1987; Fenske et al., 1985; Harris et al., 1991 Harris et al., 1990; Sheinkopf & Siegel, 1998).

Although the general efficacy of DTT for helping children with ASD to acquire new skills has not been disputed, this approach does have significant limitations. The two most frequently cited limitations of DTT are lack of initiation of skills acquired in DTT in the absence of previously learned contingencies, and limited generalization of those skills across settings, people, and materials, given that DTT is an adult-directed intervention and the teaching environment in DTT is highly structured. (Harris, Wolchik, & Weitz, 1981; Lovaas, Koegel, Simmons, & Long, 1973; Rogers-Warren & Warren, 1980; Spradlin & Siegel, 1982).

Given these limitations, alternative methods are required to promote initiation and generalization of skills to new settings, using more natural learning environments and reinforcers (Hart & Risley, 1968; Kaiser, Ostrosky, & Alpert, 1993; McGee, Krantz, & McClannahan, 1985; Spradlin & Siegel, 1982).

Incidental Teaching (IT)

One alternative instructional procedure that facilitates initiation and generalization of skills is incidental teaching (IT). The term "incidental teaching" refers to instruction that focuses on teaching children directly whenever the child shows interests in the teaching materials or the motivation to request an item or activity in the natural environment (Hart & Risley, 1968, 1975; McGee, Krantz, Mason, & McClannahan, 1983). Although teaching opportunities are provided in the

natural daily environment in IT, it is essential that teachers carefully select target behaviors to meet each child's individual needs and abilities, and arrange the environment to provide the opportunities for the child to initiate the behavior that has been targeted for intervention. In IT, materials or activities selected by the child, dependent on each child's interests and motivation, are also used as the naturally occurring reinforcers for the child's behavior. For example, to teach an appropriate request, the teacher arranges the environment by placing each child's preferred snacks or toys in a manner visible to the child but out of the child's reach, to encourage the child to initiate making requests. Once the child demonstrates motivation to request the item via gaze shift, gesturing, word approximation, or using words, depending on the child's abilities, the teacher provides a prompt to initiate a more elaborate communicative response. When the child emits such a response with or without prompting, the child receives the desired item as a reinforcer.

One of the limitations of IT is that it provides fewer learning opportunities than does DTT, especially for those children with low rates of initiation, resulting in a slower rate of target skill acquisition. To address this shortcoming, variations of IT such as modified incidental teaching (MIT) have been developed to increase the number of learning opportunities by using adult initiations in a natural setting (Rogers-Warren & Warren, 1980; Warren, McQuarter, & Rogers-Warren, 1984). In MIT, when the child shows motivation to request an item, the adult begins by asking the child to make the request: "What do you want?" When the child responds correctly with or without prompting, the child receives the desired item as a reinforcer.

Evidence Base

IT and MIT have been shown to enhance the generalization and initiation of receptive and expressive language skills (Charlop-Christy & Carpenter, 2000; Farmer-Dougan, 1994; Hart & Risley, 1975; McGee et al., 1983; McGee et al., 1985; Miranda-Linne & Melin, 1992; Neef, Walters, & Egel, 1984; Rogers-Warren & Warren, 1980; Warren et al., 1984), as well as social interaction skills (McGee, Almeida, Sulzer-Azaroff, & Feldman, 1992) in children with ASD. In addition, some studies have reported that IT results in greater generalization of acquired expressive language skills than DTT (Delprato, 2001; McGee et al., 1985; Miranda-Linne & Melin, 1992).

Pivotal Response Training (PRT)

Another ABA approach to enhance initiation and generalization of skills in children with ASD is Pivotal Response Training (PRT, Koegel & Koegel, 1995; Koegel, Koegel, Harrower, & Carter, 1999; Koegel, O'Dell, & Koegel, 1987). PRT is a naturalistic behavioral intervention based on principles of ABA and developed by Lynn and Robert Koegel and Laura Schreibman at the University California in Santa Barbara (UCSB). "Pivotal response" in PRT refers to responses that seem to be central to many different aspects of functioning in children with ASD, such that changes in these skills appear to influence many different behaviors in children (Koegel, Koegel, Harrower, et al., 1999; Prizant & Rubin, 1999). In PRT, the focus is on pivotal responses such as motivation, responsivity to multiple cues, self management, and self initiation, instead of teaching individual target behaviors one at a time and serially as is done in DTT (Koegel, Koegel, Shoshan, & McNerney, 1999).

Similar to IT, the teaching environment is less structured than that in DTT, and play settings are used in PRT. During training, a child is allowed to choose the toys or activities to be used in training, to enhance the child's motivation (Koegel et al., 1987). Motivation can also be improved by varying the nature of the intervention task, and interspersing tasks that the child has previously mastered with new acquisition tasks (Koegel, Koegel, Harrower, et al., 1999). In PRT, all of the child's attempts to respond correctly (rather than reinforcing only successful attempts) were reinforced using more naturally occurring reinforcers directly related to the task (Koegel, Koegel, Harrower, et al., 1999; Koegel, O'Dell, & Dunlap, 1988). For example, when the child says "open" in the presence of the box in which small snacks are deposited, the child's response is reinforced by the adult opening the box and getting the snacks. In addition, adequate modeling of the target behavior (such as demonstrating turn-taking) is provided in PRT. In sum, procedures used in PRT to increase child motivation include child choice of learning stimuli, task variation and interspersal of maintenance tasks among new learning trials, reinforcement of response attempts, the use of natural and direct reinforcers, and turn-taking.

Evidence Base

PRT has been shown to increase the initiation and generalization of language skills, improve the intelligibility of speech sounds, and to decrease maladaptive behavior in children with ASD (Koegel, Camarata, Koegel, Ben-Tall, & Smith, 1998; Koegel, Koegel, & Surratt, 1992; Koegel et al., 1988; Koegel et al., 1987; Koegel & Williams, 1980). In addition, PRT has been adapted to teach manipulative, symbolic, and sociodramatic play (Stahmer, 1995, 1999; Thorp, Stahmer, & Schreibman, 1995), peer interaction (Pierce & Schreibman, 1995), responding to and initiating joint attention (Whalen & Schreibman, 2003), and object imitation (Ingersoll & Gergans, 2007; Ingersoll, Lewis, & Kroman, 2007; Ingersoll & Schreibman, 2006). In addition, a recent study (Baker-Ericzén, Stahmer, & Burns, 2007) has reported the effectiveness of PRT in community settings on improvements in adaptive functioning on the Vineland Adaptive Behavior Scales (Sparrow, Balla, & Cicchetti, 1984).

Previous studies comparing PRT and DTT have suggested that PRT can be more effective than DTT, at least in terms of increased generalization and maintenance of the target behavior (Delprato, 2001; Koegel et al., 1998; Koegel et al., 1992; Koegel et al., 1988; Koegel et al., 1987; Laski, Charlop, & Schreibman, 1988). In addition, research has shown that when PRT is implemented in parent training, the child (Koegel et al., 1988; Prizant & Rubin, 1999) as well as the parent (Schreibman, Kaneko, & Koegel, 1991) exhibit more positive emotions during instruction, and parent–child interactions in the unstructured family setting are rated happier and less stressful, as compared to those of parents and children trained with DTT (Koegel, Bimbela, & Schreibman, 1996).

Verbal Behavior (VB)

Verbal Behavior (VB) is based on ABA principles but is focused on the acquisition of functional language skills in children with ASD. VB is based on B.F. Skinner's analysis of verbal behavior. Skinner (1957) has classified verbal behaviors into core functional units (i.e., verbal operant), such as mand, tact, echoic, and intraverbal.

A mand is defined as a verbal operant in which the response is evoked by a specific establishing operation and reinforced by a characteristic consequence (Skinner, 1957). An establishing operation (EO; Michael, 1982, 1993, 2000) or motivating operation (MO; Laraway, Snycerski, Michael, & Poling, 2003) is defined as an environmental event that momentarily increases or decreases the reinforcing value of consequences, and increases or decreases the frequency of any behavior that has been associated with consequences in the past. For example, a child's mand "Juice" is reinforced by receiving the juice. In addition, when the child is thirsty (a condition in which the EO is present), the reinforcing value of juice will increase and the mand "Juice" will be emitted more frequently compared to when the child is not thirsty. Tact is a verbal operant in which a given response form is evoked or at least strengthened by a particular object or event, or by a property of an object or event (Skinner, 1957) (for example, when a child looks at a picture card of juice, the child labels the card "Juice"). An echoic is a verbal behavior whose form is controlled by someone else's verbal behavior with point-to-point correspondence (for example, the adult says, "Juice" and the child says, "Juice"). An intraverbal is defined as a verbal behavior that is under the stimulus control of another verbal behavior but does not show point-to-point correspondence (for example, the child says "Juice" in response to the adult's question "What is something you drink?").

Language assessment and intervention programs for children with ASD have been developed based on Skinner's (1957) analysis of verbal behavior (Partington & Sundberg, 1998; Spradlin, 1963; Sundberg, 1983), which are known as VB. The VB approach shares similarities with incidental teaching and PRT in that the natural environment and naturally occurring consequences are used in teaching. VB is different from other ABA-based interventions in that it primarily focuses on functional analysis of a child's verbal behaviors and teaching multiple functions of language (i.e., mands, tacts, echoic, and intraverbal). A major focus of early VB training is on mands, on the basis that the mand is essential to human communication (Bijou & Baer, 1965; Skinner, 1957), and that mand training is effective in providing the child with some control over the environment (Sundberg & Partington,

1998). In mand training, a child is taught to request desired items, activities, and information by using the child's current EO and delivering specific reinforcement (Sundberg, 1993; Sundberg & Michael, 2001; Sundberg & Partington, 1998).

Evidence Base

A number of studies suggest that interventions based upon Skinner's analysis of verbal behavior are effective for increasing the functional use of verbal behavior in children with ASD. Mand training is effective in establishing the use of mands (Duker, Dortmans, & Lodder, 1993; Hartman & Klatt, 2005; Yamamoto & Mochizuki, 1988), decreasing various maladaptive behaviors (Carr & Durand, 1985; Shafer, 1994), and increasing the effectiveness of language training for other verbal operants such as tact (Arntzen & Almas, 2002; Carroll & Hesse, 1987; Nuzzolo-Gomez & Greer, 2004). In addition, many studies have focused on establishing tacts in children with ASD (Naoi, Yokoyama, & Yamamoto, 2007; Partington, Sundberg, Newhouse, & Spengler, 1994; Sundberg, Endicott, & Eigenheer, 2000).

Intervention studies based on VB have shown that a form of verbal behavior established as one verbal operant does not always result in the child using that form as the other verbal operant in the absence of direct instruction (Arntzen & Almas, 2002; Carroll & Hesse, 1987; Lamarre & Holland, 1985; Ross & Greer, 2003; Tsiouri & Greer, 2003; Twyman, 1995; Williams, & Greer, 1993), as suggested by Skinner (1957). Multiple Exemplar Instruction (MEI) has been applied to teach two verbal operants across establishing and reinforcement conditions for each function, for a subset of forms. MEI have been shown to be effective in establishing two operants (e.g., mand and tact) in children with ASD (Arntzen & Almas, 2002; Greer, Yuan, & Gautreaux, 2005; Nuzzolo-Gomez & Greer, 2004).

Picture Exchange Communication System (PECS)

The Picture Exchange Communication System (PECS) was developed by Frost and Bondy (1994) as an augmentative and alternative communication (AAC)

approach for those children with ASD who have limited or no verbal communication skills.

Using PECS, a child approaches communicative partners (e.g., parents or teachers) in order to spontaneously initiate communicative interaction by using a picture card to request a desired item or to comment on something the child observes. PECS is similar to VB in that this approach was inspired by Skinner's analysis of verbal behavior (1957), and focuses on the function rather than the form of behavior. Typically, requesting skills are the first skills taught to children with ASD (Bondy & Frost, 2002).

PECS training can be broken down into six phases (Bondy & Frost, 1994). In the first phase of PECS training, one of a child's favorite items (such as a food item or toy) is placed in sight but out of reach. If the child looks interested in the item, the adult partner gives the child a picture card. The child is then physically prompted by holding the child's hand and guiding it to hand the picture card back to the partner. Upon receipt of the picture card, the communicative partner provides the item depicted on the card to the child as a positive reinforcer. In the second phase of PECS training, the distance between the communicative partner and the child is increased so that the child has to move toward the communicative partner in order to make the exchange. In the third phase, the child is taught to discriminate, selecting the picture card corresponding to a desired item from among multiple cards. During the fourth phase, the child is taught to construct simple sentences on sentence strips such as "I want ____" to communicate. In the fifth phase, the communicative partner asks the child "What do you want?" and the child is taught to respond to this direct question. In the sixth phase, the child is taught to comment on something the child observes using sentences such as "I see ____." The skills required in PECS are broken down into small components, consistent with the ABA approach. This procedure is useful in identifying which phase of the skill the child is struggling with. Furthermore, prompts are given to ensure skill mastery (Yokoyama, Naoi, & Yamamoto, 2006).

One of the advantages of PECS is that it capitalizes on simple motor skills that are easy to acquire or already in a child's behavioral repertoire, including reaching for, picking up, and handing over a card. Therefore, PECS can be rapidly utilized by children with severely limited behavioral repertoires to ensure

some degree of effective communication from the very beginning of the intervention. In addition, unlike sign language, pictures used in PECS are easily understood by most members of the community without explicit training, and can be used in a variety of settings, including home, classroom, and the broader community (Berkowitz, & Buyrberry, 1989).

Evidence Base

Several initial reports have suggested that a large number of children acquire PECS rapidly, with a corresponding decrease in maladaptive behaviors, and some children do eventually develop spoken language following PECS training (Bondy & Frost, 1994, 1998; Peterson, Bondy, Vincent, & Finnegan, 1995; Schwartz, Garfinkle, & Bauer, 1998).

Subsequent to these studies, more controlled experimental studies have addressed the effects of PECS on speech development, social communication, and maladaptive behaviors in children with ASD and related disabilities. Studies using single subject designs have demonstrated that children with ASD master PECS rapidly, and show increases in spontaneous and advanced speech, other social-communicative behaviors such as eye contact and joint attention, and decreases in various maladaptive behaviors following the acquisition of PECS (Charlop-Christy, Carpenter, Le, LeBlanc, & Kellet, 2002; Ganz & Simpson, 2004; Yokoyama et al., 2006). In addition, a group of children with ASD who received 15 h of PECS training over a period of about 5 weeks through the third phase of PECS training (discrimination training), showed significant increases in speech production when compared to a group of children with ASD who did not receive PECS training (Carr & Felce, 2007a). Furthermore, communicative interactions increased significantly between children and teachers in the PECS group but not in the control group (Carr & Felce, 2007b).

Using a randomized controlled trial, Howlin, Gordon, Pasco, Wade, and Charman (2007) showed that initiations and use of PECS in the classroom increased in a group of ASD children whose teachers received expert training and consultancy in the use of PECS. However, these positive effects were not maintained after consultations for teachers ceased. In addition, there were no observed increases in speech, communication, and social interaction, and problem behaviors did not decrease following PECS teacher training. Howlin et al. (2007) suggested that the main consideration for generalizing and maintaining communication with PECS is the ongoing monitoring of the environment. For example, pictures used in PECS need to be continually modified to reflect the changing needs of the child.

In addition, when PECS is used with children who have nonEnglish speaking backgrounds, linguistic differences such as word order may impact on the use of PECS. For example, although Japanese sentences can be written either in vertical or horizontal lines, almost all textbooks used in Japanese language classes in schools are written in the vertical orientation. Therefore, it is possible that vertical sentence strip orientation may be easy to acquire in Japanese children with ASD (Koita & Sonoyama, 2004; Koita, Sonoyama, & Takeuchi, 2003).

TEACCH

Another intervention program that enjoys empirical support is the Treatment and Education of Autistic and related Communication handicapped CHildren (TEACCH). The TEACCH program was founded in the early 1970s by Schopler at the University of North Carolina at Chapel Hill, as a statewide program in North Carolina. The core feature of the TEACCH program is understanding and accepting the existing strengths and weaknesses of each child with ASD, and the main emphasis of the TEACCH program is on structuring the environment to accommodate the characteristics of each individual with ASD, as well as improving the functioning of the child by structured teaching (Lord & Schopler, 1994; Mesibov, 1994, 1996; Schopler, 1989, 1997). The TEACCH program includes the development of an individualized and family centered plan based on the characteristics and learning profiles of each child with ASD, rather than using a standard curriculum.

Structured teaching involves structuring the physical environment of the child (for example, providing individual work system and group activity areas with clear physical and visual boundaries to facilitate learning and minimize visual and auditory distractions; Schopler,

Brehm, Kinsbourne, & Reichler, 1971). In addition, structured teaching also involves making the start and end of each task understandable and predictable by manipulating spatial orientation (e.g., starting on work in a tray placed to the left of the child and placing the finished task on the finished tray on the right; Mesibov, Schopler, & Hearsey, 1994; Schopler, Mesibov, & Hearsey, 1995). In addition, based on relative strengths in visual skills when compared to the difficulties in auditory processing evidenced by many children with ASD, the TEACCH program involves use of a visual schedule to tell the child with ASD what activities will occur and in what sequence. Visual schedules are also used to facilitate transitioning of the child from one activity to another with less adult support.

Evidence Base

A few studies have been conducted to validate the effectiveness of TEACCH. Ozonoff and Cathcart (1998) examined the effectiveness of home-based intervention based on TEACCH for young children with ASD. Children in the TEACCH treatment group had significantly higher gains on various subtests of the Psychoeducational Profile-Revised (PEP-R, Schopler, Reichler, Bashford, Lansing, & Marcus, 1990), including imitation, gross and fine motor skills, and nonverbal conceptual skills, as well as in overall PEP-R scores as compared to those in a no treatment control group. Another study conducted by Panerai, Ferrante, and Zingale (2002) compared the TEACCH program to a nonspecific integration program for children with ASD. Scores on the PEP-R and the Vineland Adaptive Behavior Scale were higher for children in the TEACCH treatment group than in the control group. The TEACCH program has been widely used outside the United States including Asian countries such as China and Japan, and one empirical study has reported the effectiveness of using the TEACCH program with Chinese children (Tsang, Shek, Lam, Tang, & Cheung, 2007).

Other aspects of TEACCH, such as the individual work system, have been shown to be effective in increasing on-task behavior, the number of tasks completed, play materials utilized, and reductions in teacher prompting (Hume & Odom, 2007; Lord & Schopler, 1989).

Future Research Agenda

This chapter reviewed research findings on behavioral interventions for children with ASD. There are a number of intervention approaches based on ABA principles including DTT, IT, PRT, VB, and PECS. Among them, IT, PRT, and VB are similar in that natural environment and naturally occurring consequences are used in teaching. Both VB and PECS are based on analysis of verbal behavior by Skinner (1957) and focus on teaching requesting skills from the beginning of intervention. In addition, PECS and TEACCH are similar in that both approaches utilize visual strategies based on relative strength in visual skills for children with ASD.

Given that there is great heterogeneity among children with ASD, every child with ASD may benefit from different interventions. It is important to individualize interventions based on assessments of the specific strengths and needs of children with ASD and their families. In addition, it is important to note that interventions for children with ASD focus on not only individual characteristics of children with ASD, but also on interactions between the child and the environment. Therefore, it is not sufficient simply to encourage a child to adopt socially appropriate functional behaviors to make changes in the child's environment. In addition, the environment of the child should be structured to accommodate individual characteristics of each child with ASD to make appropriate behaviors that are likely to occur and to avoid maladaptive behaviors. To ensure this, collaboration between parents and teachers of children is indispensable.

In addition to individual differences of children with ASD, it is important to consider the cultural and linguistic differences of children and families (Bridges, 2004; Dyches, Wilder, Sudweeks, Obiakor, & Algozzine, 2004; Trembath, Balandin & Rossi, 2005; Wilder, Dyches, Obiakor, & Algozzine, 2004).

Cultural differences in child-rearing beliefs and practices, and community and parental attitudes to disorder may affect parents' interactions with their children and expectations for their children, and such differences may affect what behavior is likely to be selected to be taught and what intervention strategies are likely to be preferred by parents of children with ASD (Fung & Roseberry-McKibbin, 1999; Hwa-Froelich & Vigil, 2004; Rodriguez & Olswang, 2003; Rossi & Balandin, 2005; Vigil & Hwa-Froelich, 2004; Wilder et al., 2004).

For example, parents' socialization goals often reflect cultural backgrounds. For example, certain cultures place an emphasis on early child independence, while other cultures place greater value on children's interdependence on family members and structured, adult-directed teaching is preferred (Rodriguez & Olswang, 2003; Simmons & Johnston, 2007). In addition, cultural differences in the degree of family involvement and interdependence in childcare may affect how and where interventions are implemented. Parents from cultural backgrounds that value strong family cohesion tend to access special services less frequently and rely more on support from their extended family (Bailey, Skinner, Rodriguez, Gut, & Correa, 1999; Lian, 1996; Pruchno, Patrick, & Burant, 1997; Rogers-Dulan & Blancher, 1995). Socioeconomic backgrounds and maternal employment may also affect the degree of family involvement and the degree of expectations placed on teachers or other professionals to implement interventions for children with ASD.

Although most intervention strategies targeting verbal behavior reviewed in this chapter are based on studies of children in English-speaking countries, the cross-linguistic differences in pronunciation, spelling, grammar, and syntax may also affect the methods and priorities for teaching verbal skills. For example, Chinese is a tonal language, which means changes in tone of a word or syllable changes the word's meaning. Given the common difficulties in receptive and expressive prosody in children with ASD (e.g., Peppé, McCann, Gibbon, O'Hare, & Rutherford, 2007), specific intervention strategies that address this difficulty may need to be developed for Chinese-speaking children with ASD.

It is necessary to examine the applicability of interventions with empirical evidence supporting their effectiveness for children with ASD who live in other countries outside the United States. In addition to the cultural and linguistic differences mentioned above, other factors that may interact with child and family characteristics and impact the effectiveness of specific intervention strategies include the quality and quantity of government support for special education, the availability of well-trained professionals, and access to public and private special services. Furthermore, shortage of information regarding interventions for children with ASD can lead to parents and teachers misunderstandings about, or overreliance on, particular interventions and strategies. Although little is known about the effects of cultural, linguistic, and country factors on the effectiveness of interventions, these factors must also be taken into account when planning intervention programs for children with ASD.

References

American Psychiatric Association. (1994). *Diagnostic and statistical manual of mentaldisorders* (4th ed.). Washington, DC: Author.

Anderson, S., Avery, D., DiPietro, E., Edwards, G., & Christian, W. (1987). Intensive home-based early intervention with autistic children. *Education & Treatment of Children, 10,* 352–366.

Arntzen, E., & Almas, I. (2002). Effects of mand-tact versus tact-only training on the acquisition of tacts. *Journal of Applied Behavior Analysis, 35,* 419–422.

Ayllon, T., & Haughton, E. (1964). Modification of symptomatic verbal behavior of mental patients. *Behaviour Research and Therapy, 2,* 87–97.

Baer, D., Peterson, R., & Sherman, J. (1967). The development of imitation by reinforcing behavioral similarity to a model. *Journal of the Experimental Analysis of Behavior, 10,* 405–416.

Bailey, D., Skinner, D., Rodriguez, P., Gut, D., & Correa, V. (1999). Awareness, use, and satisfaction with services for Latino parents of young children with disabilities. *Exceptional Children, 65,* 367–381.

Baker-Ericzén, M., Stahmer, A., & Burns, A. (2007). Child demographics associated with outcomes in a community-based pivotal response training program. *Journal of Positive Behavior Interventions, 9,* 52–60.

Berkowitz, S., & Buyrberry, J. (1989). Functionality of two modes of communication in the community by students with developmental disabilities: A comparison of signing and communication books. *Journal of the Association for Persons with Severe Handicaps, 14,* 227–233.

Bijou, S., & Baer, D. (1965). *Child development II: Universal stage of infancy.* New York: Appleton-Century-Crofts.

Bondy, A., & Frost, L. (1994). The picture exchange communication system. *Focus on Autistic Behavior, 9,* 1–19.

Bondy, A., & Frost, L. (1998). The picture exchange communication system. *Seminars in Speech and Language, 19,* 373–389.

Bondy, A., & Frost, L. (2002). *A picture's worth: PECS and other visual communication strategies in autism.* Bethesda, MD: Woodbine House.

Bosch, S., & Fuqua, R. (2001). Behavioral cusps: A model for selecting target behaviors. *Journal of Applied Behavior Analysis, 34,* 123–125.

Bridges, S. (2004). Multicultural issues in augmentative and alternative communication and language: Research to practice. *Topics in Language Disorders, 24,* 62–75.

Carr, E. (1977). The motivation of self-injurious behavior: A review of some hypotheses. *Psychological Bulletin, 84,* 800–816.

Carr, E., Dunlap, G., Horner, R., Koegel, R., Turnbull, A., Sailor, W., et al. (2002). Positive behavior support: Evolution of an applied science. *Journal of Positive Behavior Interventions, 4,* 4–16.

Carr, E., & Durand, V. (1985). Reducing behavior problems through functional communication training. *Journal of Applied Behavior Analysis, 18,* 111–126.

Carr, D., & Felce, J. (2007a). Increase in production of spoken words in some children with autism after PECS teaching to phase III. *Journal of Autism and Developmental Disorders, 37,* 780–787.

Carr, D., & Felce, J. (2007b). The effects of PECS teaching to phase III on the communicative interactions between children with autism and their teachers. *Journal of Autism and Developmental Disorders, 37,* 724–737.

Carr, E., Kologinsky, E., & Leff-Simon, S. (1987). Acquisition of sign language by autistic children III: Generalized descriptive phrases. *Journal of Autism and Developmental Disorders, 17,* 217–229.

Carroll, R., & Hesse, B. (1987). The effect of alternating mand and tact training on the acquisition of tacts. *The Analysis of Verbal Behavior, 5,* 55–65.

Charlop-Christy, M., & Carpenter, M. (2000). Modified incidental teaching sessions: A procedure for parents to increase spontaneous speech in their child with autism. *Journal of Positive Behavior Interventions, 2,* 98–112.

Charlop-Christy, M., Carpenter, M., Le, L., LeBlanc, L., & Kellet, K. (2002). Using the picture exchange communication system (PECS) with children with autism: Assessment of PECS acquisition, speech, social-communicative behavior, and problem behavior. *Journal of Applied Behavior Analysis, 35,* 213–231.

Coe, D., Matson, J., Fee, V., Manikam, R., & Linarello, C. (1990). Training nonverbal and verbal play skills to mentally retarded and autistic children. *Journal of Autism and Developmental Disorders, 20,* 177–187.

Davies, M., Howlin, P., Bernal, J., & Warren, S. (1998). Treating severe self-injury in a community setting: Constraints on assessment and intervention. *Child Psychology and Psychiatry Review, 3,* 26–32.

Delprato, D. J. (2001). Comparisons of discrete-trial and normalized behavioral intervention for young children with autism. *Journal of Autism and Developmental Disorders, 31,* 315–325.

Derby, K., Wacker, D., Sasso, G., Steege, M., Northup, J., Cigrand, K., et al. (1992). Brief functional assessment techniques to evaluate aberrant behavior in an outpatient setting: A summary of 79 cases. *Journal of Applied Behavior Analysis, 25,* 713–721.

Ducharme, J., & Van Houten, R. (1994). Operant extinction in the treatment of severe maladaptive behavior. *Behavior Modification, 18,* 139–170.

Duker, P., Dortmans, A., & Lodder, E. (1993). Establishing the manding function of communicative gestures with individuals with severe/profound mental retardation. *Research in Developmental Disabilities, 14,* 39–49.

Durand, M., & Carr, E. (1987). Social influences on 'self-stimulatory' behavior: Analysis and treatment application. *Journal of Applied Behavior Analysis, 20,* 119–132.

Dyches, T., Wilder, L., Sudweeks, R., Obiakor, F., & Algozzine, B. (2004). Multicultural issues in autism. *Journal of Autism and Developmental Disorders, 34,* 211–222.

Farmer-Dougan, V. (1994). Increasing requests by adults with developmental disabilities using incidental teaching by peers. *Journal of Applied Behavior Analysis, 27*, 553–544.

Fenske, E., Zalenski, S., Krantz, P., & McClannahan, L. (1985). Age at intervention and treatment outcome for autistic children in a comprehensive intervention program. *Analysis and Intervention in Developmental Disabilities, 5*, 49–58.

Fisher, W., Piazza, C., Cataldo, M., Harell, R., Jefferson, G., & Corner, R. (1993). Functional communication training with and without extinctions and punishment. *Journal of Applied Behavior Analysis, 26*, 23–26.

Frost, L., & Bondy, A. (1994). *The picture exchange communication system training manual.* Cherry Hill, NJ: Pyramid Educational Consultants.

Fung, F., & Roseberry-McKibbin, C. (1999). Service delivery in working with clients from Cantonese-speaking backgrounds. *American Journal of Speech-Language Pathology, 8*, 309–318.

Ganz, J., & Simpson, R. (2004). Effects on communicative requesting and speech development of the picture exchange communication system in children with characteristics of autism. *Journal of Autism and Developmental Disorders, 34*, 395–409.

Greer, R., Yuan, L., & Gautreaux, G. (2005). Novel dictation and intraverbal responses as a function of a multiple exemplar history. *The Analysis of Verbal Behavior, 21*, 99–116.

Hagopian, L., Fisher, W., Sullivan, M., Acquisto, J., & LeBlanc, L. (1998). Effectiveness of functional communication training with and without extinction and punishment: A summary of 21 inpatient cases. *Journal of Applied Behavior Analysis, 2*, 211–235.

Hanley, G., Iwata, B., & McCord, B. (2003). Functional analysis of problem behavior: A review. *Journal of Applied Behavior Analysis, 36*, 147–185.

Hanley, G., Piazza, C., & Fisher, W. (1997). Noncontingent presentation of attention and alternative stimuli in the treatment of attention-maintained destructive behavior. *Journal of Applied Behavior Analysis, 30*, 229–237.

Harris, S. L., Handleman, J. S., Gordon, R., Kristoff, B., & Fuentes, F. (1991). Changes in cognitive and language functioning of preschool children with autism. *Journal of Autism and Developmental Disorders, 21*, 281–290.

Harris, S. L., Handleman, J. S., Kristoff, B., Bass, L., & Gordon, R. (1990). Changes in language development among autistic and peer children in segregated and integrated preschool settings. *Journal of Autism and Developmental Disabilities, 20*, 23–32.

Harris, S. L., Wolchik, S., & Weitz, S. (1981). The acquisition of language skills by autistic children: Can parents do the job? *Journal of Autism and Developmental Disorders, 11*, 373–384.

Hart, B., & Risley, T. (1968). Establishing use of descriptive adjectives in the spontaneous speech of disadvantaged preschool children. *Journal of Applied Behavior Analysis, 1*, 109–120.

Hart, B., & Risley, T. (1975). Incidental teaching of language in the preschool. *Journal of Applied Behavior Analysis, 8*, 411–420.

Hartman, E., & Klatt, K. (2005). The effects of deprivation, presession exposure, and preferences on teaching manding to children with autism. *Analysis of Verbal Behavior, 21*, 135–144.

Horner, R. (2000). Positive behavior supports. *Focus on Autism and Other Developmental Disabilities, 15*, 97–105.

Horner, R., Dunlap, G., Koegel, R., Carr, E., Sailor, W., Anderson, J., et al. (1990). Toward a technology of "nonaversive" behavior support. *Journal of the Association for Persons with Severe Handicaps, 15*, 125–132.

Howlin, P. (1981). The effectiveness of operant language training with autistic children. *Journal of Autism and Developmental Disorders, 11*, 89–105.

Howlin, P., Gordon, R., Pasco, G., Wade, G., & Charman, T. (2007). The effectiveness of picture exchange communication system (PECS) training for teachers of children with autism: A pragmatic, group randomised controlled trial. *Journal of Child Psychology and Psychiatry and Allied Disciplines, 48*, 473–481.

Hume, K., & Odom, S. (2007). Effects of an individual work system on the independent functioning of students with autism. *Journal of Autism and Developmental Disorders, 37*, 1166–1180.

Hung, D. (1977). Generalization of 'curiosity' questioning behavior in autistic children. *Journal of Behavior Therapy and Experimental Psychiatry, 8*, 237–245.

Hung, D. (1980). Training and generalization of yes and no as mands in two autistic children. *Journal of Autism and Developmental Disorders, 10*, 139–152.

Hwa-Froelich, D., & Vigil, D. (2004). Three aspects of cultural influence on communication: A literature review. *Communication Disorders Quarterly, 25*, 107–118.

Ingersoll, B., & Gergans, S. (2007). The effect of a parent-implemented imitation intervention on spontaneous imitation skills in young children with autism. *Research in Developmental Disabilities, 28*, 163–175.

Ingersoll, B., Lewis, E., & Kroman, E. (2007). Teaching the imitation and spontaneous use of descriptive gestures in young children with autism using a naturalistic behavioral intervention. *Journal of Autism and Developmental Disorders, 37*, 1446–1456.

Ingersoll, B., & Schreibman, L. (2006). Teaching reciprocal imitation skills to young children with autism using a naturalistic behavioral approach: Effects on language, pretend play, and joint attention. *Journal of Autism and Developmental Disorders, 36*, 487–505.

Iwata, B., Dorsey, M., Slifer, K., Bauman, K., & Richman, G. (1994). Toward a functional analysis of self-injury. *Journal of Applied Behavior Analysis, 27*, 197–209.

Kaiser, A., Ostrosky, M., & Alpert, C. (1993). Training teachers to use environmental arrangement and milieu teaching with nonvocal preschool children. *Journal of the Association for Persons with Severe Handicaps, 18*, 188–199.

Kennedy, C., Meyer, K., Knowles, T., & Shukla, S. (2000). Analyzing the multiple functions of stereotypical behavior for students with autism: Implications for assessment and treatment. *Journal of Applied Behavior Analysis, 33*, 559–571.

Koegel, R., Bimbela, A., & Schreibman, L. (1996). Collateral effects of parent training on family interactions. *Journal of Autism and Developmental Disorders, 26*, 347–359.

Koegel, R., Camarata, S., Koegel, L., Ben-Tall, A., & Smith, A. (1998). Increasing speech intelligibility in children with autism. *Journal of Autism and Developmental Disorders, 28*, 241–251.

Koegel, R., & Koegel, L. (eds). (1995). *Teaching children with autism: Strategies for initiating positive interactions and improving learning opportunities.* Baltimore, MD: Paul H. Brookes.

Koegel, L., Koegel, R., & Dunlap, G. (eds). (1996). *Positive behavioral support: Including people with difficult behavior in the community*. Baltimore, MD: Paul H. Brookes.

Koegel, L., Koegel, R., Harrower, J., & Carter, C. (1999). Pivotal response intervention I: Overview of approach. *Journal of the Association for Persons with Severe Handicaps, 24*, 174–185.

Koegel, L., Koegel, R., Shoshan, Y., & McNerney, E. (1999). Pivotal response intervention II: Preliminary long-term outcomes data. *Journal of the Association for Persons with Severe Handicaps, 24*, 186–198.

Koegel, R., Koegel, L., & Surratt, A. (1992). Language intervention and disruptive behavior in preschool children with autism. *Journal of Autism and Developmental Disorders, 22*, 141–153.

Koegel, R., O'Dell, M., & Koegel, L. (1987). A natural language teaching paradigm for nonverbal autistic children. *Journal of Autism and Developmental Disorders, 17*, 187–200.

Koegel, R., O'Dell, M., & Dunlap, G. (1988). Producing speech use in nonverbal autistic children by reinforcing attempts. *Journal of Autism and Developmental Disorders, 18*, 525–538.

Koegel, R., & Williams, J. (1980). Direct versus indirect response-reinforcer relationships in teaching autistic children. *Journal of Abnormal Child Psychology, 8*, 537–547.

Koita, H., & Sonoyama, S. (2004). Communication training using the picture exchange communication system (PECS): Case study of a child with autistic disorder. *Japanese Journal of Behavior Analysis, 19*, 161–174.

Koita, H., Sonoyama, S., & Takeuchi, K. (2003). Communication training with the picture exchange communication system (PECS) for children with autistic disorder: The training program and current and future research. *Japanese Journal of Behavior Analysis, 18*, 120–130.

Krantz, P., & McClannahan, L. (1993). Teaching children with autism to initiate to peers: Effects of a script-fading procedure. *Journal of Applied Behavior Analysis, 26*, 121–132.

Lamarre, J., & Holland, J. (1985). The functional independence of mands and tacts. *Journal of the Experimental Analysis of Behavior, 43*, 5–19.

Laraway, S., Snycerski, S., Michael, J., & Poling, A. (2003). Motivating operations and terms to describe them: Some further refinements. *Journal of Applied Behavior Analysis, 36*, 407–414.

Laski, K., Charlop, M., & Schreibman, L. (1988). Training parents to use the natural language paradigm to increase their autistic children's speech. *Journal of Applied Behavior Analysis, 21*, 391–400.

Lian, M. (1996). Teaching Asian American children. In E. Durán (Ed.), *Teaching students with moderate/severe disabilities, including autism: Strategies for second language learners in inclusive settings* (2nd ed., pp. 239–253). Springfield, IL, England: Charles C. Thomas.

Lord, C., & Schopler, E. (1989). The role of age at assessment, developmental level, and test in the stability of intelligence scores in young autistic children. *Journal of Autism and Developmental Disorders, 19*, 483–499.

Lord, C., & Schopler, E. (1994). TEACCH services for preschool children. In S. L. Harris & J. S. Handleman (Eds.), *Preschool education programs for children with autism* (pp. 87–106). Austin, TX: Pro-Ed.

Lovaas, O. (1987). Behavioral treatment and normal educational and intellectual functioning in young autistic children. *Journal of Consulting and Clinical Psychology, 55*, 3–9.

Lovaas, O., Berberich, J., Perloff, B., & Schaeffer, B. (1966). Acquisition of imitative speech in schizophrenic children. *Science, 151*, 705–707.

Lovaas, O., Koegel, R., Simmons, J., & Long, J. (1973). Some generalization and follow up measures on autistic children in behavior therapy. *Journal of Applied Behavior Analysis, 6*, 131–165.

Mace, F., & Belfiore, P. (1990). Behavioral momentum in the treatment of escape-motivated stereotypy. *Journal of Applied Behavior Analysis, 23*, 507–514.

Matson, J., & LoVullo, S. (2008). A review of behavioral treatments for self-injurious behaviors of persons with autism spectrum disorders. *Behavior Modification, 32*, 61–76.

Matson, J., & Nebel-Schwalm, M. (2007). Comorbid psychopathology with autism spectrum disorder in children: An overview. *Research in Developmental Disabilities, 28*, 341–352.

Matson, J., & Taras, M. (1989). A 20 year review of punishment and alternative methods to treat problem behaviors in developmentally delayed persons. *Research in Developmental Disabilities, 10*, 85–104.

McEachin, J., Smith, T., & Lovaas, O. (1993). Long-term outcome for children with autism who received early intensive behavioral treatment. *American Journal on Mental Retardation, 97*, 359–372.

McGee, G., Almeida, M., Sulzer-Azaroff, B., & Feldman, R. (1992). Promoting reciprocal interactions via peer incidental teaching. *Journal of Applied Behavior Analysis, 25*, 117–126.

McGee, G., Krantz, P., Mason, D., & McClannahan, L. (1983). A modified incidental-teaching procedure for autistic youth: Acquisition and generalization of receptive object labels. *Journal of Applied Behavior Analysis, 16*, 329–338.

McGee, G., Krantz, P., & McClannahan, L. (1985). The facilitative effects of incidental teaching on preposition use by autistic children. *Journal of Applied Behavior Analysis, 18*, 17–32.

Mesibov, G. (1994). A comprehensive program for serving people with autism and their families: The TEACCH model. In J. L. Matson (Ed.), *Autism in children and adults: Etiology, assessment, and intervention* (pp. 85–97). Pacific Grove, CA: Brooks/Cole.

Mesibov, G. (1996). Division TEACCH: A program model for working with autistic people and their families. In M. C. Roberts (Ed.), *Model practices in service delivery in child and family mental health*. Hillsdale, NJ: Erlbaum.

Mesibov, G., Schopler, E., & Hearsey, K. (1994). Structured teaching. In E. Schopler & G. B. Mesibov (Eds.), *Behavioral issues in autism* (pp. 195–207). New York: Plenum Press.

Metz, J. (1965). Conditioning generalized imitation in autistic children. *Journal of Experimental Child Psychology, 4*, 389–399.

Michael, J. (1982). Distinguishing between discriminative and motivational functions of stimuli. *Journal of the Experimental Analysis of Behavior, 37*, 149–155.

Michael, J. (1993). Establishing operations. *Behavior Analyst, 16*, 191–206.

Michael, J. (2000). Implications and refinements of the establishing operation concept. *Journal of Applied Behavior Analysis, 33*, 401–410.

Miranda-Linne, F., & Melin, L. (1992). Acquisition, generalization, and spontaneous use of color adjectives: A comparison of incidental teaching and traditional discrete-trial procedures for children with autism. *Research in Developmental Disabilities, 13*, 191–210.

Naoi, N., Yokoyama, K., & Yamamoto, J. (2007). Intervention for tact as reporting in children with autism. *Research in Autism Spectrum Disorders, 1,* 174–184.

Neef, N., Walters, J., & Egel, A. (1984). Establishing generative yes/no responses in developmentally disabled children. *Journal of Applied Behavior Analysis, 17,* 453–460.

Nuzzolo-Gomez, R., & Greer, R. (2004). Emergence of untaught mands and tacts of novel adjective-object pairs as a function of instructional history. *The Analysis of Verbal Behavior, 20,* 63–76.

Ozonoff, S., & Cathcart, K. (1998). Effectiveness of a home program intervention for young children with autism. *Journal of Autism and Developmental Disorders, 28,* 25–32.

Panerai, S., Ferrante, L., & Zingale, M. (2002). Benefits of the TEACCH programme as compared with a non-specific approach. *Journal of Intellectual Disability Research, 46,* 318–327.

Partington, J., & Sundberg, M. (1998). *The assessment of basic language and learning skills (the ABLLS).* Pleasant Hill, CA: Behavior Analysts, Inc.

Partington, J. W., Sundberg, M. L., Newhouse, L., & Spengler, S. M. (1994). Overcoming an autistic child's failure to acquire a tact repertoire. *Journal of Applied Behavior Analysis, 27,* 733–734.

Peppé, S., McCann, J., Gibbon, F., O'Hare, A., & Rutherford, M. (2007). Receptive and expressive prosodic ability in children with high-functioning autism. *Journal of Speech, Language, and Hearing Research, 50,* 1015–1028.

Peterson, S., Bondy, A., Vincent, Y., & Finnegan, C. (1995). Effects of altering communicative input for students with autism and no speech: Two case studies. *Augmentative and Alternative Communication, 11,* 93–100.

Piazza, C., Moes, D., & Fisher, W. (1996). Differential reinforcement of alternative behavior and demand fading in the treating fading in the treatment of escape-maintained destructive behavior. *Journal of Applied Behavior Analysis, 29,* 569–572.

Pierce, K., & Schreibman, L. (1995). Increasing complex social behaviors in children with autism: Effects of peer-implemented pivotal response training. *Journal of Applied Behavior Analysis, 28,* 285–295.

Potoczak, K., Carr, J., & Michael, J. (2007). The effects of consequence manipulation during functional analysis of problem behavior maintained by negative reinforcement. *Journal of Applied Behavior Analysis, 40,* 719–724.

Prizant, B., & Rubin, E. (1999). Contemporary issues in interventions for autism spectrum disorders: A commentary. *The Journal of the Association for Persons with Severe Handicaps, 24,* 199–208.

Pruchno, R., Patrick, J., & Burant, C. (1997). African American and White mothers of adults with chronic disabilities: Caregiving burden and satisfaction. *Family Relations, 46,* 335–346.

Rodriguez, B., & Olswang, L. (2003). Mexican-American and Anglo-American mothers' beliefs and values about child rearing, education, and language impairment. *American Journal of Speech-Language Pathology, 12,* 452–462.

Rogers-Dulan, J., & Blancher, J. (1995). African American families, religion, and disability: A conceptual framework. *Mental Retardation, 33,* 226–238.

Rogers-Warren, A., & Warren, S. (1980). Mands for verbalization: Facilitating the display of newly trained language in children. *Behavior Modification, 4,* 361–382.

Rosales-Ruiz, J., & Baer, D. (1997). Behavioral cusps: A developmental and pragmatic concept for behavior analysis. *Journal of Applied Behavior Analysis, 30,* 533–544.

Ross, D., & Greer, R. (2003). Generalized imitation and the mand: Inducing first instances of speech in young children with autism. *Research in Developmental Disabilities, 24,* 58–74.

Rossi, C., & Balandin, S. (2005). Bilingualism, culture, and AAC. *Acquiring Knowledge in Speech, Language and Hearing, 7,* 27–29.

Schopler, E. (1989). Principles for directing both educational treatment and research. In C. Gillberg (Ed.), *Diagnosis and treatment of autism* (pp. 167–183). New York: Plenum Press.

Schopler, E. (1997). Implementation of TEACCH philosophy. In D. J. Cohen & F. R. Volkmar (Eds.), *Handbook of autism and pervasive developmental disorders* (pp. 767–795). New York: Wiley.

Schopler, E., Brehm, S., Kinsbourne, M., & Reichler, R. (1971). Effect of treatment structure on development in autistic children. *Archives of General Psychiatry, 24,* 415–421.

Schopler, E., Mesibov, G., & Hearsey, K. (1995). Structured teaching in the TEACCH system. In E. Schopler & G. B. Mesibov (Eds.), *Learning and cognition in autism* (pp. 243–268). New York: Plenum Press.

Schopler, E., Reichler, R., Bashford, A., Lansing, M., & Marcus, L. (1990). *Individualized assessment and treatment for autistic and developmentally disabled children: 1. Psychoeducational profile (PEP-R).* Austin, TX: Pro-Ed.

Schreibman, L., Kaneko, W., & Koegel, R. (1991). Positive affect of parents of autistic children: A comparison across two teaching techniques. *Behavior Therapy, 22,* 479–490.

Schroeder, G., & Baer, D. (1972). Effects of concurrent and serial training on generalized vocal imitation in retarded children. *Developmental Psychology, 6,* 293–301.

Schwartz, I., Garfinkle, A., & Bauer, J. (1998). The picture exchange communication system: Communicative outcomes for young children with disabilities. *Topics in Early Childhood Special Education, 18,* 144–159.

Shafer, E. (1994). A review of interventions to teach a mand repertoire. *Analysis of Verbal Behavior, 12,* 53–66.

Sheinkopf, S., & Siegel, B. (1998). Home based behavioral treatment of young children with autism. *Journal of Autism and Developmental Disorders, 28,* 15–23.

Sigafoos, J., & Saggers, E. (1995). A discrete-trial approach to the functional analysis of aggressive behaviour in two boys with autism. *Australia and New Zealand Journal of Developmental Disabilities, 20,* 287–297.

Simmons, N., & Johnston, J. (2007). Cross-cultural differences in beliefs and practices that affect the language spoken to children: Mothers with Indian and Western heritage. *International Journal of Language and Communication Disorders, 42,* 445–465.

Skinner, B. F. (1938). *The behavior of organisms: An experimental analysis.* New York: Appleton-Century-Crofts.

Skinner, B. F. (1953). *Science and human behavior.* New York: Macmillan.

Skinner, B. F. (1957). *Verbal behavior.* New York: Appleton-Century-Crofts.

Smith, T. (2001). Discrete trial training in the treatment of autism. *Focus on Autism and Other Developmental Disabilities, 16,* 86–92.

Smith, T., Buch, G., & Gamby, T. (2000). Parent-directed, intensive early intervention for children with pervasive developmental disorder. *Research in Developmental Disabilities, 21,* 297–309.

Sparrow, S., Balla, D., & Cicchetti, D. (1984). *Vineland adaptive behavior scales.* Circle Pines, MN: American Guidance Service.

Spradlin, J. E. (1963). Assessment of speech and language of retarded children: The parsons language sample. *Journal of Speech and Hearing Disorders. Monograph Supplement, 10,* 8–31.

Spradlin, J. E., & Siegel, G. (1982). Language training in natural and clinical environments. *Journal of Speech and Hearing Disorders, 47,* 2–6.

Stahmer, A. (1995). Teaching symbolic play skills to children with autism using pivotal response training. *Journal of Autism and Developmental Disorders, 25,* 123–141.

Stahmer, A. (1999). Using pivotal response training to facilitate appropriate play in children with autistic spectrum disorders. *Child Language Teaching and Therapy, 15,* 29–40.

Sundberg, M. (1983). Language. In J. L. Matson & S. E. Breuning (Eds.), *Assessing the mentally retarded* (pp. 285–310). New York: Grune & Stratton.

Sundberg, M. (1993). The application of establishing operations. *Behavior Analyst, 16,* 211–214.

Sundberg, M., Endicott, K., & Eigenheer, P. (2000). Using intraverbal prompts to establish tacts for children with autism. *Analysis of Verbal Behavior, 17,* 89–104.

Sundberg, M., & Michael, J. (2001). The benefits of Skinner's analysis of verbal behavior for children with autism. *Behavior Modification, 25,* 698–724.

Sundberg, M., & Partington, J. (1998). *Teaching language to children with autism or other developmental disabilities.* Danville, CA: Behavior Analysts, Inc.

Thorp, D., Stahmer, A., & Schreibman, L. (1995). Effects of sociodramatic play training on children with autism. *Journal of Autism and Developmental Disorders, 25,* 265–282.

Trembath, D., Balandin, S., & Rossi, C. (2005). Cross-cultural practice and autism. *Journal of Intellectual and Developmental Disability, 30,* 240–242.

Tsang, S., Shek, D., Lam, L., Tang, F., & Cheung, P. (2007). Brief report: Application of the TEACCH program on Chinese pre-school children with autism – Does culture make a difference? *Journal of Autism and Developmental Disorders, 37,* 390–396.

Tsiouri, I., & Greer, R. (2003). Inducing vocal verbal behavior in children with severe language delays through rapid motor imitation responding. *Journal of Behavioral Education, 12,* 185–206.

Twyman, J. (1995). The functional independence of impure mands and tacts of abstract stimulus properties. *Analysis of Verbal Behavior, 13,* 1–19.

Vigil, D., & Hwa-Froelich, D. (2004). Interaction styles in minority caregivers: Implications for intervention. *Communication Disorders Quarterly, 25,* 119–126.

Wacker, D., Steege, J., Sasso, G., Berg, W., Reimers, T., Cooper, L., et al. (1990). A component analysis of functional communication training across three topographies of severe behavior problems. *Journal of Applied Behavior Analysis, 23,* 417–429.

Warren, S., McQuarter, R., & Rogers-Warren, A. (1984). The effects of mands and models on the speech of unresponsive language-delayed preschool children. *Journal of Speech and Hearing Disorders, 49,* 43–52.

Whalen, C., & Schreibman, L. (2003). Joint attention training for children with autism using behavior modification procedures. *Journal of Child Psychology and Psychiatry and Allied Disciplines, 44,* 456–468.

Wilder, L., Dyches, T., Obiakor, F., & Algozzine, B. (2004). Multicultural perspectives on teaching students with autism. *Focus on Autism and Other Developmental Disabilities, 19,* 105–113.

Williams, G., & Greer, R. (1993). A comparison of verbal-behavior and linguistic-communication curricula for training developmentally delayed adolescents to acquire and maintain vocal speech. *Behaviorology, 1,* 31–46.

Yamamoto, J., & Mochizuki, A. (1988). Acquisition and functional analysis of manding with autistic students. *Journal of Applied Behavior Analysis, 21,* 57–64.

Yoder, P., & Layton, T. (1988). Speech following sign language training in autistic children with minimal verbal language. *Journal of Autism and Developmental Disorders, 18,* 217–229.

Yokoyama, K., Naoi, N., & Yamamoto, J. (2006). Teaching verbal behavior using the picture exchange communication system (PECS) with children with autistic spectrum disorders. *Japanese Journal of Special Education, 43,* 485–503.

Young, J., Krantz, P., McClannahan, L., & Poulson, C. (1994). Generalized imitation and response-class formation in children with autism. *Journal of Applied Behavior Analysis, 27,* 685–697.

Chapter 5
Differential Diagnosis in Autism Spectrum Disorders

Dennis R. Dixon, Mark J Garcia, Doreen Granpeesheh, and Jonathan Tarbox

While differential diagnosis is typically not one of the primary areas of discussions in ABA, we believe it has particular importance for ASD. The idiosyncratic nature of the disorder and how they affect the nature and type of ABA assessment and treatment cannot be overstated. This chapter will review basic diagnostic methods and their relevance to ABA.

Differential Diagnosis and Autism

Autism spectrum disorders (ASD) are a heterogeneous group of disorders that share common core symptoms. Differentiating among the various ASDs is an important task within research studies as well as clinical practice. The purpose of this chapter is to provide the practitioner of applied behavior analysis with practical information regarding other diagnostic considerations when providing services to children with an ASD. Central to this task is a discussion of assessment methods. Furniss (this volume) discusses assessment methods that are more common to behavior analysis. Our focus will instead be upon assessments as they serve the overall process of making diagnostic decisions.

When beginning a discussion on differential diagnosis in ASD, it is important to be aware of the philosophical perspective from which the diagnosis is made. The two major nosologies (DSM & ICD) are ultimately derived from a Kraeplinian perspective.

This diagnostic system is comprised of a checklist approach to diagnosis such that the clinician determines the underlying cause of symptoms by how they cluster together. Thus diagnoses are made based upon the presence or absence of specific symptoms. As such, diagnoses are considered dichotomously present or absent. There are significant limitations to this approach in regard to psychiatric disorders. Further, these limitations become more pronounced when applied to autism spectrum disorders. An unfortunate consequence of Kraeplinian model is that practitioners frequently begin to discuss these "disorders" as if they were discrete entities and use these terms as explanations of causality. This convention may be appropriate when discussing disorders such as Simple Phobias; yet, we see an attempt at addressing the true dimensional nature of these disorders in the different diagnoses for varying levels of severity such as specifying Mild, Moderate, Severe, or Profound for an intellectual disability (ID). Likewise using Major Depressive Disorder rather than Dysthymic Disorder is an attempt to address the true dimensional nature of depression. While these attempts help to capture some of the dimensionality of the disorder, this practice breaks down when addressing disorders that are widely spread-out along multiple dimensions.

Alternatives to the categorical approach to diagnosis have been proposed, such as a dimensional approach to diagnosis. However, the DSM-IV TR committee concluded that the benefits and limitations to the dimensional approach were equivocal to the categorical approach to diagnosis (American Psychiatric Association, 2000). While we agree with the committee's judgment as it relates to the disorders covered in the DSM as a whole, this is clearly not the case when discussing ASDs.

D.R. Dixon (✉)
Research and Development, Center for Autism and Related Disorders, Inc., 19019 Ventura Blvd. #300, Tarzana, CA, 91356, USA
e-mail: D.Dixon@centerforautism.com

J.L. Matson (ed.), *Applied Behavior Analysis for Children with Autism Spectrum Disorders*, DOI 10.1007/978-1-4419-0088-3_5, © Springer Science+Business Media, LLC 2009

A Spectrum of Symptoms

Much debate has been made concerning the discrete or continuous nature of autism and it is generally agreed that these disorders are more adequately described as falling along a spectrum of symptoms rather than disorders with discrete boundaries (Barrett, Prior, & Manjviona, 2004; Buitelaar, Van der Gaag, Klin, & Volkmar, 1999; Prior et al., 1998; Tryon, Mayes, Rhodes, & Waldo, 2006; Verté, Geurts, Roeyers, Oosterlaan, & Sergeant, 2006; Volkmar, Lord, Bailey, Schultz, & Klin, 2004). Both the DSM-IV and ICD-10 systems provide criteria upon which the Pervasive Developmental Disorders may be differentiated. However, many have questioned the utility of these diagnostic systems in regard to adequate differential diagnosis (Matson & Boisjoli, 2007; Prior et al., 1998; Tryon et al., 2006).

Researchers using cluster analysis have done much to illuminate the multidimensional and continuous nature of ASD. In studying a group of 135 children with some form of an ASD, Prior et al. (1998) conducted a cluster analysis and observed that three groups emerged: an autistic-like cluster, an Asperger's-like cluster, and a mild PDD cluster. The autistic-like cluster showed in general lower levels of functioning than the Asperger's cluster and had a tendency to self-isolate. In contrast, the Asperger's cluster had higher levels of social and communication development, showing efforts to engage others socially. The mild PDD group showed fewer problems across all domains. While Prior et al. (1998) used diagnostic titles for their clusters, they noted the lack of correspondence between clinical diagnosis and cluster membership. In other words, a child's clinical diagnosis based upon DSM criteria was not predictive of which cluster they were in. Overall, the data presented by Prior et al. (1998) support the concept of an autism spectrum rather than discrete but similar disorders. As such, the form and severity of a symptom matters much more than simply the presence or absence of the symptom.

More recently, Verté, Geurts, Roeyers, Rosseel, et al. (2006) also provided evidence that suggests placing an emphasis on the severity of symptom impairment rather than a clear categorical approach. Results of their cluster analysis indicated that their data were best described by three clusters. The authors named three clusters: High Functioning Autism (HFA), Pervasive Developmental Disorder – Not Otherwise Specified (PDD-NOS), and a combined HFA/PDD-NOS cluster.

As was reported by Prior et al. (1998), there was very little correspondence between the clusters and the participants' diagnostic category.

These studies help illustrate that the nature of autism is that of a spectrum. As such, many researchers have begun to design their diagnostic instruments to differentiate among the ASDs based upon the severity of symptoms (e.g., Lord, Rutter, & Couteur, 1994; Matson, Boisjoli, Gonzalez, Smith, & Wilkins, 2007) rather than simply the presence or absence of symptoms as described by the DSM-IV. These studies have laid a foundation on which a richer understanding of ASD can now be developed.

Definition and Diagnostic Criteria

PDD-NOS, Autism, and Asperger's disorder are the most commonly studied groups; however, this may reflect the lower incidence rate of Childhood Disintegrative Disorder (CDD) and Rett's Disorder. While epidemiological studies have found the occurrence of these disorders to be much lower than other ASDs, this may be due to other factors than diagnostic criteria. Among these other factors are practitioner knowledge of differential diagnosis and discrepant levels of services provided for the various ASDs. Discrepant funding for autism may lead some practitioners to error on the side of underdiagnosis of CDD in favor of autism so that the examinee may receive public services. Likewise, parents and caregivers may simply doctor-shop until their child receives a diagnosis of autism. It is these human factors of real-life outcomes that reveal the greatest breakdown of the categorical checklist approach to diagnosis. As long as the diagnosis remains simply a dichotomous "yes or no" then reimbursement for treatment services will also remain a dichotomous "funded or not funded."

Autism

The most recent estimates of autism prevalence place it at 0.67% or 1 in 150 children (Center for Disease Control and Prevention, 2007). The core symptoms of Autistic Disorder are communication impairments, social skills deficits, and the presence of repetitive or overly restricted behaviors. Persons diagnosed with autism show significant heterogeneity in the degree to which these (and other) symptoms are present.

Asperger's Disorder

By far, the greatest amount of attention on differential diagnosis in autism has been given to differentiating Asperger's Disorder. This topic has caused much debate, with opponents contending that Asperger's Disorder is simply an extension of high functioning autism. However, a result of this debate has been the recognition that autism is not a categorical diagnosis but rather a cluster of symptoms falling along a spectrum. While the debate still continues, the majority of researchers consider Asperger's disorder as distinct from high functioning autism (Matson & Boisjoli, 2008; Matson & Wilkins, 2008).

Numerous definitions for Asperger's disorder exist and as noted by Volkmar et al. (2004), the only clear agreement is that the DSM-IV and ICD systems are not adequate and treat Asperger's disorder as only an afterthought to the diagnosis of autism. While disorders such as Asperger's may sometimes be conceptualized as distinct from autism, there is evidence to suggest this distinction may not be accurate (Wing, 1998) and that the DSM-IV differentiation is not useful (Tryon et al., 2006). In an excellent discussion of the topic, Howlin (2003) noted that there is little evidence to suggest that autism and Asperger's are discrete disorders. Her data instead suggest that what matters is the level of language deficits and the subsequent development of the child, with differences diminishing as the child moves into adulthood. Sciutto and Cantwell (2005) noted similar findings, wherein the presence of language delays, IQ scores, and desire for social interaction were all useful for differentiating Asperger's from autism but were not sufficient by themselves. Instead, Sciutto and Cantwell suggest that clinicians add other sources of information outside of the DSM-IV's criteria when making a diagnosis of Asperger's Disorder.

PDD-NOS

Arriving at a definition for "Autistic Disorder" is much easier than for the other ASDs such as PDD-NOS wherein the disorder is primarily defined as *not* being

autism (Matson & Boisjoli, 2007; Tidmarsh & Volkmar, 2003). This diagnostic uncertainty is likely a byproduct of attempting to apply discrete boundaries to symptoms that lie along a continuum. A consequence of this is that efforts to develop more stringent diagnostic criteria have languished (Matson & Boisjoli, 2007). Overall, those who have explored this topic have primarily concluded that PDD-NOS may be defined as a more mild form of autism (Heflin & Alaimo, 2006; Buitelaar & Van der Gaag, 1998; Buitelaar et al., 1999). However, Matson and Boisjoli (2007) point out that most of these efforts lack specific details as to where along the continuum of symptoms does a person move from a diagnosis of autism to PDD-NOS. Much more empirical evidence is needed to make this distinction. Further, one must wonder if the absence of empirical evidence suggests that these disorders, particularly those that lie along the boundaries, are useful distinctions to begin with. A more useful distinction may be to simply describe autism severity or other modifiers that communicate a particular profile of ASD symptoms.

Core Symptoms

Since Kanner's (1943) initial description of autism there have been many efforts to describe the characteristics of disorder, all of which ultimately come back to the core symptoms of impaired communication, impaired social skills, and stereotypical behaviors. Each of these domains will be discussed further.

Communication Skills

The communication skills in children with an autism spectrum disorder may vary widely. For those diagnosed with autistic disorder, the impairment in communication affects both verbal and nonverbal skills. Often the child will present without any verbal communication skills. Children categorized as "high functioning" autism typically will not show as marked deficits in language skills but will still have the tendency to use language in a stereotypical or pedantic fashion. These communication deficits are even more subtle in regard to Asperger's disorder in that the reciprocal nature of conversation is what is primarily impaired.

Social Skills

As with communication skills, impairments in social skills vary widely among children with ASD and are best described as falling along a continuum (Constantino et al., 2003). While social skills have received much attention in the literature, Matson and Wilkins (2007) note that the definitions of socials skills vary widely among studies. The lack of a coherent definition of social skills within research studies has limited the generalizability of findings. Further, many disorders outside of the ASDs include impaired social interactions as a component. Thus, there is a need to further explore particular social deficits within ASD.

Recently Bishop, Gahagan, and Lord (2007) examined the nature of social deficits between a group of children with an ASD and those with Fetal Alcohol Spectrum Disorder (FASD). They found clear differences among these two groups, with ASD group showing specific deficits in eye contact, directed facial expressions, gestures, the amount of reciprocal social communication, and unusual sensory interests. They also note that social impairments such as inappropriate behaviors and difficulty with peers were ineffective to differentiate the two groups. Bishop et al. (2007) further comment:

> … what appears to be particularly unique to children with ASD, and therefore potentially most useful in differentiating children with ASD from other populations, is the reduced frequency with which they initiate common types of social interaction or respond to others' attempts to engage with them (p. 1119)

Thus, social impairments seem to be much more nuanced than simply determining if these interactions are impaired or not. Rather, what appears to be useful is noting the degree to which social interactions are impaired, the particular form of the impairment, and regardless of if the social interactions are impaired or not, the overall frequency of the child's social attempts.

Stereotypy

In a series of publications, Rapp and Vollmer (2005a, 2005b) provide an excellent discussion of stereotypy as it relates to behavioral assessment and neurobiological interpretations. Rapp and Vollmer (2005a) note the difficulty in defining stereotypies and argue for a functional approach to stereotypies. There is still controversy related to defining this class of behaviors. Rapp and Vollmer review the work by Berkson (1967) who argues for two categories of stereotypies: repetitive and nonrepetitive. Berkson has further elaborated on the characteristics of stereotypies (1983). Rapp and Vollmer add to the discussion the concept of periodicity and rhythmicity (Lewis & Baumeister, 1982; Ross, Yu, & Kroprola, 1998). In spite of these efforts, a definition of stereotypy has yet to be fully accepted and applied consistently across the literature.

Cunningham and Schreibman (2008) note the diagnostic importance of determining the function of stereotypy. The form of stereotypies may be quite varied; however, the function of stereotypy is often assumed to be automatically maintained, that is, many forms of behavior with one common function. Cunningham and Schreibman (2008) argue that this assumption may be premature and reviewed evidence supporting socially operant stereotypies. Rapp and Vollmer (2005a, 2005b) also discuss many other functions for stereotypies. Most notably though in relation to differential diagnosis, is that the function of the stereotypy is not considered when making the diagnosis of autism. The DSM-IV simply requires that stereotypies or repetitive behaviors be present. The simple present/absent dichotomy used by the DSM-IV may be problematic as it may lead to errors in diagnosis among similar diagnostic categories. For example, many individuals with intellectual disabilities engage in stereotypies. In these situations, the form, intensity, and frequency of stereotypic behavior may be useful distinctions among diagnostic groups (Bodfish, Symons, Parker, & Lewis, 2000), wherein children with autism exhibit more bizarre and socially inappropriate stereotypies than typically developing children or children with an ID (Smith & Van Houten, 1996).

Comorbid Diagnoses

The nature of a spectrum is not to have clear boundaries. Barrett et al. (2004) suggest that this does not simply apply to disorders within the autism spectrum but also among other syndromes and ASD. Recent estimates have placed the prevalence of a comorbid psychiatric disorder in children with PDD-NOS at 80% (de Bruin, Ferdinand, Meester, de Nijs, & Verheij, 2007).

Likewise, Hill and Furniss (2006) found that emotional and behavioral disturbances were scored much higher for persons with ID and autism than ID alone. Overall, autism appears to have a high level of comorbidity with psychiatric and behavior disorders including depression, anxiety, and ADHD (Matson & Nebel-Schwalm, 2007; Tidmarsh & Volkmar, 2003).

Intellectual Disability

Intellectual disability may present a challenge in regard to differential diagnosis of ASD. This is due to high level of comorbidity of ID with ASD. Some have estimated that 75% of children with an ASD diagnosis also have an ID (Rapin, 1997). Others have shown that the severity of ID is positively correlated with an ASD diagnosis (La Malfa, Lassi, Bertelli, Salvini, & Placidi, 2004). In an effort to evaluate the role of intellectual functioning on the presentation of ASD core deficits, Matson, Dempsey, LoVullo, and Wilkins (2008) contrasted groups of individuals with ID and ASD to those with ID alone. They found that for persons with ID alone, the level of intellectual functioning had a moderating effect on ASD deficits, with the largest increase observed in stereotypies. Further, for those individuals with an Autism diagnosis, the level of ID had little effect on the expression of core ASD deficits. Finally, for those individuals with a PDD-NOS diagnosis, level of ID had an effect but to a much smaller degree than for those without an ASD diagnosis. Thus, as one moves along the ASD spectrum, from autism to PDD-NOS to no ASD diagnosis at all, the effect that IQ has upon the occurrence of ASD symptoms will increase. Put another way, as IQ decreases, the occurrence of ASD symptoms increases, thus making differential diagnosis more difficult among persons with severe and profound ID.

Language Disorder

Children rarely present with a clear diagnostic profile that allows for them to be readily and accurately diagnosed. This is particularly true in the arena of language impairments. In recent years, autism treatment and research has benefited from an increased awareness of

the disorder among clinicians, however one consequence has been the tendency for clinicians to assume that a diagnosis is warranted based upon the presence of a single core symptom such as communication impairments. Or, for those children on the border between two diagnostic categories, to have the default classification of an ASD. Addressing some of these concerns, Bishop and Norbury (2002) evaluated children with language impairments and classified them by using standardized diagnostic instruments. Overall, while they found a good deal of overlap between specific language impairment and ASD, they stressed that an ASD should not be assumed based solely upon language impairments. Likewise, Noterdaeme, Sitter, Mildenberger, and Amorosa (2000) found that of the three cores symptoms of ASD, the language impaired group could be differentiated based upon the absence of stereotyped behaviors.

A number of studies have been conducted to differentiate language disorders from autism (Allen & Rapin, 1992; Bartak, Rutter, & Cox, 1975; Cantwell, Baker, & Rutter, 1978; Rapin, 1996; Shields, Varley, Broks, & Simpson, 1996a, 1996b; Tuchman, Rapin, & Shinnar, 1991). In all these studies, differentiation is made as one would expect: along the core symptoms of autism and the defining characteristic of language disorder. Expanding upon this literature, Barrett et al. (2004) studied two groups that are not readily differentiated because they lie along the borders of both diagnostic categories, that being mild autism and language impairments with social deficits. They found that the groups could be distinguished based upon the frequency of repetitive behaviors, pragmatic language, and engaging in joint attention during play sessions. Interestingly, no differences were observed on formal assessments of vocabulary and comprehension skills.

Barrett et al. (2004) also found that one of the most useful observations to differentiate among diagnostic groups was the frequency and severity of repetitive behaviors. Thus, it may be the case that when the task is to determine which diagnostic group a person belongs to, an emphasis should be placed on assessing/evaluating the nonoverlapping symptoms rather than on teasing out subtle differences in severity or form of dysfunction in the overlapping symptoms. As Barrett et al. (2004) suggest, it may also be the case that no meaningful distinction can be made among groups for some children.

Attention Deficit/Hyperactivity Disorder

There is a good deal of symptom overlap between
PDD-NOS and ADHD. Distinguishing when differential diagnosis or when making a dual diagnosis is
appropriate may be essential for appropriate treatment
(Yoshida & Uchiyama, 2004). Koyama, Tachimori,
Osada, and Kurita (2006) have examined cognitive
profiles of these two groups to see if systematic differences were present. They found that overall, children
with PDD-NOS or ADHD showed differences centered on communication skills, with PDD-NOS group
scoring significantly lower on measures of verbal comprehension, vocabulary, and general comprehension.
Luteijn et al. (2000) have also explored the social and
communicative impairments in children with PDD-
NOS, ADHD, or PDD-NOS and ADHD. They found
that PDD-NOS group experienced significantly more
social problems and engaged in more withdrawn
behavior. However, the two groups did not differ in
regard to overall autism symptoms or attention problems. Instead the differences were in regard to how the
core deficits were expressed. Both groups showed
some form of autistic-like social problems, but the
PDD-NOS group showed the tendency to withdraw or
engage in peculiar behavior. Hence, we see again that
what differentiates ASD from other disorders is not
simply a dichotomous decision regarding a symptoms
presence or absence, but rather a more qualitative look
at that behavior. For instance, both the child with
ADHD and the child with ASD will show attention
problems. Yet the differentiation between the two
groups is observed in why the child stops paying attention or is distracted and what type of behavior is
engaged in when the child is off-task.

Assessing ASD Spectrum

Central to the task of differential diagnosis in ASD are
diagnostic assessments, and in recent years, the development of these tools has significantly increased.
Nonetheless, these diagnostic tools focus almost exclusively on autism and ignore other autism spectrum disorders (Matson, 2007a). In essence, what has happened
is that the other disorders classified by the DSM-IV as
"Pervasive Developmental Disorders" have begun to

be defined as *not being* autism; or rather, to what
degree and along what symptoms does the disorder
differ from autism. In this system, autism is the central
disorder from which all other spectra emerge.

As discussed earlier, core symptoms of autism date
back to Kanner's original description (1943), in which a
group of children were described who engaged in repetitive behaviors, showed a lack of eye contact, and had
poor verbal skills. While the symptoms were loosely
described at first, these observations have become more
systematic over the years and formal assessment measures have been developed (Matson, 2007a). As the
prevalence of this disorder has become realized, diagnostic instruments have proliferated. However, the vast
majority of these scales have not been developed to
address disorders across the full spectrum. This has left
a gap in the tools available for clinicians to use (Matson,
Nebel-Schwalm, & Matson, 2007).

While the development of numerous diagnostic
instruments is beneficial in that research and concepts
regarding ASD are greatly stimulated, a downside is
that many of these instruments are never developed
fully and their psychometric properties are not explored
(Matson, 2007a). The glut of underdeveloped assessment instruments impact is twofold. First, it obfuscates
the status of assessment instruments such that users both
new and old to the area have a difficult time sifting
the wheat from the chaff. A result is that instruments
with little to no evidence of adequate psychometric
properties are presented on equal par with those that
have years of demonstrated validity and reliability.
Second, due to the confusion, researchers and clinicians
may insist on using the "gold standard" assessments
even when another instrument may be more appropriate
to answer their clinical or research question. Both of
these errors will result in the best tool for their purposes
not being used.

To control for both of these errors, diagnostic instruments must be evaluated according to their published
psychometric data and thoughtful consideration of
how well the instrument meets the assessment needs.
Test users must know the characteristics of the instruments they use to diagnose. In an excellent review of
diagnostic instruments with published psychometric
data, Matson, Nebel-Schwalm, and Matson (2007)
present a list of 21 identified scales and the research
that has evaluated their use. Due to space limitations
we provide and in depth review of the most commonly
used scales in the ASD research literature.

Assessment Tools

Autism Behavior Checklist

The Autism Behavior Checklist (ABC; Krug, Arick, & Almond, 1980) is among the first measures of this kind and is used both in the USA and Sweden. It is a checklist of 57 items used alone or as part of a larger battery, the Autism Screening Instrument for Educational Planning (ASIEP-3; Krug, Arick, & Almond, 2008). The ASIEP is now in its third iteration but the ABC has not yet been revised. The ABC is designed to be completed independently by a parent or a teacher and then interpreted by a clinician. Administration time is approximately 20 min. The target group for this measure are children with severe disabilities ages 3 years to school age. While it is still used and there is a wide literature base, researchers investigating the psychometrics have questioned its utility beyond gross assessment of ASD (Ozonoff, Goodlin-Jones, & Solomon, 2005; Rellini, Tortolani, Trillo, Carbone, & Montecchi, 2004).

Krug et al. (1980) present the first psychometric evaluation of the ABC. Item selection was based on a three part approach, a literature review, expert consultation, and practitioner administration. First, was a literature review of Rimland (1964); Creak (1964); Ruttenberg, Dratmann, Fraknoi, and Wemar (1966); Rendle-Short and Clangy (1968); Lotter (1974) Lovaas, Freitag, Gold, and Kassorla (1965), Lovaas, Koegel, Simmons, and Long (1973); and Kanner (1943). From these researchers, items were developed and sent for expert review. Once comments were returned from the expert group, the revised items were formed into a 57 item checklist with 5 rationally derived factors (Sturmey, Matson, & Sevin, 1992). Items were grouped into factors labeled sensory, relating, body and object use, language, social, and self help.

Next, the checklist was sent to practitioners to administer and return for statistical analysis. This resulted in 1049 completed protocols. Ages sampled ranged from 18 months to 35 years. Item analysis was conducted to determine critical items. Gamma and phi scores were calculated; gamma scores indicate the consistent ordinal relationship of scores across variables and phi scores indicate association between binary variables. From these characteristics, items were assigned weightings of 1–4, with 4 being the highest predictor of ASD. Total scores range from 0 to 120 with cutoff scores of 68 or above considered a high probability of autism, 53–67 range considered questionable autism, and less than 53 are considered unlikely to have autism. However, some researchers have questioned these recommended cutoff scores (Sevin, Matson, Coe, Fee, & Sevin, 1991; Volkmar et al., 1988; Wadden, Bryson, & Rodger, 1991; Yirmiya, Sigman, & Freeman, 1994).

Reliability and validity of the ABC were reported to be good. Reliability for the Total Score (TS) internal consistence is reported with a Split-Half analysis, $r = 0.87$, and a Pearson Product Moment, $r = 0.94$ for the complete checklist. However, Volkmar et al. (1988) found less robust results (split half: 0.74). Interrater reliability for TS was calculated using 42 raters scoring 14 children; each child was rated simultaneously by three raters. Agreement among raters was 95%. Again, Volkmar et al. (1988) found dissimilar results with agreement at 0.70. Validity reports include criterion-related validity using comparison of the measures total score of the entire sample of individuals with an ASD to a random sample of 62 children drawn from the larger group of individuals with ASD. They found that 86% of this second group scored within 1 standard deviation of the mean for the larger group and 14% scored within 1.5 standard deviations. However, some researchers are underwhelmed with this evidence (see Lerea, 1987; Parks, 1983).

Criterion-related validity was examined through an Analysis of Variance to compare individuals with and without an ASD on the factors of sex, age, living setting, language development, and student-teacher ratio. The authors found that almost all of the permutations were statistically significant except analyses investigating children with an ASD and those with severe emotional disturbances. These individuals had total scores similar to individuals categorized as ASD on 3 of the 15 analyses. Lastly, reliability analysis was investigated for both intra and interrater reliability. Intrarater reliability was good (split half: 0.87; complete: 0.94). Interrater reliability was evaluated using 42 raters scoring 14 children; each child was rated simultaneously by three raters. Agreement was at 95%.

Discriminant validity was assessed by separating the ABC protocol into four groups to represent the following classifications: ASD ($n = 172$), ID ($n = 423$), severely emotionally disturbed ($n = 254$), deaf-blind ($n = 100$), and neural normal ($n = 100$). They found that 55 of the 57 items were useful to distinguish ASD from the four non-ASD groups. Individuals with an ASD scored higher on all 5 factors and had a total score average of 77. Individuals from the ID, severely emotionally disturbed, and deaf-blind groups scored alike and had a total score average of 42. Lastly, individuals from the neural normal group had a total score average of 0. Another analysis of criterion-related validity was conducted on a sample formed of 62 randomly selected individuals ages 3 to 23 years from the original group of individuals with an established diagnosis of ASD. They found that 86% of this second group scored within 1 standard deviation of the mean for the larger group and 14% scored within 1.5 standard deviations. Conversely, Volkmar et al. (1988), found only 57% of individuals with ASD were correctly classified as "probably autistic", 23% as "questionably autistic", and 62% as "neural normal". Wadden et al. (1991) also found low sensitivity and specificity using the original cutoff scores. However, when the cutoff score was lowered to 44, these researchers found that 87% of individuals with ASD were correctly classified as well as 96% of the neural normal. Most recently, Eaves, Campbell, and Chambers (2000) used the lower cutoff score recommended by Krug, Arick, and Almond (1993) and found that the ABC correctly classified 80% of the participants in their sample.

In sum, the ABC has a large body of published research. Noted attributes are its simplicity, administration time, and ease of scoring. Published data for different age groups are available. The scale can be used as a parent interview or may be completed independently by parents. Perhaps its best use is as an index of ASD symptoms or a screening instrument. Noted weaknesses are its limited utility with children under the age of 3 years, possible overidentification of autism in children with intellectual disabilities and possible underidentification of "high functioning" school-age children with an ASD.

Autism Diagnostic Interview – Revised

The Autism Diagnostic Interview – Revised (ADI-R; Lord et al., 1994) is a semi-structured interview of caregivers of individuals with autism. The ADI-R is the second edition of the Autism Diagnostic Interview (Le Couteur et al., 1989). Overall, administration time for the ADI-R is 1.5 to 2.5 h. The reported uses of

ADI-R are to aid in the diagnosis of autism, treatment planning, and differential diagnosis among other developmental disabilities (Rutter, Couteur, & Lord, 2003). The ADI-R produces an algorithm that is used for determining diagnosis. The algorithm is based upon ICD-10 and DSM-IV diagnostic criteria. The algorithm is calculated from the individual's total score across all symptoms queried without regard for severity within particular symptom domains.

In regard to user training, the manual requires users to meet three components. First, extensive familiarity with ASDs and behavioral manifestations of ASD symptoms. Second, adequate interviewing skills to obtain detailed information. Third, skill at coding behaviors to meet the ADI-R item format. The manual also stipulates that there are two levels of training for use of the ADI-R. The first level is for clinical or non-research use of the ADI-R. This is considered a less precise level of training as it requires the user only to meet the aforementioned criteria and to have read the manual, and studied training videos produced by Western Psychological Services. A more rigorous level of training is required by the test developers if the user intends the results of the ADI-R to be used in research. A large part of this additional training is the requirement to attend approved training programs, and submit videotaped interviews with coding samples.

As a revision of the ADI, the ADI-R builds off of the original psychometric properties reported by Le Couteur et al. (1989) The revised version was streamlined in order to reduce administration time and a new algorithm was developed to identify cut-off scores with the highest sensitivity and specificity. The scale was further streamlined in the WPS version, but the manual notes that the algorithm remains the same (Rutter et al., 2003). Lord et al. (1994) report the algorithm to have a high level of sensitivity and specificity (both above 0.9).

Initial psychometric data on the reliability and validity of the ADI-R are presented by Lord et al. (1994) A total of 20 children, 10 with autism and 10 "mentally handicapped or language-impaired" were evaluated with the ADI-R. The ADI-R showed adequate to good interrater reliability, internal consistency, and stability of scores over a 6-month period. For the validity analyses, the sample size was increased to 50, with 25 participants per group. Validity of the diagnostic algorithm was tested by evaluating differences among diagnostic groups on the individual items included in the algorithm. Significant differences between groups were found for all items.

The ADI-R's utility for distinguishing between autism and other developmental disabilities was further evaluated by Mildenberger, Sitter, Noterdaeme, and Amorosa (2001). In their study, they examined the ADI-R's classification rates among children with an autism or a receptive language disorder diagnoses. They found that 1 of 11 children with autism was not classified as having autism. Further, they found that 1 of 16 children with a receptive language disorder was falsely classified as having autism. Overall, these data show that the ADI-R is useful for differential diagnosis among these symptomatically similar disorders.

The results by Mildenberger et al. (2001) are contrasted though with the results of Bishop and Norbury (2002). While the purpose of the study by Bishop and Norbury was not to evaluate the psychometric properties of the ADI-R but rather to explore the overlap of symptoms along the borders of two diagnostic groups, their results do offer important information regarding the differential diagnosis process using the ADI-R. They found the classification process among children with an ASD and children with specific language impairment to be much more complicated than was found by Mildenberger et al. (2001). Particularly, Bishop and Norbury found that the ADI-R and the ADOS-G had poor agreement among diagnoses.

The evaluation of autism in very young children is of increasing importance as the impact of early intervention on ASD treatments has been realized. As such, the psychometric properties of diagnostic scales must be evaluated in samples of young children. Lord, Storoschuk, Rutter, and Pickles (1993) evaluated the ADI-R in 51 children with autism and 43 children with a non-ASD developmental disorder. They found that the groups differed significantly on all items of the ADI-R. The ADI-R also showed good sensitivity with 1 of the 51 children with autism not meeting the full ADI-R criteria. Lord and her colleagues further reported interrater reliability to be good.

The stability of ADI-R diagnostic scores in young children has also been evaluated by Cox et al. (1999) They found that the stability of an autism diagnosis from the ADI-R was good for the period between 20 and 42 months of age. Also, they found that the ADI-R had good specificity, with all of the children identified as having autism at 20 months eventually receiving a diagnosis by 42 months. In contrast, the ADI-R showed poor

sensitivity for children at 20 months. They reported that only 50% of the children who eventually received an autism diagnosis at 42 months were identified at 20 months by the ADI-R. Further, they report that for children who fell on the autism spectrum but who did not meet criteria for an ICD-10 diagnosis of autism, the sensitivity was even lower. In their study, none of the children who went on to receive diagnoses of Asperger's Disorder or other PDDs were identified by the ADI-R.

More recently, Moore and Goodson (2003) evaluated the stability of an autism diagnosis using the ADI-R and clinical judgment from 2 years to 4–5 years of age. They found that 14 of the 16 children identified at age two as having autism continued to be similarly classified at age 4 to 5. They note though that parent report and recall on the ADI-R may not have been adequate alone and that they felt the need to augment their diagnostic decisions with clinical judgment. Hence, these results do not reflect the ADI-R classification stability alone, but only in conjunction with clinical judgment.

The stability of diagnosis in young children using the ADI-R was again evaluated by Charman et al. (2005) over a 5-year period. In their study they assessed 26 children at age 2 and again at age 7. Their results showed much greater variability in diagnostic stability than that reported by previous studies (e.g., Cox et al., 1999; Lord, 1995; Moore & Goodson, 2003), with 17 of the 26 (65%) participants receiving the same diagnostic classification at 7 years of age as they had received at 2 years. Diagnostic stability was somewhat better with a shorter time period, which is seen at the 4–5 year period with 19 of the 26 (73%) participant receiving the same diagnosis as they received at 2 years of age. Probably the most interesting finding by Charman and colleagues though is that there was considerable variability over time in the ADI-R classification results wherein the 17 classified as having autism at 7 years of age were not necessarily the same who were classified at age 4–5 as having autism. Instead, many of their participants moved across diagnostic categories over the assessment phases. They also note that the variability in symptom severity increased with age.

The ADI-R is often considered the gold-standard for making a diagnosis of autism. Indeed, the National Database for Autism Research (NDAR) requires both the ADI-R and ADOS to be included in the submission of any clinical research data (National Institutes of Health, 2008). However, the ADI-R requires a substantial amount of training to administer.

The simple cost of attending training seminars is likely to limit researchers' willingness to use this instrument, particularly those with a limited research budget. Likewise, ADI-R requires a significant amount of time to administer. This too can often exceed the resources available for conducting a study. Thus, while ADI-R has shown excellent psychometric properties, the overall requirements for using the scale in clinical research are a significant drawback.

Autism Diagnostic Observation Schedule – Generic

The Autism Diagnostic Observation Schedule – Generic (ADOS-G; Lord, Rutter, DiLavore, & Risi, 1999) is a semi-structured assessment that uses direct observation and interaction with individuals who may have an ASD. Administration of ADOS-G consists of a series of interactions with the individual that are designed to elicit a wide rage of social responses that the examiner can use to determine the presence or absence of ASD symptoms. As with ADI-R, ADOS-G requires substantial training for administration. As stated by Lord "use of the ADOS-G is clearly related to the skill of the examiner" (Lord et al., 2000). Administration time for the ADOS should last approximately 30 min (Lord et al., 2000).

The ADOS-G is the latest permutation of the Autism Diagnostic Observation Schedule (ADOS; Lord et al., 1989), which was originally constructed as a companion instrument to the ADI (Lord et al., 2000). As need arose for an instrument appropriate for use in younger children, ADOS was extended to be used with children as young as 2 years old. This version of ADOS became the Pre-Linguistic Autism Diagnostic Observation Schedule (PL-ADOS; DiLavore, Lord, & Rutter, 1995). However, Lord et al. (2000) note that the PL-ADOS tended to underdiagnose children with autism who had some expressive language skills. Thus, the ADOS-G was designed to fill the gap in development between the PL-ADOS and the ADOS.

The development process of ADOS-G has been well described (Lord et al., 2000). Interrater reliability at the item-level was good for all modules except for module 4, which required elimination of a number of items. Overall after the elimination of items with poor interrater reliability, the interrater reliability of items

in the ADOS-G modules were very high. Domain scores showed high interrater and test-retest reliability for all domains. In regard to validity, all modules of ADOS-G showed excellent specificity and sensitivity for those with autism (95% correct classification) and those outside autism spectrum (92%). However, for those with PDD-NOS, only 33% were classified as having a nonautism ASD. Thus, ADOS-G appears to be excellent for the use of differentiating autism and PDD-NOS from nonspectrum disorders, but less robust ability to differentiate within the autism spectrum.

Less robust results have been found by Noterdaeme et al. (2000) for the previous version of ADOS. These authors found that for differentiating between autism and a language disorder, ADOS had excellent specificity, wherein none of the children with a language disorder was falsely classified as having autism. Conversely, they found ADOS to have poor sensitivity, with only 3 of 11 children with autism meeting the cut-off for stereotyped behaviors. These authors note though that the correct classification rates may have been better if the ADOS-G algorithm had been available for their study.

DiLavorre, Lord, and Rutter (1995) describe the development of PL-ADOS and initial psychometric evaluations. They found interrater reliability to range from moderate to excellent for all domains. In regard to differential diagnosis, DiLavorre et al. (1995) found similar results to those already reported, that is, showing excellent specificity with very few false positives, but an overall weaker sensitivity to classify those with autism as having autism. Specific to PL-ADOS, this weakness was observed in regard to children who had autism but also had some level of verbal skills. As mentioned, this weakness was one of the reported purposes of developing the ADOS-G (Lord et al., 2000).

Overall, ADOS-G is an excellent diagnostic instrument. As with the ADI-R though, the appropriate use of this instrument requires significant training. The limitations noted for using ADI-R in clinical research also apply to ADOS-G. However, ADOS-G takes significantly less time than ADI-R, which improves the overall usability of the instrument. Further, ADOS is one of the few assessment measures that has the rater score from direct observations. Whether or not this results in improved diagnostic ability is an empirical question that has gone untested (Matson, 2007a). Nonetheless, this format may have particular appeal with many clinicians who feel that scoring from observations may yield a more precise and nuanced diagnostic evaluation.

Autism Spectrum Disorders – Diagnostic

The Autism Spectrum Disorders – Diagnostic (ASD-D; Matson & González, 2007) is an informant based rating scale. The scale may be administered directly by a trained test user to an informant or it may be given to the parent or caregiver to complete independently (Matson & González, 2007). The ASD-D takes approximately 30–45 min to complete. The ASD-D is part of a larger battery of assessments that include the diagnostic instrument, an assessment for comorbid disorders (ASD-C), and an assessment for problem behaviors (ASD-PB). Each of these assessments has a version developed specifically for use with children. The ASD battery has received much recent attention, however, for the purpose of differential diagnosis; we will focus on those studies that discuss ASD-D.

The reliability and factor structure of ASD-D was evaluated in 192 adults with varying levels of ID (Matson, Wilkins, & González, 2008). Matson and his colleagues present data from the overall development process of ASD-D. In this initial study, items were first evaluated for interrater and test-retest reliability. Those items that were retained were then evaluated for a lack of variance and if there was a significant difference in endorsement between ASD and non-ASD groups. Finally, an exploratory factor analysis was conducted on the remaining items. Overall, reliability coefficients at the item level were moderate yet statistically significant. The relatively low reliability coefficients are to be expected as individual items rarely have high coefficients (Crocker & Algina, 1986). The exploratory factor analysis yielded 3 factors, which loosely reflect the three core symptom clusters in ASD, namely, communication deficits, social skill deficits, and stereotypical behavior. Each of these factors showed high coefficients of internal stability.

Normative data and cut-off scores for the ASD-D are presented on adults with intellectual disabilities (Matson, Boisjoli, et al., 2007). The best cut-off score was determined through calculating receiver operating characteristics (ROC). Results showed that the optimal cut-off point for classification between adults with an intellectual disability and autism and those only with an intellectual disability, resulted in sensitivity at 0.86 and specificity at 0.62, which yielded a total correct classification rate of 73.7%. The task became much harder though when trying to differentiate between

autism and PDD-NOS. For the differentiation of autism from PDD-NOS, the authors found that the total score cut-off points were ineffective. Instead, individual cut-off scores for each factor were used. With this method, the authors were able to effectively differentiate between the autism and PDD-NOS groups.

Further evidence supporting the validity of the ASD-D is presented by Matson, Wilkins, Boisjoli, and Smith (in press). A variation of the multitrait-multimethod matrix (Campbell & Fiske, 1959) is presented in which 307 adults with IDs were evaluated through a diverse battery of assessments. The ASD-D was shown to have good convergent and discriminant validity. The psychometric properties of the child version of the ASD-D has been independently evaluated in two studies (Matson, González, Wilkins, & Rivet, 2008; Matson, González, & Wilkins, in press). The ASD-DC showed excellent internal consistency (0.99), good interrater reliability (0.67), and good test-retest reliability (0.77; Matson, González et al., 2008.

The ASD-DC has been shown to have excellent sensitivity (92.5) and specificity (79.3) in differentiating atypical development from ASD (Matson, González, & Wilkins, in press). Differentiating between typical and atypical development showed less robust sensitivity (55.2) but excellent specificity (95.9). For the purpose of differentiating between PDD-NOS and Asperger's, the ASD-DC showed excellent sensitivity (92.9) and specificity (80.0). Differentiating between PDD-NOS and autism also showed excellent sensitivity (83.3) but less robust specificity (58.3).

The ASD-D is a relatively new instrument that has seen a tremendous amount of studies considering the amount of time it has been available. Overall, the ASD-DC shows strong psychometric foundations. This is a promising scale for differential diagnosis, particularly among children. A strength of this instrument is its development to assess symptoms across the autism spectrum.

The Childhood Autism Rating Scale

The Childhood Autism Rating Scale (CARS; Schopler, Reichler, & Renner, 1988) was developed by the Treatment and Education of Autistic and Related Communication handicapped Children (TEACCH) program. It is an update from an earlier version entitled the Childhood Psychosis Rating Scale (Reichler & Schopler, 1971). Updates for the CARS included new psychometric evaluations, new or updated items, and lessening of restrictions on which professionals were qualified to administer the instrument. Administration time is approximately 30 min. Given its age; it has the benefit of many published studies reporting psychometric data and demonstrating its utility. It was designed to be an observational instrument used to assess ASD and distinguish children with autistic disorder from children with other developmental disorders.

The CARS comprises 15 items, which are summed to generate a total score that is used to discern where on the continuum of "Mildly-Moderately Autistic" to "Severely Autistic" or "Non-Autistic" a rating corresponds. Item inclusion was based on five prominent works on the diagnosis and classification of ASD: Kanner (1943), Creak (1961), the National Society for Autistic Children (1978), Rutter (1978), and the Diagnostic and Statistical Manual of Mental Disorders Third Edition – Revised (American Psychiatric Association, 1987). Of note though is that this sampling of sources leaves the measure unsupported as a whole by any of the five works.

As noted, classification is divided into one of three ranges: Mildly moderately autistic, severely autistic, or nonautistic. The authors recommended that CARS be used as an initial aid in the classification process and have designed it as an observational assessment or an archival review (i.e., chart or record review). It is designed to be administered after minimal training. Additionally, the authors provide adjusted cutoff scores for adolescent and adults.

The CARS has had significant attention in the research and clinical community since its inception. Original authors Schopler and Reichler with colleagues DeVellis and Daly (1980) present some of the original psychometrics and rationale for the CARS. They note that item inclusion and the rationale for the CARS came from their clinical experience and observations. They found that in their clinical experience, Kanner's (1943) criteria were excluding children who had been diagnosed with an ASD and that Creak's (1964) criteria were excluding young children. Thus, their paper was intended to establish utility and content validity of CARS by comparing it to other diagnostic criteria: Rimland (1971), Rutter (1978) and Ritvo and Freeman (1978). Using a sample of 450 children, participants were diagnosed with various criteria from Rimland,

Rutter, and Ritvo and Freeman. Overall they found that these measures alone or combined under identified those with ASD. Whereas Rutter emphasized insistence on sameness and stereotyped behaviors, Ritvo and Freeman emphasized sensory peculiarities. Both these systems alone or combined under identified those with ASD.

Psychometric data provided by the author were developed from a sample of approximately 1,600 children with an ASD ranging in age from below 6 to above 10. Most were Caucasian (67%) males (75%). Seventy-one percent of their sample had IQ scores below 70. Reliability and validity were reported to be good. Internal consistency for the total score (TS) was excellent (0.94). Interrater reliability ($n=280$) for the TS was 0.71, with the items ranging from 0.55 (Level and Consistency of Intellectual Response) to 0.93 (Relating to People). The 1-year test-retest reliability ($n=91$) was reported as 0.88. Criterion-related validity was examined through comparison of the CARS TS to concurrent clinical ratings. Correlations were good for all contrasts ($r>0.8$).

Garfin and McCallon (1988) also examined CARS scores among different age groups. Investigation of age differences was prompted by researchers who suggested that the presentation of ASD may become less pronounced over time (e.g., Rutter, Greenfeld, & Lockyer, 1967). Twenty-two matched adolescents and children with autism were assessed. These participants were matched on ethnicity, sex, IQ and prescreening checklist scores. No statistically significant difference was found between these age groups and the authors concluded that CARS was insensitive to developmental changes in their sample. However it should be noted that the scores tended to be lower for adolescents by 2 points. It is recommended in CARS manual to lower the cutoff scores by 2 for adolescents and adults. Garfin and McCallon (1988) also examined the discriminant validity of CARS. Twenty adolescents with autism were matched with adolescents without an autism diagnosis. They found that CARS scores were able to discriminate between these two groups.

Stone et al. (1999) used CARS scores to examine the reliability and stability of autism diagnoses of children under the age of 3. The CARS was the primary dependent variable used to assess interrater reliability among experienced clinicians. Percent agreement for differentiating those with and without ASD was 88% ($n=65$). However, percent agreement was lower when differentiating those with Autism and PDD-NOS (64%) and ranged from 38 to 82% depending upon the rater. Stability of scores over a 12 month test-retest interval ($n=37$) showed similar results in that there was greater stability for those classified with autism ($r=0.80$) versus those classified with PDD-NOS ($r=0.42$). The authors concluded that based on CARS scores that autism was a more stable diagnosis.

The factor structure of the CARS was examined by Magyar and Pandolfi (2007). Using archival data for 164 children, principal component and principal factor analyses were calculated. Four factors were identified that accounted for 57% of the variance. These factors were labeled Social Communication, Social Interactions, Stereotypies and Sensory Abnormalities, and Emotional Regulation. The authors cite these results as support for the use of the CARS and point out that this measure is still relevant despite being constructed according to the 1980 version of the Diagnostic and Statistical Manual of Mental Disorders.

In all, CARS has been shown to have clinical utility. This measure is widely used and has a substantial literature base. This measure requires minimal training to administer. However, the rater should be knowledgeable of developmental sequences and chronology. It has the benefit of cutoff scores for both adolescents and adults. Areas of concern though are its dated normative group, which was collected only from one state. Further, it includes items that are no longer considered primary behavioral presentations of ASD.

Gilliam Autism Rating Scale

The Gilliam Autism Rating Scale (GARS; Gilliam, 1995) is a 56-item questionnaire that is divided into four subscales. These subscales include Social Interaction, Communication, Stereotyped Behaviors, and Developmental Disturbance. Each scale is a measure of the child's current and typical behavior. The developmental disturbances scale is an exception in that it rates past severe maladaptive behaviors. All items are summed and the total for each subscale is converted into standard scores.

Psychometric data provided by the author (Gilliam, 1995) were developed from a sample of approximately 1,100 children with an ASD ranging in age from 3 to 22 years. Reliability and validity were reported to be excellent. The reported internal consistency (coefficient alphas) ranged from 0.88 to 0.96. Item-total point biserial correlation coefficients for all items were above 0.35 with median values ranging from 0.61 to 0.69. The 1-week test-retest reliability was 0.88 for the Autism Quotient (AQ) and the subscales were all above 0.80. Discriminant validity analyses using AQ correctly classified 90% of the individuals. Concurrent validity with Autism Behavior Checklist was 0.94 and ranged from 0.37 to 0.92 for the subscales. Interrater reliability ($n=57$) for AQ was 0.88 and ranged from 0.73 to 0.82 for the subscales.

Reviews of this measure have been critical but not dismissive. South et al. (2002) evaluated GARS with 119 children, mostly Caucasian males. The mean age was 6 with a range of 3–10.5. All children were diagnosed by recognized autism experts and pooled from five research centers throughout the United States. South and colleagues concluded that their sample scored significantly different from that described by Gilliam (1995). Their sample scored well below the reference mean, classifying only 52% of the sample as "probably autistic." While reliability among the scales was good, convergent validity was reported as poor, and adaptive function appeared to be negatively correlated with the measure. A final critique by South et al. (2002) was that several parents reported confusion about phrasing of items; this was addressed in the second edition.

Lecavalier (2005) provides an extensive evaluation of the GARS. Analyses were completed using 284 children with ASD from 29 school districts in Ohio. The majority of this sample was Caucasian males with a mean age of 9 years and a range of 3–21 years. The factor structure was analyzed and suggested a three-factor solution; however items did not necessarily hang together in the subscale they are assigned. Approximately half the items were associated with only one factor derived from Lecavalier's analysis. As reported by South et al. (2002), Lecavalier reported a significant portion of the sample (62%) was classified only as "probably autistic" suggesting low sensitivity of the measure. Inter-rater reliability ($n=63$) was reported to be low as well with intra class correlations ranging form 0.31 to 0.48. These are considered poor to fair (Cichetti, 1994).

Content validity review of the items indicated an overemphasis of stereotypies, echolalia, and repetitive motor mannerisms. Conversely, an under-emphasis was suggested in the content areas of social and communication, and associated challenging behaviors of pica, self-injury, and unreasonable fears. Evaluation of the participant characteristic (sex, age, and level of function) found that the overall level of functioning was negatively correlated with the GARS, similar to that reported by South et al. (2002).

The most positive review of the GARS is provided by Eaves, Woods-Groves, Williams, and Fall (2006). This group assessed the psychometrics of the GARS and the Pervasive Developmental Disorders Rating Scale (PDDRS). Analyses were completed using 134 children with ASD and children with an other developmental disability from five southeastern states and Washington, DC. The majority of this sample was Caucasian males and this group included a large sample of African Americans (40%). The mean age was 9.75 years with a range of 3–26 years. Construct validity was analyzed through comparison with the PDDRS. Cronbach's alpha was 0.94 with the subscales ranging from 0.74 to 0.90. Correlation with the PDDRS was 0.84. and the validity coefficients for the subscales ranged from 0.09 to 0.84. Discriminant Validity analysis was significant and the effect size was reported to be 0.19 for the GARS. As reported by South et al. (2002) and Lecavalier (2005) a significant portion of the sample was classified only as "probably autistic" suggesting low sensitivity of the measure. However, when Eaves et al. adjusted the cutoff to 85 from 100 and ran predictive validity analyses, sensitivity was reported as 0.83, specificity as 0.68 and positive predictive value as 0.81.

The GARS was recently revised in 2006 and consequently more information is currently available for the GARS than the GARS-2. We were unable to identify any published studies that evaluated this revision. The reasons for this revision were based on test reviews, feedback, new research, and clinical observations (Gilliam, 2006). Revisions include a new normative sample, rewritten items and greater clarification of the scoring guidelines.

The GARS-2 is a rating scale in which parents or caregivers are interviewed concerning the examinee's behavior. Administration time is approximately 20 min. This assessment requires minimal training to complete but requires training and experience with ASD for interpretation of results. This measure comprises 42 items divided into three subscales (Stereotyped Behaviors, Communication, and Social Interaction).

These subscales were based on definitions of autism provided by the Autism Society of America and the DSM-IV-TR (American Psychiatric Association, 2000) however items do not necessarily correspond to the subscales they are placed.

Psychometric data provided by the author (Gilliam, 2006) were developed from a sample of approximately 1,100 children with an ASD ranging in age from 3 to 22 years. Gilliam reported that reliability and validity were good. Reliability for the Autism Index (AI) internal consistency is reported as a coefficient alpha of 0.94 with the subscales of Stereotypic Behaviors at 0.84, Communication at 0.86, and Social Interaction at 0.94. The 1-week test-retest reliability ($n=37$) was reported as 0.84 for the AI, 0.64 for Communication, 0.82 for Social Interaction, and 0.83 for Stereotyped Behaviors subscales. Validity analyses include content validity, criterion-related validity and construct-identification validity. Item-discrimination coefficients ranged from 0.35 to 0.64. Concurrent validity with the Autism Behavior Checklist was 0.64. Inter-item correlation for the AI and the subscales ranged from 0.53 to 0.64. Correlations for the subscales ranged from 0.46 to 0.59. Predictive validity was reported for a group of those with ASD, intellectual disability (ID), multiple disabilities, and no disabilities. Sensitivity is reported to range from 1.00 for nondisabled, 0.85 for ID, and 0.84 for multiple-disabilities. Specificity ranged from 0.84 to 0.87 and positive predictive values ranged from 0.84 to 0.85. Inter-rater reliability is not provided.

Overall, the GARS has been widely used but has had mixed results by researchers. Positive features of the GARS include quick administration and scoring. The GARS has been widely used and accepted. This measure can be used as an index of severity of autism for selected populations, as well as used as a measure of specific behaviors (e.g., repetitive motor behaviors). Lecavalier suggested that it may show good discriminant validity with lower functioning individuals. A final critique was that Lecavalier questions the utility of the subscale Developmental Disturbances as it did not appear to have acceptable psychometrics (i.e., poor diagnostic validity, low convergent validity, and poor internal consistency).

The GARS-2 has been developed to address some of the limitations reported by researchers. This measure uses a mulitmethod approach where the assessment is completed using interviews with the parents, direct observation of the child, and an evaluative portion where the examiner completes "Key Questions" used to synthesize the examiners diagnostic conclusions. Other highlights for this measure are its recent publication date with current normative data, published in 2006. This measure is shown to distinguish individuals aged 3 through 22 years with autism from others who have severe behavioral problems, it can be used as an index of severity of autism, it can be used as a measure of specific behaviors (e.g., repetitive motor behaviors), and has been shown discriminant validity with lower functioning individuals. Weaknesses of this measure include a lack of published research independent of the manual, the age range does not address DSM criteria of symptom presentation before age 3, the normative data are not broken down by age, gender, or level of functioning and it does not provide for alternate forms of communication for those who are nonverbal.

Checklist for Autism in Toddlers

The Checklist for Autism in Toddlers (CHAT; Baron-Cohen, Allen, & Gillberg, 1992) is a rating scale primarily developed to serve as a screening tool to detect ASD at an early age. As such, the scale is relatively quick to administer (5–15 min) by a trained clinician. The goal is to identify children by 18 months based upon developmental milestones. Two additional iteration of the CHAT, the Modified version (M-CHAT) and the Quantitative version (Q-CHAT) have also been developed.

The original CHAT comprises 14 items scored dichotomously and derived from 5 milestone areas typically occurring by 15 months of age in neural normal children. These milestone areas are typically negatively impacted by ASD: social play, social interest, pretend play, joint-attention, and protodeclarative pointing. An additional 4 areas were included that are reported to be unaffected by an ASD: functional play, protoimperative pointing, motor development, and rough and tumble play. Of these, two critical milestones were hypothesized to be paramount in identifying children with ASD. The first is pretend play and the second is joint-attention. One way a child may demonstrate joint attention is by using protodeclarative pointing; pointing to indicate to another person an object of interest, versus protoimperative pointing; pointing to simply indicate a desire for

that object. Another way a child may show joint attention is by gaze monitoring; looking in the direction of one's gaze. Failure to attain these milestones by 18 months is the core indicator of ASD. Presence of these developmental achievements are first assessed by an interview with the parent and then corroborated with behavioral observation as a guard against drawbacks of self-report.

The initial psychometric properties of the CHAT were based on a London, UK group of 91 children, 17–21 months old. Fifty of these children were randomly selected from children attending wellness check ups. The other 41 children were recruited from a pool of children with older siblings identified as having an ASD. From this sample 4 children of the siblings-with-an-ASD group were identified as also having an ASD. At the 2.5 year follow up these four children still evidenced criteria for an ASD, demonstrating discriminate validity for the CHAT. In addition, none of the children from the randomly selected group developed an ASD. Further these researches found that the reliability between the parents report and the corroborating observation by clinicians was in agreement 92% of the time.

In a follow-up study, Baron-Cohen et al. (1996) examined the sensitivity and specificity of the CHAT using a sample of 16,000 children attending an 18 month medical check up. These authors described that for their sample the ADI-R significant score cutoff was lowered for the "Repetitive Behavior" section to increase differentiation among their groupings. According to the authors, children with an ASD scored well above the cutoff on "Reciprocal Social Interactions" and "Communication" sections but only approached the cutoff score for "Repetitive Behavior." Using this approach it was found that they could differentiate children with an ASD from children with another developmental delay or those considered of typical development. From their sample, 12 children were identified as having an ASD and 10 of these 12 children were still diagnosed with an ASD at the 3.5-years follow up.

On the basis of this research Baron-Cohen et al. (1996) concluded that the CHAT could identify ASD at an early age and that this could be done with specific CHAT items. All children in their sample with an ASD fail 3 of 5 CHAT items designed specifically to assess pretend play, protodeclarative pointing, and gaze monitoring. Most importantly, gaze monitoring was indicated as the key difference among children with ASD, children with other developmental disabilities and children described as neural normal. Using these as the criteria to identify ASD, the authors were able to assert that the CHAT accurately identified 83% of children with an ASD. In addition, the false positive rate was 17% for this group. At the 3.5-year follow up, 100% of the earlier identified children still warranted an ASD diagnosis. A significant portion also failed additional items, 50% failed item 2 regarding social interest in others and 90% failed item 6 regarding use of protoimperative pointing. In identifying children with other developmental disabilities, these authors report that they consistently failed only CHAT items related to pretend play and/or protodeclarative pointing. Using these as the criteria, CHAT accurately identified 68% of children with other developmental disabilities. Finally, children described as neural normal were able to demonstrate all the milestones assessed by the CHAT.

More recently Baron-Cohen et al. (2000) reported on additional psychometric evaluations of the CHAT. With their sample of 50 children meeting ICD-10 criteria for autism and 44 children meeting criteria for other pervasive developmental disorders, they examined the specificity, sensitivity, and predictive validity of CHAT. In this study, data is reported for assessments at 18, 20, and 42 months. Using their previously established methods, these researchers first sought to differentiate children with high, medium, and low risk for an ASD. Interestingly they found that a small proportion of children with severe ASD features traversed diagnostic categories by the final 42 month assessment. Traversing diagnostic categories was not the case for low-risk group. Once the child demonstrated the milestone skill, there was no regression of skill in this sample group. As with their previous research, children with high risk for autism failed 3 of 5 CHAT items designed specifically to assess pretend play, protodeclarative pointing, and gaze monitoring. As well as, children with a low risk demonstrated all the milestone skills. However, children with a medium risk failed only protodeclarative pointing, which is different than reported in the 1996 study where gaze monitoring was indicated as the key difference among children with ASD. Overall, Baron-Cohen et al. reported that the CHAT has excellent specificity (100%), low sensitivity (21%), and good predictive positive value (75%) and excellent negative predictive value (100%). An examination of the long-term data from the Baron-Cohen et al. (1992, 1996) sampled

children at the 6 year follow-up. Using 94 children, at age 7, they calculated the sensitivity for identifying children classified as high, medium, and low for both autism and PDD. The overall specificity was analogous to that reported by Baron-Cohen et al. (1996).

The Modified Checklist for Autism in Toddlers (M-CHAT; Robins, Fein, Barton, & Green, 2001) is designed to assess children 16 and 30 months of age as part of a wellness check-up. Recognizing that the American health care system does not provide the same level of access to services as the UK, these authors planned a redesign that was easy, objective, and reliable for a parent checklist alone. In an effort to increase sensitivity without reducing specificity, they added a structured follow-up interview to the assessment process for children who obtained significant scores. By this interview, the false positive rate was reduced. The primary difference with the M-CHAT is the inclusion of new items in addition to the first 9 items from the original CHAT. Areas covered include sensory, motor activity, social interaction, joint attention, and language/communication abnormalities. From the accompanying test instructions the authors advise that the M-CHAT continue to be studied, and may be revised in the future.

Robins et al. (2001) report on the M-CHAT psychometric research based on a sample derived largely from Connecticut, USA. Participants ($n=1,122$) were recruited from wellness checkup visits and early intervention provider nomination ($n=171$). Item development came from literature, other measures designed for older children, and clinical experience. Evaluation of specificity, sensitivity, and predictive validity was completed by assessing children divided into one of four groups. As expected, no child with significant scores from the initial parent completed M-CHAT was found to have typical development. These researchers found that each of their four groups scored differently. Children with nonsignificant scores failed in only 0.5 items followed by the group of children ruled out via telephone interview who failed in 3.4 items. The third group, children found to have language or global delays but not an ASD, failed in 6.4 items. This is contrasted to the group of children with an ASD who failed in 10.3 items. Identification and differentiation was most successful when the structured follow-up interview conducted via telephone was part of the screening process. A cutoff of 3 on either the initial parent completed M-CHAT or follow-up telephone interview yielded a sensitivity value of 0.97, specificity value of 0.99, positive predictive value of 0.68, and negative predictive value of 0.99. Internal consistency was assessed using a sample of 480 participants, Cronbach's alpha was 0.85. Through canonical discriminant function analysis six critical items were identified. These pertained to protodeclarative pointing, following a point, bringing objects to show parent, interest in other children, imitation, and responding to name. The authors advise that children who fail in more than 3 items or 2 of the critical items are to be referred to a trained diagnostician of ASD with experience in diagnosis of very young children.

The quantitative CHAT (Q-CHAT; Allison et al., 2008) is the latest iteration of the CHAT. This new version is comprised of 25 items, now scored on a 5-point scale (0–4). Allison et al. report that it is the result of recognition that the original CHAT is most sensitive to the classic presentation of autism but not with Asperger Syndrome. This is likely because Asperger Syndrome is typically diagnosed at an older age then CHAT is designed to assess, specifically school age to adolescents and adulthood. Their research sample included 779 children classified without an ASD and 160 children diagnosed with an ASD. In this latter group, children diagnosed with an ASD had a mean score of 52 on Q-CHAT whereas for children classified without an ASD the mean score was 27. The test-retest reliability, calculated with intraclass correlation, was 0.82.

In summary, CHAT in all it iterations is regarded positively. Specific to CHAT, this measure has been shown to have excellent positive and negative predictive validity and specificity. It is quick to administer and uses a multimethod assessment approach. The most notable detraction for those outside of Europe is that the normative data is from UK and may not apply to other countries. However, in the absence of evidence that there are regional differences in autism presentation, this is unlikely. Other concerns are that the original CHAT may not be applicable to children with severe disabilities as this group was excluded in the normative process. The use of a dichotomous rating approach presents additional concerns in that it gives credit for minimal use of the skill reported which may lead to false negatives along with parent inaccurate reporting. This measure is susceptible to maturation/age effects and less able to identify late onset ASD especially when assessment is completed early in life. As mentioned above, CHAT has limited sensitivity in detecting Asperger Syndrome, that said the Q-CHAT is designed to address this concern. The recent construction of Q-CHAT provides it with current diagnostic theory, definitions, and psychometrics. Unlike the previous version, it uses a dimensional rating approach which accounts for minimal use of the skill reported. The M-CHAT has several benefits of which the most important are its quick administration. However, the M-CHAT does generate a high false positive rate, uses a dichotomous rating approach, and may not be applicable to children with severe language impairment or motor deficits as these groups were excluded in the normative process. Overall, these findings suggest that this scale is best used as a screening instrument.

PDD Behavior Inventory

The PDD Behavior Inventory (PDDBI; Cohen & Sudhalter, 1999) is a parent or teacher completed rating scale. Administration time for the standard form is reported to be 20–30 min. An extended form is available for the assessment of behaviors not specifically associated with making an ASD diagnosis. The extended form takes approximately 45 min to administer. The authors state that no formal training or degree is required to administer the PDDBI; however, they state that interpretation of results should only be undertaken by someone with graduate training in a related field (Cohen & Sudhalter, 1999). According to the authors, the purpose of creating the PDDBI was due to limitations in the existing assessment instruments, most particularly in the area of measuring changes over time (Cohen & Sudhalter, 1999). Further, PDDBI was developed to measure both adaptive and maladaptive behaviors, not simply focus upon behavior deficits or excesses.

Cohen, Schmidt-Lackner, Romanczyk, and Sudhalter (2003) present data on 311 children between the ages of 1 to 17 years. The authors evaluated reliability and factor structure of PDDBI. The scale showed good internal consistency with coefficient alpha scores ranging from 0.79 to 0.97 for the parent version and 0.73 to 0.97 for the teacher version. Interrater reliability was weak between parents and teachers for maladaptive behaviors but was adequate for adaptive behaviors. Reliability scores improved when teachers were contrasted with other teachers, showing acceptable reliability for all subscale scores. Results of principal components factor analyses confirmed most of the subscales of the PDDBI. However, Cohen et al. (2003) note that items grouped in the "verbal" adaptive subscales did not match the results of the factor analysis and may require reassignment from the a priori subscale.

Cohen (2003) has also reported on the criterion-related validity of PDDBI. In his study, 84 children between 3 and 6 years were assessed with PDDBI, ADI-R, CARS, Nisonger Child Behavior Rating Form (Aman, Tasse, Rojahn, & Hammer, 1996), Vineland Adaptive Behavior Scales (Sparrow, Ballya, & Cicchetti, 1984), and the Griffiths Mental Development Scales (Griffiths, 1984). Results of PDDBI were contrasted to each of these scales. For purposes of evaluating PDDBI for differential diagnosis, the contrasts with ADI-R and CARS are the most important. The PDDBI subscales and overall autism score showed statistically significant yet relatively low correlation coefficients with ADI-R algorithm scores and current behavior scores. While the coefficients may be reduced due to different scoring methods between PDDBI and ADI-R (Cohen, 2003), this does not explain the statistically significant yet relatively low correlation coefficients found between CARS and PDDBI ($r=0.53$ for parent ratings; $r=0.50$ for teacher ratings).

Overall PDDBI is a promising tool for use in differential diagnosis of ASDs. Cohen and his colleagues have invested substantial time developing and examining this instrument. The conceptual foundations of PDDBI fit well within the current understanding of autism as a spectrum disorder and scores are not relative to only one diagnosis (Autistic Disorder). Further, normative data is presented in the manual and scores are based upon standardized t-scores. However, relatively few studies have been conducted to explore the psychometric properties of PDDBI.

Social Responsiveness Scale

The Social Responsiveness Scale (SRS; Constantino & Gruber, 2005) measures the severity of autism spectrum symptoms as they occur in natural social settings. The SRS has been developed for use with children 4 to 18 years of age and places an emphasis on measuring symptoms across the full spectrum, particularly in the subthreshold for autistic disorder range. Administration time is reported to be 15–20 min. The SRS is a 65-item questionnaire that covers social awareness, social cognition, social communication, social motivation, and autistic mannerisms. While scores are provided for these five subscales, the primary interpretation of SRS centers on the total score of 65 items.

Constantino and Gruber (2005) have posited that reciprocal social behaviors are the *sine qua non* of all autism spectrum conditions. Essentially, what this does is center the distinguishing characteristics of ASD on reciprocal social behaviors, which would suggest the best tool for differential diagnosis is one that is focused upon the social aspects of this disorder. It is fitting then that SRS, which has primarily been developed as a diagnostic tool and screening instrument, focuses on social skills.

The SRS has been developed for use with children 4 to 18 years of age. Administration time is reported to be 15–20 min (Constantino & Gruber, 2005). The SRS development included a fairly large standardization sample ($N=1636$), which was a combination of five studies conducted throughout North America. Concerning the psychometric properties, internal consistency was excellent with all alpha coefficients above 0.9. Interrater reliability was also good with values ranging from 0.75 to 0.91. Temporal stability was measured over an average test-retest delay of 17 months. Ratings for males were more stable than for females, but both were in the acceptable-to-good range. Validation of the SRS was in regard to its use as a diagnostic instrument, as such, contrasts were made with other diagnostic scales (e.g. ADI-R). The SRS has shown good agreement with these diagnostic scales (Constantino & Gruber, 2005). Recently the utility of the SRS to assess for ASD symptoms rapidly has also been demonstrated (Constantino et al., 2007).

Due to the recent emphasis on early detection and diagnosis of autism, a preschool version of the SRS has been developed for children 36 to 48 months of age (Pine, Luby, Abbacchi, & Constantino, 2006). Test-retest reliability over a 1-month period fell in the acceptable range ($r=0.7$). No further examinations have been reported for this version.

The SRS has been used as a dependent variable in a number of research studies. Constantino and Todd (2003) report on autistic traits within the general population by measuring symptoms among twins. The continuous nature of SRS scores allowed for the full range of symptom severity to be examined. In another study evaluating autistic traits within twins, Constantino and Todd (2005) report on the presence of sub-threshold scores within parents of children with ASD showing greater SRS scores. The notion of genetic susceptibility has further been examined by Constantino et al. (2006) who evaluated SRS scores in proband sibling pairs. As with earlier studies, they found symptom scores to be continuously distributed with highest scores among siblings of children with autism. Constantino et al. (2004) used SRS and ADI-R to evaluate the factor structure of autism symptoms. They found that autism symptoms were best represented as falling along a single continuum and that varying degrees of severity across social communication, and stereotypical behavior domains was what best distinguished diagnostic clusters. The SRS has been used to assess ASD symptoms in non-ASD populations. Most recently, Pine, Guyer, Goldwin, Towbin, and Leibenluft (2008) reported on autism symptoms within children with mood and anxiety disorders.

Overall, SRS is a promising diagnostic instrument for ASD. While the items center on measuring social behaviors, these items have been shown to have good diagnostic utility. The scale has been included in many research studies, yet few have specifically examined the psychometric properties of the scale. Constantino and his colleagues have laid a good foundation in the development of this scale and it certainly warrants further attention by researchers.

General Assessment Discussion

Each of the diagnostic tools discussed have some evidence supporting their use for differential diagnosis. However, not all have equal support. Both ADOS and ADI-R have substantial research supporting their use. Yet, when comparing their psychometric properties to other scales discussed, they do not stand-out of the crowd as much as one would assume based upon their widespread use. Nonetheless, these scales are certainly accepted as the gold-standard by the research community. Further, while adequate psychometric properties are a requisite characteristic, it is not the only thing upon which to judge the utility of a diagnostic tool. For instance, all of these scales require some level of time to complete. The ADI-R is by far the lengthiest of these tools whereas the CHAT is the briefest.

A goal should be to create the most efficient tool in terms of administration time and training without losing excellent reliability and validity (Matson, 2007a). The best of both worlds will likely be between these two poles. Thus, one must judge the degree to which sensitivity and specificity are improved, if at all, with increased administration and training requirements.

For majority of studies discussed, diagnostic classifications made by targeted instrument are contrasted with clinical diagnoses based upon DSM-IV or ICD-10 criteria. Rarely though are the results of these instruments contrasted with one another. This is important to evaluate because conclusions about the diagnosis of a particular child may differ based upon which instrument was used.

The ADI-R and the CARS have been contrasted most frequently. The first report was by Lord (1995) who studied the stability of a diagnosis from 2 to 3 years of age. She reported a high level of agreement among the two instruments, but showing CARS to be less accurate in terms of over-diagnosis of autism. Later, Pilowsky, Yirmiya, Shulman, and Dover (1998) evaluated 70 individuals with suspected autism and found overall diagnostic agreement between CARS and ADI-R to be approximately 85%. Similar levels of diagnostic agreement between CARS and ADI-R have also been found (Stone et al., 1999). Most recently, Saemundsen, Magnússon, Smári, and Sigurdardóttir (2003) found a high correlation between ADI-R and CARS scores. Further, diagnostic classifications were also compared, showing an overall agreement of 67% when suggested diagnostic cut-off scores were used. However, when less stringent cut-off scores were used the agreement steadily increased to 83% and then to 94%. These authors also found similar results to Lord (1995) wherein CARS was more inclusive than ADI-R, with the suggested cut-off score classifying more children with autism than ADI-R.

Bishop and Norbury (2002) found poor agreement between diagnoses based upon ADI-R and ADOS-G. Part of this disagreement may be due to the format of the instrument, one being based upon caregiver report and one based upon direct observation. The tendency for the behavior analyst is undoubtedly to favor direct observation over caregiver report. However, this bias may not be without its faults. First, while observations allow for the child's behavior to be directly observed and scored, there is still a large degree of judgment as to what constitutes behavior indicative of ASD.

This is presumably the basis for requiring lengthy training and expertise in ASD to use measures such as the ADOS. It is not as simple as operationally defining a few discrete behaviors from which frequency data may be collected. An additional step of making inferences about generalized behavior repertoires from a limited sample of behaviors is required. It is this step of inference that is presumably effected by training and overall experience with ASDs. Further, the observations are typically made over a relatively short period during which a series of activities are used by the examiner to observe how the child responds. These "presses" have been expertly designed to elicit symptoms of autism, yet they are still a limited sample of the child's behavior. Indirect measures that use caregiver report have the advantage of sampling a much larger range of settings and occasions. Nonetheless, caregiver report measures are not without limitations either. It may be the case that the best diagnostic sensitivity and specificity may be found by incorporating both direct observation and caregiver report (Lord et al., 2006).

Matson, Nebel-Schwalm, and Matson (2007) have commented on the disparity between the argument for broader diagnostic methods that incorporate clinician judgment and what is actually practiced in research studies. Wherein the former suggests that clinical judgments are crucial to good diagnostic practices and the latter rarely includes these judgments in their studies. In one of the few empirical evaluations of diagnostic stability, Lord et al. (2006) found that clinicians identified children as having autism only 1% of the time when the ADI-R and PL-ADOS did not. Further, they found that 15% of children were classified as having autism when ADI-R or PL-ADOS had classified them as having autism. While the argument for incorporating clinician judgment has some rationale appeal, the question is an empirical one. Clinical judgment may add a level of confidence for the one making the diagnosis; however, the available literature does not support the notion that it is required for a stable or valid diagnosis. It is also likely that by adding in clinician judgment the overall reliability of the diagnostic decisions will change with and increases in variability depending upon the clinician's experience and expertise.

It is noteworthy that rarely do test developers present data describing the early stages of assessment development that includes the process of item selection and reliability at the item-level. This level of transparency is to be encouraged. Test manuals are rarely subject to peer-review. Thus while presenting this information in the test manual is applauded, it is not a substitute for publication of this process in a peer-reviewed journal.

The impact of differential diagnostic methods goes beyond simply determining which type of classification to place a child within. The area of ASD intervention research is also greatly impacted. As noted by Matson (2007b), one of the greatest limitations in ASD treatment research is in regard to assessment methods. An insistence upon using scales designed upon a categorical rather than quantitative approach has limited researchers in reporting actual changes in core symptoms of autism. Instead, what is common is to treat secondary outcomes such as changes in IQ scores as the primary dependent variable. This has led to some confusion and erroneous assumptions about what is actually being treated through intensive ABA programs. The actual core symptoms must be measured as the primary dependent variable for these studies.

Further, some ASD treatment outcome studies report diagnostic changes such as moving from an Autistic Disorder diagnosis to the less severe diagnosis of PDD-NOS. However, almost none of the measures discussed above have been evaluated outside the strict autism diagnosis. PDD-NOS and other ASD diagnoses have largely gone without development of assessment tools. Diagnostic tools such as ASD-D or PDDBI, which take into account the full spectrum of severity, will do much to advance treatment outcome studies by allowing a more sensitive measure of diagnostic change.

Conclusion and Future Directions

The implications of ASD differential diagnosis process for professionals in ABA have not been sufficiently discussed in general literature. At the current time, it is often the case that the professionals who diagnose ASDs are largely or completely separate from those who treat those who receive the diagnosis. For example, a family may go to a clinical psychologist for the diagnosis process and then later to an ABA provider for the treatment process. Unfortunately the field of clinical psychology, from which many professional diagnosticians hail, and the field of ABA, from which many ASD treatment providers hail, have historically suffered from a disconnect and this disconnect continues to exist to a significant degree. The historical and philosophical roots of this disconnect are beyond the scope of this chapter but we will briefly discuss some of its clinical implications here. In what follows, we will discuss the relevance of ASD differential diagnosis to the ABA professional and, in so doing, suggest some directions for future research and professional activity.

Prescriptive Function of Diagnosis

One of the reasons cited in favor of making a diagnosis is that diagnosis should prescribe treatment. If one is to base treatment prescription on the basis of which treatments possess the most scientific support, a diagnosis of autistic disorder or PDD NOS today would result in prescribing treatment in the form of early intensive behavioral intervention (Myers & Plauché Johnson, 2007; Rogers & Vismara, 2008). In the most basic sense, this system works; many thousands of children receive such diagnoses and many thousands then go on to receive appropriate intervention. However, each child is of course an individual, possessing highly unique arrays of problem behavior and unique deficits in behavioral skills repertoires. This is particularly so, given the fact that ASDs are pervasive in nature and affect many areas of human functioning. Comprehensive behavioral intervention programs must be tailored to the unique characteristics of each child and cannot, therefore, be a "cookie-cutter" approach. Given the combined complexities of the behavioral repertoires of each individual child and the behavioral intervention programs required for each child, a simple label of autistic disorder or PDD NOS does very little to actually prescribe treatment.

As we discussed earlier, a significant limitation to many of the diagnostic tools currently available and to the general diagnostic perspective is a tendency toward binary classification of the presence or absence of a disorder, and away from more qualitative evaluations of individuals' repertoires. It is hoped that future development of the diagnostic process will occur along the lines of providing more detailed information regarding individual client characteristics and repertoires. One area that differential diagnosis may come to provide more specific information on is about specific

behavioral repertoires. For example, a diagnosis of Autistic Disorder requires significant impairment in communication and ABA treatment providers therefore focus heavily on language. It is likely though that the effectiveness of ABA treatment providers would be enhanced if they were given more detailed information regarding which particular areas of language a particular client might excel in and which areas may require more focused treatment.

A second area where the diagnostic process might be enhanced to provide more prescriptive information is in the area of comorbid disorders. As discussed earlier in the chapter, scientific literature on comorbidities between ASDs and other psychiatric disorders is still in its infancy, but further development in this area may be of use to ABA professionals. For example, if the differential diagnosis process resulted in identifying severe attention deficits in a particular child with an ASD, then an ABA professional may benefit from focusing treatment on establishing a generalized repertoire of attending to relevant stimuli, more so than might be the case in a child with an ASD who does not suffer from such deficits. Similarly, if a child with an ASD suffers from a specific phobia, an ABA professional might do well to either address the phobia with focused treatment early on (if such treatment is within the realm of competence for the professional) or to avoid situations that might provoke challenging behaviors, which may otherwise simply be interpreted as noncompliance with instruction.

A third area in which the diagnostic process could be more prescriptive for treatment is to be found in further development of autism phenotypes. A complete discussion of further phenotyping of ASDs is beyond the scope of this chapter but many are calling for research of this type. It is possible that further subtypes of autism exist on the basis of physiological distinctions or behavioral distinctions (e.g., salience of different stimulus modalities, aberrations in basic behavioral processes such as conditioned reinforcement or habituation). Knowledge of distinctions between children in potential subcategories of ASDs may be critical to ABA professional because such distinctions may impact directly on how ABA treatment can be modified or further customized to optimize learning and avoid challenging behaviors. It is hoped that future research on further phenotyping ASDs will include the systematic production of information that will be of direct use to the treating clinician.

Funding for Treatment

A somewhat controversial topic is the issue of how ASD diagnoses interact with differential economic contingencies at the local, state, and federal levels. There is currently little or no funding available for ABA treatment for individuals with ASDs in most areas of the United States, and indeed, the rest of the world. In the small number of regions in which there is public funding available for such treatment, the availability of funding depends, of course, on an ASD diagnosis. However, funding contingencies often require a diagnosis of autistic disorder, excluding all other ASDs. At the present time, the vast majority of ABA treatment providers are either in private practice, are nonpublic schools, nonpublic agencies, or university-based clinics. In other words, comprehensive ABA treatment is not typically provided as a normal part of public schooling. Unfortunately, comprehensive ABA treatment is highly labor-intensive and costs are usually prohibitive in cases where public funding is not available. Therefore, in many areas, a clear contingency is in place; if a child receives a diagnosis of Autistic Disorder, then that child may receive effective treatment. If the child receives a diagnosis of another sort, then they may not. This contingency clearly places a high degree of importance on the validity of autism diagnosis. For this reason, diagnosticians must not compromise the assessment methods they employ. This places an even greater importance upon using instruments with sound psychometric properties that are also appropriate for measuring symptoms across the autism spectrum.

In conclusion, the process of differential diagnosis in ASDs is unfortunately separated to a large degree from the treatment process. Nevertheless, it has many implications for treatment. A shift in diagnostic philosophy and therefore practical tools from mere classification to a greater degree of emphasis on prescriptive evaluation of client characteristics would likely be useful to both the diagnostician and the provider of treatment and it is hoped that future research will progress in this direction.

References

Allen, D. A., & Rapin, I. (1992). Autistic children are also dysphasic. In H. Naruse & E. M. Ornitz (Eds.), *Nerobiology of infantile autism* (pp. 157–168). Amsterdam: Excerpta Medica.

Allison, C., Baron-Cohen, S., Wheelwright, S., Charman, T., Richler, J., Pasco, G., et al. (2008). The Q-CHAT (Quantitative CHecklist for Autism in Toddlers): A normally distributed quantitative measure of autistic traits at 18–24 months of age: Preliminary report. *Journal of Autism and Developmental Disorders, 38*, 1414–1425.

Aman, M. G., Tasse, M. J., Rojahn, J., & Hammer, D. (1996). The Nissonger CBRF: A child behavior rating form for children with developmental disabilities. *Research in Developmental Disabilities, 17*, 41–57.

American Psychiatric Association. (1987). *Diagnostic and statistical manual of mental disorders – revised* (3rd ed.). Washington, DC: Author.

American Psychiatric Association. (2000). *Diagnostic and statistical manual of mental disorders – fourth edition text revision (DSM-IV-TR)*. Washington, DC: Author.

Baron-Cohen, S., Allen, J., & Gillberg, C. (1992). Can autism be detected at 18 months?: The needle, the haystack and the CHAT. *British Journal of Psychiatry, 161*, 839–843.

Baron-Cohen, S., Cox, A., Baird, G., Swettenham, J., Nightingale, N., Morgan, K., et al. (1996). Psychological markers in the detection of autism in infancy in a large population. *British Journal of Psychiatry, 168*, 158–163.

Baron-Cohen, S., Wheelwright, S., Cox, A., Baird, G., Charman, T., Swettenham, J., et al. (2000). Early identification of autism by the CHecklist for Autism in Toddlers (CHAT). *Journal of the Royal Society of Medicine, 93*, 521–525.

Barrett, S., Prior, M., & Manjiviona, J. (2004). Children on the borderlands of autism: Differential characteristics in social, imaginative, communicative and repetitive behaviour domains. *Autism, 8*, 61–87.

Bartak, L., Rutter, M., & Cox, A. (1975). A comparative study of infantile autism and specific developmental receptive language disorder I: The children. *British Journal of Psychiatry, 126*, 127–145.

Berkson, G. (1967). Abnormal stereotyped motor acts. In J. Zubin & H. Hunt (Eds.), *Comparative psychology* (pp. 76–94). New York: Grune and Stratton.

Berkson, G. (1983). Repetitive stereotyped behaviors. *American Journal of Mental Deficiency, 88*, 239–246.

Bishop, S., Gahagan, S., & Lord, C. (2007). Re-examining the core features of autism: A comparison of autism spectrum disorder and fetal alcohol spectrum disorder. *Journal of Child Psychology and Psychiatry, 48*, 1111–1121.

Bishop, D. V. M., & Norbury, C. F. (2002). Exploring the borderlands of autistic disorder and specific language impairment: A study using standardized diagnostic instruments. *Journal of Child Psychology and Psychiatry, 43*, 917–929.

Bodfish, J. W., Symons, F. J., Parker, D. E., & Lewis, M. H. (2000). Varieties of repetitive behavior in autism: Comparisons to mental retardation. *Journal of Autism and Developmental Disorders, 30*, 237–243.

Buitelaar, J. K., & Van der Gaag, R. (1998). Diagnostic rules for children with PDD-NOS and multiple complex developmental disorders. *Journal of Child Psychology and Psychiatry, 39*, 911–919.

Buitelaar, J. K., Van der Gaag, R., Klin, A., & Volkmar, F. (1999). Exploring the boundaries of pervasive developmental disorder not otherwise specified: Analyses of data from the DSM-IV autistic disorder field trial. *Journal of Autism and Developmental Disorders, 29*, 33–43.

Campbell, D. T., & Fiske, D. W. (1959). Convergent and discriminant validation by the multitrait-multimethod matrix. *Psychological Bulletin, 56*, 81–105.

Cantwell, D., Baker, L., & Rutter, M. (1978). A comparative study of infantile autism and specific developmental receptive language disorder IV: Analysis of syntax and language function. *Journal of Child Psychology and Psychiatry, 19*, 351–362.

Center for Disease Control and prevention. (2007). Prevalence of autism spectrum disorders autism and developmental disabilities monitoring network, six sites, United States, 2000; Prevalence of autism spectrum disorders autism and developmental disabilities monitoring network, 14 sites, United States, 2002; and Evaluation of a methodology for a collaborative multiple source surveillance network for autism spectrum disorders autism and developmental disabilities monitoring network, 14 sites, United States, 2002. *Surveillance Summaries, 56*, 1–40.

Charman, T., Taylor, E., Drew, A., Cockerill, H., Brown, J., & Baird, G. (2005). Outcome at 7 years of children diagnosed with autism at age 2: Predictive validity of assessments conducted at 2 and 3 years of age and pattern of symptom change over time. *Journal of Child Psychology and Psychiatry, 46*, 500–513.

Cichetti, D. V. (1994). Guidelines, criteria, and rule of thumb for evaluating normed and standardized assessment instruments in psychology. *Psychological Assessment, 6*, 284–290.

Cohen, I. L. (2003). Criterion-related validity of the PDD Behavior Inventory. *Journal of Autism and Developmental Disorders, 33*, 47–53.

Cohen, I. L., Schmidt-Lackner, S., Romanczyk, R., & Sudhalter, V. (2003). The PDD Behavior Inventory: A rating scale for assessing response to intervention in children with pervasive developmental disorder. *Journal of Autism and Developmental Disorders, 33*, 31–45.

Cohen, I. L., & Sudhalter, V. (1999). *PDD Behavior Inventory: Professional manual*. Lutz, FL: Psychological Assessment Resources.

Constantino, J. N., Davis, S. A., Todd, R. D., Schindler, M. K., Gross, M. M., et al. (2003). Validation of a brief quantitative measure of autistic traits: Comparison of the social responsiveness scale with the Autism Diagnostic Interview – Revised. *Journal of Autism and Developmental Disorders, 33*, 427–433.

Constantino, J. N., & Gruber, C. P. (2005). *The social responsiveness scale manual*. Los Angeles: Western Psychological Services.

Constantino, J. N., Gruber, C. P., Davis, S., Hayes, S., Passanante, N., & Przybeck, T. (2004). The factor structure of autistic traits. *Journal of Child Psychology and Psychiatry, 45*, 719–726.

Constantino, J. N., Lajonchere, C., Lutz, M., Gray, T., Abbacchi, A., et al. (2006). Autistic social impairment in the siblings of children with pervasive developmental disorders. *American Journal of Psychiatry, 163*, 294–296.

Constantino, J. N., LaVesser, P. D., Zhang, Y., Abbacchi, A. M., Gray, T., & Todd, R. D. (2007). Rapid quantitative assessment of autistic social impairment by classroom teachers. *Journal of the American Academy of Child and Adolescent Psychiatry, 46*, 1668–1676.

Constantino, J. N., & Todd, R. D. (2003). Autistic traits in the general population: A twin study. *Archives of General Psychiatry, 60*, 524–530.

Constantino, J. N., & Todd, R. D. (2005). Intergenerational transmission of subthreshold autistic traits in the general population. *Biological Psychiatry, 57*, 655–660.

Cox, A., Klein, K., Charman, T., Baird, G., Baron-Cohen, S., et al. (1999). Autism spectrum disorders at 20 and 42 months of age: Stability of clinical and ADI-R diagnosis. *Journal of Child Psychology and Psychiatry, 40*, 719–732.

Creak, M. (1961). Schizophrenia syndrome in childhood: Progress report of a working party. *Cerebral Palsy Bulletin, 3*, 501–504.

Creak, M. (1964). *Infantile autism*. Englewood Cliffs, NJ: Prentice-Hall.

Crocker, L., & Algina, F. (1986). *Introduction to classical & modern test theory*. Belmont, CA: Wadsworth.

Cunningham, A. B., & Schreibman, L. (2008). Stereotypy in autism: The importance of function. *Research in Autism Spectrum Disorders, 2*, 469–479.

de Bruin, E. I., Ferdinand, R. F., Meester, S., de Nijs, P. F. A., & Verheij, F. (2007). High rates of psychiatric co-morbidity in PDD-NOS. *Journal on Autism and Developmental Disorders, 37*, 877–886.

DiLavore, P., Lord, C., & Rutter, M. (1995). Pre-linguistic autism diagnostic observation schedule. *Journal of Autism and Developmental Disorders, 25*, 355–379.

Eaves, R. C., Campbell, H. A., & Chambers, D. (2000). Criterion-related and construct validity of the pervasive developmental disorders rating scale and the Autism Behavior Checklist. *Psychology in the Schools, 37*, 311–321.

Eaves, R. C., Woods-Groves, S., Williams, T. O., Jr., & Fall, A. (2006). Reliability and validity of the "Pervasive Developmental Disorders Rating Scale" and the "Gilliam Autism Rating Scale". *Education and Training in Developmental Disabilities, 41*, 300–309.

Garfin, D. G., McCallon, D., & Cox, R. (1988). Validity and reliability of the Childhood Autism Rating Scale with autistic adolescents. *Journal of Autism and Developmental Disorders, 18*, 367–378.

Gilliam, J. E. (1995). *Gilliam autism rating scale*. Austin, TX: Pro-Ed.

Gilliam, J. E. (2006). *Gilliam autism rating scale* (2nd ed.). TX: Pro-ed.

Griffiths, R. (1984). *The abilities of young children: A comprehensive system of mental measurement for the first eight years of life* (revised edition). Bucks, UK: A.R.I.C.D. The Test Agency Limited.

Heflin, L. J., & Alaimo, D. F. (2006). *Students with autism spectrum disorders*. Columbus, OH: Pearson Prentice Hall.

Hill, J., & Furniss, F. (2006). Patterns of emotional and behavioural disturbance associated with autistic traits in young people with severe intellectual disabilities and challenging behaviours. *Research in Developmental Disabilities, 27*, 517–528.

Howlin, P. (2003). Outcome in high-functioning adults with autism with and without early language delays: Implications for the differentiation between autism and Asperger syndrome. *Journal of Autism and Developmental Disorders, 33*, 3–13.

Kanner, L. (1943). Autistic disturbance of affective contact. *Nervous Child, 2*, 217–250.

Koyama, T., Tachimori, H., Osada, H., & Kurita, H. (2006). Cognitive and symptom profiles in high-functioning pervasive developmental disorder not otherwise specified and attention-deficit/hyperactivity disorder. *Journal of Autism and Developmental Disorders, 36*, 373–380.

Krug, D. A., Arick, J., & Almond, P. (1980). Behavior checklist for identifying severely handicapped individuals with high levels of autistic behavior. *Journal of Child Psychology and Psychiatry, 21*, 221–229.

Krug, D. A., Arick, J., & Almond, P. (1993). *Autism Screening Instrument for Educational Planning (ASIEP)*. Austin, TX: Pro-Ed.

Krug, D. A., Arick, J. R., & Almond, P. J. (2008). *Autism Screening Instrument for Educational Planning: Third Edition (ASIEP-3)*. Austin, TX: Pro-Ed.

La Malfa, G., Lassi, S., Bertelli, M., Salvini, R., & Placidi, G. F. (2004). Autism and intellectual disability: A study of prevalence on a sample of the Italian population. *Journal of Intellectual Disability Research, 48*, 262–267.

Le Couteur, A., Rutter, M., Lord, C., Rios, P., Robertson, S., Holdgrafer, M., et al. (1989). Autism diagnostic interview: A semistructured interview for parents and caregivers of autistic persons. *Journal of Autism and Developmental Disorders, 19*, 363–387.

Lecavalier, L. (2005). An evaluation of the Gilliam Autism Rating Scale. *Journal of Autism and Developmental Disorders, 35*, 795–805.

Lerea, L. E. (1987). The behavioral assessment of autistic children. In D. J. Cohen, A. M. Donnellan & R. Paul (Eds.), *Handbook of autism and pervasive developmental disorders* (pp. 273–288). New York: Wiley.

Lewis, M. H., & Baumeister, A. A. (1982). Stereotyped mannerisms in mentally retarded persons: Animal models and theoretical analyses. In N. R. Ellis (Ed.), *International review of research in mental retardation* (pp. 123–161). New York: Academic Press.

Lord, C. (1995). Follow-up of two-year-olds referred for possible autism. *Journal of Child Psychology and Psychiatry, 36*, 1365–1382.

Lord, C., Risi, S., DiLavore, P. S., Shulman, C., Thurm, A., & Pickles, A. (2006). Autism from 2 to 9 years of age. *Archives of General Psychiatry, 63*, 694–701.

Lord, C., Risi, S., Lambrecht, L., Cook, E. H., Leventhal, B. L., et al. (2000). The autism diagnostic observation schedule-generic: A standard measure of social and communication deficits associated with the spectrum of autism. *Journal of Autism and Developmental Disorders, 30*, 205–223.

Lord, C., Rutter, M., DiLavore, P. C., & Risi, S. (1999). *Autism diagnostic observation schedule*. Los Angeles: Western Psychological Services.

Lord, C., Rutter, M., Goode, S., Heemsbergen, J., Jordan, H., Mawhood, L., et al. (1989). Autism diagnostic observation schedule: A standardized observation of communicative and social behavior. *Journal of Autism and Developmental Disorders, 19*, 185–212.

Lord, C., Rutter, M., & Le Couteur, A. (1994). Autism Diagnostic Interview – Revised: A revised version of a diagnostic interview for caregivers of individuals with possible pervasive developmental disorders. *Journal of Autism and Developmental Disorders, 24*, 659–686.

Lord, C., Storoschuk, S., Rutter, M., & Pickles, A. (1993). Using the ADI-R to diagnose autism in preschool children. *Infant Mental Health Journal, 14*, 234–252.

Lotter, V. (1974). Factors related to outcome in autistic children. *Autism and Childhood Schizophrenia, 4*, 263–276.

Lovaas, I. O., Freitag, G., Gold, V. J., & Kassorla, I. C. (1965). Recording apparatus and procedure for observation of behaviors of children in free play setting. *Journal of Experimental Child Psychology, 2*, 108–120.

Lovaas, I. O., Koegel, R., Simmons, J. Q., & Long, J. S. (1973). Some generalization and follow-up measures on autistic children in behavior therapy. *Journal of Applied Behavioral Analysis, 6*, 131–166.

Luteijn, E. F., Serra, M., Jackson, S., Steenhuis, M. P., Althaus, M., Volkmar, F., et al. (2000). How unspecified are disorders of children with a pervasive developmental disorder not otherwise specified? A study of social problems in children with PDD-NOS and ADHD. *European Child & Adolescent Psychiatry, 9*, 168–179.

Magyar, C. I., & Pandolfi, V. (2007). Factor structure evaluation of the childhood autism rating scale. *Journal of Autism and Developmental Disorders, 37*, 1787–1794.

Matson, J. L. (2007a). Current status of differential diagnosis for children with autism spectrum disorders. *Research in Developmental Disabilities, 28*, 109–118.

Matson, J. L. (2007b). Determining treatment outcome in early intervention programs for autism spectrum disorders: A critical analysis of measurement issues in learning based interventions. *Research in Developmental Disabilities, 28*, 207–218.

Matson, J. L., & Boisjoli, J. A. (2007). Differential diagnosis of PDD-NOS in children. *Research in Autism Spectrum Disorders, 1*, 75–84.

Matson, J. L., & Boisjoli, J. A. (2008). Strategies for assessing Asperger's syndrome: A critical review of data based methods. *Research in Autism Spectrum Disorders, 2*, 237–248.

Matson, J., Boisjoli, J., González, M., Smith, K., & Wilkins, J. (2007). Norms and cut off scores for the autism spectrum disorders diagnosis for adults (ASD-DA) with intellectual disability. *Research in Autism Spectrum Disorders, 1*, 330–338.

Matson, J. L., Dempsey, T., LoVullo, S. V., & Wilkins, J. (2008). The effects of intellectual functioning on the range of core symptoms of autism spectrum disorders. *Research in Developmental Disabilities, 29*, 341–350.

Matson, J. L., & González, M. (2007). *Autism spectrum disorders – child version: Administrator's manual*. Baton Rouge, LA: Disability Consultants.

Matson, J.L., González, M.L., & Wilkins, J. (2009). Validity study of the Autism Spectrum Disorders-Diagnostic for Children (ASD-DC), *Research in Autism Spectrum Disorders, 3*, 196–206.

Matson, J. L., González, M. L., Wilkins, J., & Rivet, T. T. (2008). Reliability of the Autism Spectrum Disorders-Diagnostic for Children (ASD-DC). *Research in Autism Spectrum Disorders, 2*, 533–545.

Matson, J. L., & Nebel-Schwalm, M. S. (2007). Comorbid psychopathology with autism spectrum disorder in children: An overview. *Research in Developmental Disabilities, 28*, 341–352.

Matson, J. L., Nebel-Schwalm, M. S., & Matson, M. L. (2007). A review of methodological issues in the differential diagnosis of autism spectrum disorders in children. *Research in Autism Spectrum Disorders, 1*, 38–54.

Matson, J. L., & Wilkins, J. (2007). A critical review of assessment targets and methods for social skills excesses and deficits for children with autism spectrum disorders. *Research in Autism Spectrum Disorders, 1*, 28–37.

Matson, J. L., & Wilkins, J. (2008). Nosology and diagnosis of Asperger's syndrome. *Research in Autism Spectrum Disorders, 2*, 288–300.

Matson, J. L., Wilkins, J., Boisjoli, J. A., & Smith, K. R. (2008). The validity of the autism spectrum disorders diagnosis for intellectually disabled adults (ASD-DA), *Research in Developmental Disabilities, 29*, 537–546.

Matson, J. L., Wilkins, J., & Gonzalez, M. (2008). Early identification and diagnosis in autism spectrum disorders in young children and infants: How early is too early? *Research in Autism Spectrum Disorders, 2*, 75–84.

Mildenberger, K., Sitter, S., Noterdaeme, M., & Amorosa, H. (2001). The use of the ADI-R as a diagnostic tool in the differential diagnosis of children with infantile autism and children with receptive language disorder. *European Child & Adolescent Psychiatry, 10*, 248–255.

Moore, V., & Goodson, S. (2003). How well does early diagnosis of autism stand the test of time? *Autism, 7*, 47–62.

Myers, S. M., & Plauché Johnson, C. (2007). Management of children with autism spectrum disorders. *Pediatrics, 120*, 1162–1182.

National Institutes of Health (2008). National database for autism research: Data submission. Retrieved September 11, 2008 from http://ndar.nih.gov/ndarpublicweb/datasubmission.go

National Society for Autistic Children. (1978). National Society for Autistic Children definition of the syndrome of autism. *Journal of Autism and Developmental Disorders, 8*, 162–167.

Noterdaeme, M., Sitter, S., Mildenberger, K., & Amorosa, H. (2000). Diagnostic assessment of communicative and interactive behaviours in children with autism and receptive language disorder. *European Child & Adolescent Psychiatry, 9*, 295–300.

Ozonoff, S., Goodlin-Jones, B. L., & Solomon, M. (2005). Evidence-based assessment of autism spectrum disorders in children and adolescents. *Journal of Clinical Child and Adolescent Psychology, 34*, 523–540.

Parks, S. L. (1983). The assessment of autistic children: A selective review of available instruments. *Journal of Autism and Developmental Disorders, 13*, 255–267.

Pilowsky, T., Yirmiya, N., Shulman, C., & Dover, R. (1998). The Autism Diagnostic Interview – Revised and the childhood autism rating scale: Differences between diagnostic systems and comparison between genders. *Journal of Autism and Developmental Disorders, 28*, 143–151.

Pine, D. S., Guyer, A. E., Goldwin, M., Towbin, K. A., & Leibenluft, E. (2008). Autism spectrum disorder scale scores in pediatric mood and anxiety disorder. *Journal of the American Academy of Child and Adolescent Psychiatry, 47*, 652–661.

Pinc, E., Luby, J., Abbacchi, A., & Constantino, J. N. (2006). Quantitative assessment of autistic symptomatology in preschoolers. *Autism, 10*, 344–352.

Prior, M., Eisenmajer, R., Leekam, S., Wing, L., Gould, J., Ong, B., et al. (1998). Are there subgroups within the autism spectrum? A cluster analysis of a group of children with autistic spectrum disorder. *Journal of Child Psychology and Psychiatry, 39*, 893–902.

Rapin, I. (1996). Practitioner review: Developmental language disorders: A clinical update. *Journal of Child Psychology and Psychiatry, 37*, 643–655.

Rapin, I. (1997). Autism. *New England Journal of Medicine, 337*, 97–104.

Rapp, J. T., & Vollmer, T. R. (2005a). Stereotypy I: A review of behavioral assessment and treatment. *Research in Developmental Disabilities, 26*, 527–547.

Rapp, J. T., & Vollmer, T. R. (2005b). Stereotypy II: A review of neurobiological interpretations and suggestions for an integration with behavioral methods. *Research in Developmental Disabilities, 26*, 548–564.

Reichler, R. J., & Schopler, E. (1971). Observation on the nature of human relatedness. *Journal of Autism and Childhood Schizophrenia, 1*, 283–296.

Rellini, E., Tortolani, D., Trillo, S., Carbone, S., & Montecchi, F. (2004). Childhood Autism Rating Scale (CARS) and Autism Behavior Checklist (ABC) correspondence and conflicts with DSM-IV criteria in diagnosis of autism. *Journal of Autism and Developmental Disorders, 34*, 703–708.

Rendle-Short, J., & Clangy, H. G. (1968). Infantile autism. *Medical Journal of Australia, 1*, 921–922.

Rimland, B. (1964). *Infantile autism*. Englewood Cliffs, NJ: Prentice-Hall.

Rimland, B. (1971). The differentiation of childhood psychoses: An analysis of checklists for 2,218 psychotic children. *Journal of Autism and Childhood Schizophrenia, 1*, 161–174.

Ritvo, E. R., & Freeman, B. J. (1978). National Society for Autistic Children definition of autism. *Journal of Autism and Developmental Disorders, 8*, 162–167.

Robins, D. L., Fein, D., Barton, M. L., & Green, J. A. (2001). The modified checklist for autism in toddlers: An initial study investigating the early detection of autism and pervasive developmental disorders. *Journal of Autism and Developmental Disorders, 31*, 131–144.

Rogers, S. J., & Vismara, L. A. (2008). Evidence-based comprehensive treatments for early autism. *Journal of Clinical Child & Adolescent Psychology, 37*, 8–38.

Ross, L. L., Yu, D., & Kropla, W. C. (1998). Stereotyped behavior in developmentally delayed or autistic populations: Rhythmic or non rhythmic? *Behavior Modification, 22*, 321–334.

Ruttenberg, B. A., Dratmann, M. L., Fraknoi, J., & Wemar, C. (1966). An instrument for evaluating autistic children. *American Academy of Child Psychiatry, 5*, 453–478.

Rutter, M. (1978). Diagnosis and definition of childhood autism. *Journal of Autism and Developmental Disorders, 8*, 139–161.

Rutter, M., Greenfeld, D., & Lockyer, L. (1967). A five to fifteen year follow-up study of infantile psychosis II: Social and behavioural outcome. *British Journal of Psychiatry, 113*, 1183–1199.

Rutter, M., Le Couteur, A., & Lord, C. (2003). *Autism Diagnostic Interview Revised: WPS edition manual*. Los Angeles: Western Psychological Services.

Saemundsen, E., Magnússon, P., Smári, J., & Sigurdardóttir, S. (2003). Autism Diagnostic Interview – Revised and the childhood autism rating scale: Convergence and discrepancy in diagnosing autism. *Journal of Autism and Developmental Disorders, 33*, 319–328.

Schopler, E., Reichler, R. J., DeVellis, R. F., & Daly, K. (1980). Toward objective classification of childhood autism: Childhood Autism Rating Scale (CARS). *Journal of Autism and Developmental Disorders, 10*, 91–103.

Schopler, E., Reichler, R. J., & Renner, B. R. (1988). *The childhood autism rating scale.* Los Angeles: Western Psychological Services.

Sciutto, M. J., & Cantwell, C. (2005). Factors influencing the differential diagnosis of asperger's disorder and high-functioning autism. *Journal of Developmental and Physical Disabilities, 17*, 345–359.

Sevin, J. A., Matson, J. L., Coe, D. A., Fee, V. E., & Sevin, B. M. (1991). A comparison and evaluation of three commonly used autism scales. *Journal of Autism and Developmental Disorders, 21*, 417–432.

Shields, J., Varley, R., Broks, P., & Simpson, A. (1996a). Hemispheric function in developmental language disorders and high-level autism. *Developmental Medicine and Child Neurology, 38*, 473–486.

Shields, J., Varley, R., Broks, P., & Simpson, A. (1996b). Social cognition in developmental language disorders and high-level autism. *Developmental Medicine and Child Neurology, 38*, 487–495.

Smith, E. A., & Van Houten, R. (1996). A comparison of the characteristics of self-stimulatory behaviors in normal children and child with developmental delays. *Research in Developmental Disabilities, 17*, 254–268.

South, M., Williams, B. J., McMahon, W. M., Owley, T., Filipek, P. A., et al. (2002). Utility of the Gilliam Autism Rating Scale in research and clinical populations. *Journal of Autism and Developmental Disorders, 32*, 593–599.

Sparrow, S. S., Ballya, D. A., & Cicchetti, D. V. (1984). *Vineland adaptive behavior scales: Interview edition, survey form manual.* Circle Pines, MN: American Guidance.

Stone, W. L., Lee, E. B., Ashfod, L., Brissie, J., Hepburn, S. L., et al. (1999). Can autism be diagnosed accurately in children under 3 years? *Journal of Child Psychology and Psychiatry, 2*, 219–226.

Sturmey, P., Matson, J., & Sevin, J. (1992). Analysis of the internal consistency of three autism scales. *Journal of Autism and Developmental Disorders, 22*, 321–328.

Tidmarsh, L., & Volkmar, F. R. (2003). Diagnosis and epidemiology of autism spectrum disorders. *Canadian Journal of Psychiatry, 48*, 517–525.

Tryon, P. A., Mayes, S. D., Rhodes, R. L., & Waldo, M. (2006). Can Asperger's disorder be differentiated from autism using DSM-IV criteria? *Focus on Autism and Other Developmental Disabilities, 21*, 2–6.

Tuchman, R. F., Rapin, I., & Shinnar, S. (1991). Autistic dysphasic children I: Clinical characteristics. *Pediatrics, 88*, 1211–1218.

Verté, S., Geurts, H. M., Roeyers, H., Oosterlaan, J., & Sergeant, J. A. (2006). Executive functioning in children with an autism spectrum disorder: Can we differentiate within the spectrum? *Journal of Autism and Developmental Disorders, 36*, 351–372.

Verté, S., Geurts, H. M., Roeyers, H., Rosseel, Y., Oosterlaan, J., & Sergeant, J. A. (2006). Can the children's communication checklist differentiate autism spectrum subtypes? *Autism, 10*, 266–287.

Volkmar, F. R., Cicchetti, D. V., Dykens, E., Sparrow, S. S., Leckman, J. F., & Cohen, D. J. (1988). An evaluation of the Autism Behavior Checklist. *Journal of Autism and Developmental Disorders, 18*, 81–97.

Volkmar, F. R., Lord, C., Bailey, A., Schultz, R. T., & Klin, A. (2004). Autism and pervasive developmental disorders. *Journal of Child Psychology and Psychiatry, 45*, 135–170.

Wadden, N. P., Bryson, S. E., & Rodger, R. S. (1991). A closer look at the Autism Behavior Checklist: Discriminant validity and factor structure. *Journal of Autism and Developmental Disorders, 21*, 529–541.

Wing, L. (1998). The history of Asperger syndrome. In E. Schopler, G. B. Mesibov & L. J. Kunce (Eds.), *Asperger syndrome or high-functioning autism?* (pp. 11–28). New York: Plenum.

Yirmiya, N., Sigman, M., & Freeman, B. J. (1994). Comparison between diagnostic instruments for identifying high-functioning children with autism. *Journal of Autism and Developmental Disorders, 24*, 281–291.

Yoshida, Y., & Uchiyama, T. (2004). The clinical necessity for assessing Attention Deficit/Hyperactivity Disorder (AD/HD) symptoms in children with high-functioning Pervasive Developmental Disorder (PDD). *European Child & Adolescent Psychiatry, 13*, 307–314.

Chapter 6
Communication

Jeff Sigafoos, Ralf W. Schlosser, Mark F. O'Reilly, and Giulio E. Lancioni

Communication impairment is a core deficit associated with autism spectrum disorder (ASD). Therefore, it should not be surprising that this topic has become a major thrust of assessment and treatment in applied behavior analysis (ABA). The types of communication skills to target for intervention and the behavioral assessment methods that can be used to identify these target behaviors are reviewed in this chapter. We also review historical and contemporary trends in the provision of communication intervention for individuals with ASD. An analysis of the strengths and weaknesses of the literature will be discussed. Communication makes up one of the three core blocks of symptoms that make up ASD. Therefore, it should not be surprising that this topic has become a major thrust of assessment and treatment in the ABA literature. Types of behavior targets and methods used to do so, along with a review of the relevant research on key interventions, will be covered. An analysis of the strengths and weaknesses of the literature will be discussed.

Introduction

Communication is a major area of need for children with autism spectrum disorder (ASD). This need stems from the fact that ASD is associated with significant, persistent, and often unique types of communication deficits and excesses (Osterling, Dawson, & McPartland, 2001). Significant and distinctive impairments in speech, language, and communication development are among the first and most obvious characteristics of ASD (Landa,

2007). In fact, the nature and extent of the child's communication impairment figures heavily in the definition, diagnosis, and classification of autism and related developmental disorders (American Psychiatric Association, 2000; World Health Organization, 2007).

Given that ASD is defined in part by the nature and extent of communication impairment, it is inevitable that practitioners will be confronted with the challenge to design and implement effective communication interventions for children who are diagnosed within the autism spectrum of developmental disorders. Indeed, delayed or impaired communication development is one of the main reasons why children with ASD, or those who are suspected of having ASD, are referred for assessment and treatment (Tager-Flusberg, Paul, & Lord, 2005). To accept such referrals, practitioners require an understanding of the nature and types of communication impairment associated with ASD and competence in the provision of evidence-based communication intervention for this population.

This chapter aims to guide practitioners in designing and implementing effective communication intervention for children with ASD. To this end, we first describe the nature and types of communication impairment associated with ASD. Following this, we review historical antecedents that have influenced contemporary practice. This review sets the stage for describing several trends that have influenced contemporary approaches to communication intervention for children with ASD. These trends include the use of multimodal communication, functional curriculum, and flexible teaching arrangements. An emerging trend is the integration of intervention procedures based on applied behavior analysis (ABA) with principles of evidence-based practice. Our focus on ABA-based interventions is justified because this approach has strong empirical support and a long history of success for improving communication behavior in children with ASD (Charlop-Christy,

J. Sigafoos (✉)
School of Educational Psychology, Victoria University of Wellington, PO Box 17-310, Karori, Wellington, New Zealand
e-mail: jeff.sigafoos@vuw.ac.nz

J.L. Matson (ed.), *Applied Behavior Analysis for Children with Autism Spectrum Disorders*,
DOI 10.1007/978-1-4419-0088-3_6, © Springer Science+Business Media, LLC 2009

Malmberg, Rocha, & Schreibman, 2008; Landa, 2007; LeBlanc, Esch, Sidener, & Firth, 2006; Lovaas, 1977, 2003; Machalicek et al., 2008). In light of this strong empirical support, ABA-based procedures are a key component in evidence-based communication intervention for children with ASD. By integrating contemporary ABA-based approaches with the evolving evidence-based practice movement, practitioners may be more successful in addressing the communication needs of children with ASD (Ogletree, 2007).

Communication Impairment in Children with ASD

Practitioners are likely to require competence in using a wide range of ABA-based procedures to address the communication needs of children with ASD (Ogletree, 2007). The need for wide-ranging competence stems from two related facts: First, ASD is not a homogenous condition, but rather covers three more specific conditions: (a) Autistic Disorder, (b) Asperger syndrome, and (c) Pervasive Developmental Disorder Not Otherwise Specified (PDD-NOS) (National Institute of Child Health and Human Development, 2007). While each of these conditions is associated with communication impairment, the nature and severity of impairment differs in certain general ways across these three diagnostic categories. Specifically, communication impairment is comparatively subtle in Asperger syndrome and PDD-NOS (e.g., lack of conversational turn-taking), but more obvious and pronounced in Autistic Disorder (American Psychiatric Association, 2000). Second, even within each of these three categories, individual children will present with varying degrees of speech development and communication impairment (Anderson et al., 2007). Many children with a diagnosis of Autistic Disorder – perhaps up to 50% – are essentially mute, for example, while others may acquire speech that appears nonfunctional and largely echolalic (Charlop-Christy et al., 2008; National Research Council, 2001). Table 6.1 provides a summary of the general nature of communication impairment associated with Autistic Disorder, Asperger syndrome, and PDD-NOS.

The nature and types of each child's communication deficits and excesses are important factors to consider in treatment planning. Children with little or no speech, for example, also tend to be those with more severe intellectual disability. These children are generally more difficult to teach and consequently might initially require more intensive and structured one-to-one intervention in order to acquire new communication skills (Duker, Didden, & Sigafoos, 2004).

It is often the case that intervention for children without speech and more severe communicative impairment will initially focus on teaching basic requesting and rejecting skills, such as requesting access to preferred objects or rejecting the offer of a nonpreferred object (Reichle, York, & Sigafoos, 1991). Such skills are highly functional for the child in that they provide a means to access reinforcement and exert some degree of control over the environment. These are considered beginning communication skills because they are among the first to emerge in typically developing children (Carpenter, Mastergeorge, & Coggins, 1983).

Developmental studies show that prior to the emergence of speech, typically developing children will often use a variety of prelinguistic acts (e.g., vocalizations, facial expressions, gestures) to request and reject objects

Table 6.1 Overview of communication deficits and excesses associated with ASD[a]

Disorder	Description of communication deficits and excess
Autistic disorder	Speech is substantially delayed and about 50% of children fail to acquire speech. Those that acquire speech often have fluency problems and use it in a nonfunctional, stereotyped, or ritualistic manner. The child may simply repeat others (echolalia) or perseverate on words or phrases. Spontaneous communication is often lacking. Communicative attempts are mainly for instrumental (e.g., requesting), rather than social (e.g., conversational) purposes. The child may fail to respond to other's speech indicating significant deficits in receptive language.
Asperger syndrome	Speech is not obviously delayed, but social deficits are apparent during communicative interactions. The child may pursue preferred topics of conversation in detail and shows deficits in many of the paralinguistic aspects of communication, such as personal space, use of facial expression and gestures to convey meaning, and grammatical intonation. The child may have considerable difficulty in conversational exchanges, such as knowing when and how to terminate conversations appropriately.
PDD-NOS	Communication impairments are similar to but less severe than in Asperger syndrome. Conversations often focus on a limited range of idiosyncratic topics. The child may not seem to enjoy conversation with others and may appear anxious and awkward when engaged in social communication.

[a]Based on American Psychiatric Association (2000), Anderson et al. (2007), and Landa (2007)

and activities (Bates, Camaioni, & Volterra, 1975). These types of informal and idiosyncratic prelinguistic acts tend to become less frequent as children acquire speech and more formal communicative gestures. For children with ASD who fail to acquire speech and more formal gestures, it is necessary to directly teach alternative forms of communication to replace existing prelinguistic acts. For this purpose, the alternative form or mode of communication could involve the use of manual signs, picture-exchange, pointing to graphic symbols on a communication board, or use of an electronic speech-generating device (Beukelman & Mirenda, 2005; Reichle et al., 1991; Schlosser, 2003).

This replacement-based treatment approach is often indicated because the reliance on informal or idiosyncratic prelinguistic acts can be limiting and socially stigmatizing for the child (Keen, Sigafoos, & Woodyatt, 2001). For example, children with ASD who lack speech will often communicate a request by leading an adult's hand to a desired item. This autistic leading is obviously limited to situations where an adult is in close proximity. Autistic leading can also be stigmatizing and socially unacceptable, especially when used by older children and when attempting to communicate with unfamiliar listeners. Some prelinguistic acts are also unacceptable (e.g., tantrums, self-injury) and must therefore be replaced with more appropriate forms of communication. Even when the form of the prelinguistic act is not necessarily problematic (e.g., vocalizing, facial expression), such behaviors can often be difficult for listeners to interpret, and hence the child may fail to gain reinforcement unless they learn more easily recognized forms of communication.

Other types of communicative impairments, such as echolalia, signal a higher level of speech development and better prognosis in terms of outcomes from ABA-based intervention approaches. Children who acquire some speech before the age of 5 years, for example, typically show better gains from intensive behavioral intervention than children who remain nonspeaking (Lovaas, 1987; McEachin, Smith, & Lovaas, 1993; Sallows & Graupner, 2005). For children who present with speech, more advanced communication interventions are indicated. Advanced communication interventions emphasize the acquisition of new and more complex speech and language skills as well as bringing existing speech under appropriate stimulus control (Lovaas, 2003).

One of the more perplexing communication impairments associated with ASD is the lack of spontaneous communication (Halle, 1987). Even when the child has acquired a large repertoire of communicative responses, it is often the case that these responses rarely occur in natural routines unless the child is prompted to communicate by an adult. This prompt dependency obviously makes communication less functional for the child. For example, instead of requesting a drink when thirsty, the child may only make such requests when an adult approaches with a preferred beverage and explicitly prompts the child to make a request (e.g., "Tell me what you want?"). This lack of spontaneous communication is surprising especially in relation to requesting preferred objects. In such cases, the lack of spontaneous requesting does not appear to stem from any lack of motivation. Instead, the lack of spontaneity may stem from narrow stimulus control, as noted by Halle (1987). That is, the child may have learned to communicate only under very precise training conditions that include prompts from adults.

Fortunately, research in ABA has generated a number of effective procedures that can be used to establish more spontaneous communication in children with ASD. These procedures include (a) training in the natural environment so that natural cues become discriminative stimuli for communication, and (b) the use of transfer of stimulus control procedures (Halle, 1987). The aim of these latter procedures is to transfer control of responding from the trainer's prompts to more natural environmental cues (Carmen, 1986). Wolery and Gast (1984) described several procedures that have proven effective for the purpose of obtaining a transfer for stimulus control, including (a) most-to-least prompting, (b) graduated guidance, (c) system of least prompts, (d) time delay, (e) stimulus shaping, and (f) stimulus fading. Duker et al. (2004) provided detailed definitions and examples of each of these transfer of stimulus control techniques. Several studies have shown how these techniques can be applied to develop more spontaneous communication in children with ASD. Hamilton and Snell (1993), for example, used the system of least prompts to transfer control of requesting behavior from verbal prompts to a mere expectant look from the trainer. Similarly, Woods (1984) transferred control of naming responses from verbal prompts ("What do you see there?") to merely being in the presence of the stimulus. In this study, transfer of stimulus control was achieved by using a time delay procedure (i.e., waiting 7 s before delivering the verbal prompt).

Given the variability in symptoms illustrated in Table 6.1, communication intervention for children with ASD will often require a highly individualized and appropriately sequenced approach. An important step in developing an individualized communication intervention sequence is to assess the nature and severity of the child's communication impairments. A range of procedures can be used to assess the nature and severity of communication impairment in children with ASD. Sigafoos, Schlosser, Green, O'Reilly, and Lancioni (2008) described three approaches that have been developed to assess communication and related social skills of individuals with ASD. Table 6.2 provides a summary of these three major approaches for assessing communication skills in children with ASD.

Assessment of the child's communication deficits and excesses is used to assist in the identification of treatment priorities and intervention requirements (Matson & Wilkins, 2007). When assessment data reveal that a child lacks acceptable ways to indicate likes and dislikes, for example, then logical intervention targets include teaching appropriate requesting and rejecting skills (Sigafoos, Drasgow, Reichle, et al., 2004). In contrast, if the child's speech is largely echolalic, then an intervention aimed at replacing echolalia with functional speech (e.g., verbal labeling responses) is indicated (Foxx, Schreck, Garito, Smith, & Weisenberger, 2004).

As part of the assessment process it is often helpful to consider the influence of communication impairment on other areas of adaptive behavior functioning. Researchers have noted that the communication domain and the social skills domain, for example, have a considerable degree of overlap (Sigafoos et al., 2008). Successful communication often requires the child to have good social skills and vice versa. With regard to this, it may be noted that an important, yet subtle mark of social competence, is the extent to which the child engages in appropriate paralinguistic behavior (e.g., eye contact, standing at an appropriate distance, making appropriate facial expressions) during communicative interactions (Landa, 2007). There is also considerable evidence showing that problematic forms of behavior,

such as tantrums, aggression, and self-injury, often serve a communicative function for children with ASD (Bott, Farmer, & Rhode, 1997; Chung, Jenner, Chamberlain, & Corbett, 1995; Sigafoos, 2000). Self-injury, for example, is often maintained by positive reinforcement in the form of attention from adults and access to preferred objects, or by negative reinforcement in the form of escape from nonpreferred tasks (Iwata et al., 1994). In such cases, self-injury can be conceptualized as an inappropriate form of communicative requesting and rejecting, respectively (Durand, 1993).

Matson, Terlonge, and Minshawi (2008) described a variety of assessment procedures that have been developed to identify the communicative function, if any, of problem behaviors in children with developmental disabilities. These procedures include the use of rating scales, informant interviews, and descriptive, and functional analyses. These types of behavioral assessments can assist practitioners in identifying the function or purpose of the child's problem behavior. Information of this type is then used to develop treatment programs that aim to replace problem behavior with more appropriate forms of communicative behavior that would serve the same function or purpose for the child.

Given the overlap between skill areas, improvement of the child's communication skills will often have a positive impact on other areas of adaptive behavior functioning. This collateral effect has been demonstrated with respect to problem behavior. Specifically, numerous studies have shown that problem behavior maintained by positive and negative reinforcement can be reduced by teaching more appropriate forms of communicative requesting and rejecting (Carr & Durand, 1985, Durand, 1993; Durand & Merges, 2001; Richmond, 2006; Wacker et al., 2005).

In light of the discussion, it has long been known that communication training alone is not always suffi-

Table 6.2 Assessment approaches

Approach	Description
Behavioral observation	Direct observation of the child's behavior during structured or unstructured communicative opportunities. For example, a preferred object may be placed in view, but out of reach to determine how the child attempts to request access to the item. Repeated opportunities are presented over a number of days and under varying conditions to obtain a representative sample of behavior.
Role-play tests	The child is involved in various simulated scenarios and observed for the presence/absence of specific communication and social skills. To assess assertiveness skills for example, an adult might pretend to misunderstand the child and wait to see if and how the child attempts to correct the misunderstanding.
Rating scales, behavior checklists, and interview protocols	Information is solicited from third-party informants (e.g., parents or teachers) on the frequency or presence/absence of specific communication behaviors. To assess echolalia, for example, the practitioner might ask: "When asking your child a question, how likely is s/he to immediately repeat the last few words that you speak?" A number of reliable and valid rating scales, checklists, and interview protocols have been developed to assess communication deficits and excesses of children with ASD (see Sigafoos et al., 2008 for a review).

cient to positively impact other areas of adaptive behavior functioning (Lovaas, 1977). Sigafoos et al. (2009), for example, have recently shown that merely teaching a useful communication response does not automatically produce collateral improvement in paralinguistic aspects of communication, such as appropriate social orientation and eye contact toward the communicative partner. This study involved an adolescent boy with diagnoses of autistic disorder and Down syndrome. The boy had no speech and was socially withdrawn. To address his communication needs, the boy was first taught to request access to preferred items by exchanging a picture communication symbol. Although the child learned to make requests by exchanging communication symbols for corresponding items, he never approached and rarely even looked at his communicative partner while doing so. Improved social interaction with the partner was eventually obtained by adding a social skills training component that required the child to first approach the trainer before making a request.

The results of this study illustrate the potential value of integrating communication intervention and paralinguistic skills training. The more general implication is that learning outcomes might be enhanced when communication intervention becomes part of, not apart from, a more comprehensive treatment program. The roots of comprehensive, ABA-based treatment programs can be found in pioneering studies from the 1960s.

Historical Perspective

Following Kanner's (1943) recognition of the condition that is now known under the umbrella term of ASD, a range of mainly psychiatric and pharmacological treatments were evaluated, including electric convulsive shock, subshock insulin, amphetamines, and antidepressants (Bender, Goldschmidt, & Siva Sankar, 1962). While most of these treatment efforts were broadly targeted, some were more specifically directed at communication impairment. Freedman, Ebin, and Wilson (1962), for example, gave what was considered a promising new therapeutic drug, (LSD-25) to 12 "autistic schizophrenic" children in the hope of developing their speech. Unfortunately, the "hoped for change from muteness to speech did not occur" (p. 44). The other psychiatric and pharmacological treatments trialed during this period proved equally ineffective.

Alongside these psychiatric and pharmacological failures, operant conditioning principles – on which contemporary ABA-based approaches are based – were just beginning to be applied for therapeutic purposes. Fuller (1949), for example, increased an arm lifting response in an 18-year-old man with profound/multiple disabilities by reinforcing each occurrence of the response with a sip of milk. This demonstration was significant in showing that a person with profound disabilities and a total absence of speech could nonetheless learn a simple gesture-mode requesting response. More generally, the results of this study suggested that there was potential value in using operant conditioning principles (e.g., shaping, differential reinforcement) for wider therapeutic purposes, such as the treatment of ASD.

A major advance in the realization of operant conditioning's potential followed several years later when Lovaas, Berberich, Perloff, and Schaeffer (1966) applied shaping and differential reinforcement to teach imitative speech to children with autism. In this pioneering work, Lovaas et al. showed that children who were initially unable to speak could learn to imitate single words through an intensive behavioral treatment program. The program involved three phases. First, the children were reinforced with food, drinks, and praise for making any type of vocalization. As the frequency of vocalizations increased, the children were then required to vocalize contingently, that is, within a few seconds of the trainer's spoken model (e.g., ball, mama). In the third phase, reinforcement was withheld until the child's vocalizations were closer and closer approximations of the trainer's models. The results of this initial study demonstrated that operant conditioning principles could be effectively applied to develop imitative speech in mute children with autism.

The 1970s gave rise to a number of comprehensive research-based programs for teaching speech to children autism and mental retardation (Guess, Sailor, & Baer, 1974; Kent, 1974; Lovaas, 1977). These programs were comprehensive in the sense that they included intervention phases that moved beyond imitation training to teach a variety of additional communication skills to children with developmental disabilities. Training typically began by first teaching a large imitative vocabulary. After this, intervention expanded to address other communication targets, such as receptive labeling, expressive labeling, requesting objects, and various grammatical constructions (e.g., plurals, past tense).

Imitative speech proved extremely useful for facilitating the acquisition of these additional communication skills. To teach expressive labeling, for example, the teacher might hold up an item (e.g., a ball) and ask: "What is this?" If the child failed to respond correctly, the trainer modeled the correct response (e.g., "Say ball."). This imitative prompt was typically faded by either reducing the volume or giving only a partial prompt (e.g., "ba__."). In light of the fact that many children with ASD failed to learn imitative speech even with intensive intervention, comparable procedures were adapted for teaching the use of manual signs and symbol-based or picture-based communication systems (Carr, 1982; Evans & Spittle, 1981).

Alongside the development of these programs, researchers made significant conceptual advances that have ushered in new and more effective ways of evaluating interventions and new and more effective ways of using behavioral learning and conditioning principles in applied settings. These advances helped to establish a distinct identity for ABA as an applied science focused on the causes of socially significant behavior change. As ABA evolved, it became characterized by a number of features (Baer, Wolf, & Risley, 1968, 1987). These features include a focus on clinically significant behavior change, direct measurement of target behaviors, and

interventions that are derived from foundational principles of learning, especially operant conditioning. Table 6.3 relates the main distinguishing features of ABA to the communication domain.

Contemporary Perspective

Since the 1960s, applied intervention research in ABA has produced a technology that has proven adaptable and effective for teaching a range of life-enhancing behaviors to children with ASD and related developmental disabilities. O'Reilly et al. (2007) identified several generic elements to this technology, including: (a) analysis of target skills into teachable responses (i.e., task analysis), (b) implementing well-established instructional strategies to ensure the response occurs at the right time and under the right conditions (e.g., graduated guidance, least-to-most-prompting), (c) effective use of reinforcement to strengthen correct responses, and (d) integrating responses into a larger behavioral chain (e.g., multiword communication responses). Intervention research in ABA continues to yield new and more effective applications of this generic technology for the treatment of children with ASD.

Table 6.3 Dimensions of ABA applied to the communication domain[a]

Dimension	Description	Application to communication
Applied	ABA focuses on changing socially important behaviors.	Focus on teaching communicative behaviors that enhance functioning and quality of life.
Behavioral	ABA requires direct observation and measurement of behavior.	Objectively define communicative behaviors in ways that make them observable and measurable.
Analytic	ABA requires a convincing demonstration of the effects of an independent variable (intervention) on one or more dependent variables (behavior).	Include repeated measures of communicative behavior prior to, during, and after intervention to determine if the intervention did in fact produce behavior change.
Conceptual	ABA is based on, derived from, and consistent with empirically validated principles of learning (e.g., shaping, chaining, stimulus discrimination training, differential reinforcement).	Identify the fundamental learning principles or mechanisms that underlie effective communication intervention.
Technological	ABA interventions are objectively described in sufficient detail to enable independent replication.	Provide a step-by-step description of the intervention procedures to facilitate replication by stakeholders (parents, teachers, etc.).
Generalized outcomes	ABA interventions will be more effective when behavior change is maintained and appropriately generalized to new settings, materials, and people.	Incorporate strategies to promote maintenance and generalization into their communication interventions.
Effective	ABA interventions are considered to be effective only if they yield clinically significant behavior change.	Intervention is effective to the extent that it produces large and meaningful changes in the child's communication repertoire.

[a]Based on Baer, Wolf, & Risley (1987)

With specific reference to communication intervention, Snell, Chen, and Hoover (2006) identified a number of well-established instructional principles that have demonstrated success in teaching communication skills to children with ASD and other developmental disabilities. Snell et al. classified these principles as antecedent-based and consequent-based strategies. The antecedent-based strategies include various response prompting techniques and environmental manipulations that are typically implemented at the beginning of teaching trials. Environmental manipulations and response prompting strategies aim to motivate the child to communicate and, when necessary, directly prompt the target behavior. Examples of antecedent-based strategies include:

1. Response prompting – use of verbal, gesture, model, or physical assistance to evoke a correct response from the child.
2. Proximity – place discriminative stimuli in conspicuous locations.
3. Multiple stimuli – include several examples of discriminative stimuli during training (e.g., when teaching the child to label or tact common objects (e.g., books, chairs, and utensils.), it would be important to use a variety of exemplars to represent each object class. These exemplars should vary systematically to sample the range of variation found within the class).
4. Capture motivation – follow the child's lead, wait for the child to initiate a request by reaching for or leading you to an object, make use of preferred stimuli and activities.
5. Embedded instruction – provide opportunities for communication during a range of typical routines, such as mealtimes, play, and recess.

Consequent-based strategies include differential reinforcement and error-correction. Such techniques are typically implemented in response to the child's communicative behavior or attempts. Reinforcement and error correction aim to promote learning and strengthen correct communication responses. Examples of consequent-based strategies include:

1. Specific reinforcement – provide reinforcement that is relevant to the child's response (e.g., if the child requests a "Drink," then use a preferred beverage as a reinforcer. the child comments on the environment (e.g., "It's raining.") then respond accordingly ("Yes, I see, it is raining out there. Thanks for letting me know.").

2. Contingent and immediate reinforcement – specific reinforcement should be delivered immediately, but only after the child makes a correct communicative response.
3. Error correction – incorrect communicative attempts should be interrupted and corrected using an effective response prompt.

In practice, antecedent-based and consequent-based strategies need to be combined and used in flexible ways that are responsive to the child's ongoing behavior. If a child begins to make the wrong sign, for example, this error should be interrupted and the correct sign prompted and then reinforced. The more general principle of communication intervention is that each and every communicative opportunity should be arranged so as to increase the probability of correct unprompted responses and ensure the child receives an appropriate type and amount of reinforcement for appropriate communicative behavior. Intervention can be considered complete only when the child has acquired a large repertoire of communication skills that are evoked and maintained by the same contingencies of reinforcement that operate in the home, school, and community.

As illustrated by Snell et al. (2006), contemporary approaches for enhancing communication skills of children with ASD remain firmly rooted in the technology of ABA (Ogletree, 2007; O'Reilly et al., 2007). However, this generic technology has been refined through continued research. From this research new procedures and innovative applications of well-established instructional principles have emerged. In addition, compared to many of the programs developed in the 1960s and 1970s, contemporary ABA-based approaches to communication intervention are characterized by four trends: (a) multimodal communication, (b) functional curriculum, (c) flexibly structured teaching arrangements, and (d) evidence-based practice.

Multimodal Communication

Communication modes fall into two categories: speech and nonspeech modes. Although parents understandably want their child to acquire speech, this can be difficult to teach to some children (Charlop-Christy et al., 2008). Because of this difficulty, a child with ASD might receive months or even years of speech-based communication that could ultimately prove ineffective and only then might s/he be considered for a nonspeech communication mode.

Contemporary practitioners, in contrast, are much more likely to adopt a multimodal approach to communication intervention (Loncke, Campbell, England, & Haley, 2006). Multimodal intervention combines speech and nonspeech modes of communication. The potential advantage of such an approach is that if the child ultimately fails to acquire speech, s/he will nonetheless have acquired an effective nonspeech mode of communication. Nonspeech modes of communication are also generally easier to teach than speech, and thus the child may be more successful during the early stages of intervention. This early success might, in turn, increase the child's motivation to learn and willingness to participate in future intervention sessions (Sundberg, 1980).

The contemporary focus on multimodal communication intervention does not discount the importance of speech as a preferred mode of communication. Procedures to promote speech and language development are clearly indicated for children with ASD. It is important to note that ABA is an evolving science and future innovations could mean that many more children with ASD will be able to learn to speak. For example, a growing number of studies suggest that a novel stimulus-stimulus pairing procedure is a promising way to increase vocalizations in children with ASD (Miguel, Carr, & Michael, 2002; Sundberg, Michael, Partington, & Sundberg, 1996; Yoon & Bennett, 2000). The technique involves first gaining the child's attention. Next, the trainer produces a speech sound (e.g., ah, eee, baa). While producing the speech sound the trainer also delivers a reinforcer to the child. The intent of this procedure is to condition vocalizations as a source of automatic reinforcement for the child. This does appear to happen, in that after 300–400 conditioning trials of this type the majority of participating children have begun to spontaneously imitate the target sounds. However, it is important to note that the procedure has so far been used with a rather limited number of children. Thus while the generality of this stimulus-stimulus pairing technique remains to be established, innovations of this type could perhaps open the door for teaching functional speech to mute children who were previously considered unlikely to acquire any appreciable amount of speech.

Even with such advances, there is no evidence to suggest that multimodal communication hinder efforts to teach speech (Millar, Light, & Schlosser, 2006). In fact, a recent systematic review has indicated that children with autism increase their speech production as a result of intervention to teach augmentative and alternative communication (AAC), although these increases tend to be rather modest (Schlosser & Wendt, 2008). In light of this evidence, early introduction of nonspeech modes and multimodal communication intervention should be considered whenever there is significant delay or lack of speech development and certainly if the child fails to acquire speech by age 3 (National Research Council, 2001). At the same time, it is important that professionals and families maintain realistic expectations regarding speech production gains of children who have been introduced to AAC following a significant delay or lack of speech development. If gains do occur, even modest ones, they should be viewed as a bonus to AAC intervention. The primary aim of AAC intervention is to increase a person's communicative competence, regardless of what specific modalities may be used.

There is considerable debate in contemporary ABA literature as to the relative merits of different nonspeech modes of communication. Specifically, there is debate as to whether it is better to emphasize topography-based (e.g., gestures, manual signs) vs. selection-based (e.g., pointing to line drawings on a communication board) systems (Potter & Brown, 1997; Shafer, 1993). However, numerous studies have shown that both can be taught to children with ASD (Duker et al., 2004; Mirenda, 2003). In fact, comparative studies have revealed few major or consistent differences in terms of the ease and speed with which topography-based vs. selection-based modes are acquired (Potter & Brown, 1997; Schlosser & Sigafoos, 2006; Tincani, 2004; Vignes, 2007).

There is also debate as to which types of selection-based systems (e.g., picture-exchange vs. speech-generating devices) are better suited to children with ASD. Lancioni et al. (2007) recently reviewed literature on teaching these two types of aided communication systems. They identified 37 studies, published between 1992 and 2006. Collectively, these studies involved a total of 173 students with developmental disabilities. The results of these studies showed that the majority of participating students successfully acquired use of the targeted communication system, that is, either picture-exchange or use of a speech-generating device. The vast majority of the participating students acquired use of the respective communication system as a result of the implementation of ABA-based intervention procedures (e.g., response prompting, prompt fading, differential reinforcement). Furthermore, in a few studies, students ($n = 11$) were successfully taught to use both systems with comparable ease and speed. Based on their review of the evidence, Lancioni et al. concluded that both systems are promising alternatives to speech for students with developmental disabilities. However, they also noted that the literature base was currently limited. For example, these 37 studies focused mainly on teaching either generalized (e.g., "Want") or more explicit requesting responses (e.g., "Food," "Drink"). It is therefore unclear how readily such systems would be acquired when intervention aimed to teach other communicative functions, such as commenting and initiating conversations.

Still, given that a variety of nonspeech communication systems have been successfully taught to children with ASD, the decision as to which modes to use within a multimodal communication intervention may depend to some extent on the skills of the child's communicative partners, demands of the environment, and child preferences. Rotholz, Berkowitz, and Burberry (1989), for example, demonstrated that manual signed requests were less effective than symbol-based communication boards for ordering meals in restaurants. This demonstration highlights the need to ensure that the child's mode of communication is ecologically valid in the sense of being effective across a range of partners and environments. Other studies have shown that children with ASD and other types of developmental disabilities will often, but not always, show a preference for using different types of nonspeech communication systems (Sigafoos et al., 2009; Sigafoos, O'Reilly, Ganz, Lancioni, & Schlosser, 2005; Soto, Belfiore, Schlosser, & Haynes, 1993). Son, Sigafoos, O'Reily, and Lancioni (2006), for example, compared acquisition and preference for using picture-exchange vs. speech-generating devices in three preschool children with ASD. There was little difference in the rate of response acquisition, but two children demonstrated a consistent preference for picture-exchange and the third showed a preference for the speech-generating device. Given the general consistency of such results from a number of studies, Schlosser and Sigafoos (2006) concluded that "a more important clinical measure [more important than acquisition rate that is] may be a learner's preference for using some type of device over another." (p. 21). Such a recommendation can be defended from a social validity perspective in that enabling the child to express such

a preference would seem important in its own right. However, there are currently no data on whether such preferences are associated with improved outcomes from communicative intervention.

Functional Curriculum

Contemporary ABA-based approaches to communication intervention for children with ASD have been increasingly influenced by Skinner's (1957) analysis of verbal behavior (LeBlanc et al., 2006; Sundberg, 1980). Skinner defined verbal behavior as a special class of operant behavior that is effective only indirectly through the actions of other people. Unlike the direct act of opening a door (operant response) to get outside (reinforcement), the verbal equivalent (i.e., saying "Open the door.") is only effective in the presence of a listener willing and able to respond to/reinforce this communicative act. Consistent with the multimodal approach, verbal behavior in Skinner's analysis includes any response form that will effectively alter the behavior of a listener. Thus verbal behavior includes speech, writing, gestures, manual signs, exchanging pictures, or using a speech-generating device.

Because verbal behavior is effective only indirectly through the mediation of a listener, practitioners will need to consider the extent to which listeners have the skills to respond to the child's communicative behaviors in ways that will strengthen or reinforce appropriate forms of communication (e.g., speech, manual signs) and weaken or extinguish inappropriate forms of communication (e.g., tantrums, self-injury). Along these lines, a Skinnerian analysis of verbal behavior highlights the importance of managing listener responsivity to enhance intervention outcomes. Responsivity in this context can be defined as the extent to which a listener acknowledges and reacts appropriately to (i. e., reinforces) the child's communicative attempts. Data show that communicative functioning is enhanced when listeners are highly responsive to even very basic communicative attempts on the part of the child (Harwood, Warren, & Yoder, 2002). Practitioners can capitalize on such findings by training listeners to acknowledge and reinforce the child's appropriate communicative attempts. In many cases, teachers and parents may need training to learn how to respond appropriately to children's communicative attempts. At a minimum, listeners should acknowledge appropriate communicative attempts and simultaneously provide relevant reinforcement.

Skinner's (1957) analysis of verbal behavior also highlighted the value of considering the more precise operant function or purpose of communicative behavior (e.g., request, comment), rather than concentrating on the linguistic aspects of communication (nouns, verbs, grammatical rules). The classification of communication skills in terms of their [operant] function has influenced the content of contemporary ABA-based approaches to communication intervention (LeBlanc et al., 2006; Reichle et al., 1991). Functional, in this context, refers to communication skills that are effective in enabling the child to gain reinforcement and interact with others. Children with ASD often need to be taught to express wants, needs, and feelings, initiate conversations, and respond to initiations from others (Kaiser & Grim, 2006). Functional curriculum content in communication interventions for children with ASD typically includes the following general classes: (a) requesting and rejecting, (b) naming and commenting, (c) imitative responses, and (d) answering and conversational skills (Sigafoos, 1997). In Skinner's (1957) analysis of verbal behavior, these classes of communicative behavior

(or verbal operants) are referred to as mands, tacts, echoics, and intraverbals, respectively. Sigafoos, O'Reilly, Schlosser, and Lancioni (2007) outlined how the basic verbal operants defined by Skinner have been operationalized for use in communication intervention for children with ASD.

Numerous more specific skills are included within each of these general classes of verbal operants. The mand, for example, includes a range of more specific requesting and rejecting skills, such as (a) requesting preferred objects, (b) requesting missing, but needed items, (c) requesting access to preferred activities, (d) requesting help or assistance, (d) requesting information, and (e) rejecting the offer of a nonpreferred object. Tacting similarly covers a number of more specific skills, such as naming objects or actions and commenting on aspects of the environment (e.g., "That's a ball.", "That's a car.", "He is running.", "It's raining.", and "The telephone is ringing."). Table 6.4 provides examples of functional communication skills that have been taught to individuals with ASD.

Sundberg and Michael (2001) emphasized the importance of providing explicit instruction to teach each of the various classes of verbal operants defined

Table 6.4 Examples of functional communication skills taught to children with ASD

Operant class	Examples
Mand (request)	Request object (e.g., food, drinks, toys)
	Request a missing, but needed item (a spoon needed to eat)
	Request more of an object
	Request more of an activity
	Request activity (television, music, swinging)
	Request attention from adult
	Request help and assistance with a difficult task
	Request information (e.g., "Where is it?")
	Request a break from a task
Mand (reject/ protest)	Reject the offer of a nonpreferred object
	Reject the offer to participate in a nonpreferred activity
	Reject the offer of a wrong item
	Request the removal of nonpreferred items
	Request the cessation of an activity or stimulus
Tact (name/ comment)	Naming objects and actions
	Naming a property of an object (big, small, red, blue)
	Labeling the location of objects (on top, under, next to)
	Describing a previously observed object or event
Echoic (imitation)	Imitate speech
	Imitate manual signs
	Reply to greetings (Hi → Hello)
Intraverbal (answer/ classify, conversation)	Maintain conversation ("What movie did you see on the weekend?" → "The movie I saw on the weekend was...")
	Name items in categories (e.g., "What are some colors?")
	Answer questions (e.g., "What is your name?")
	Maintain conversation ("Nice day today." → "Yes, I might go out for a walk.")

by Skinner (1957). They argued that intervention should focus on teaching the child to use each response form (e.g., the manual signs for ball, water, and coat) as a mand, as a tact, as an echoic, and as an intraverbal response. This recommendation is consistent with evidence showing that mands, tacts, echoics, and intraverbals are functionally independent (Kelley, Shillingsburg, Castro, Addison, & LeRue, 2007). Teaching a child to name a spoon does not necessarily enable the child to use that object label to request a spoon when needed and vice versa. In light of this functional independence, contemporary approaches to communication intervention often include training on a range of specific functions (e.g., requesting objects, naming those same objects). This is a departure from earlier approaches that often focused on teaching a large vocabulary of nouns or object labels with the resulting expectation that these would then be used spontaneously to request, make comments, and start conversations effectively.

A potential problem with the current emphasis on teaching operant functions is that the many associated skills (e.g., requesting objects, naming objects) are often taught in isolation and out of context (LeBlanc et al., 2006). This separation may help to ensure that each function is in fact explicitly taught and acquired. However, there is evidence that generalization across the verbal operants is facilitated when training occurs simultaneously on different communicative functions (e.g., mands and tacts) becomes more integrated (Sigafoos, Reichle, Doss, Hall, & Pettitt, 1990). More generally, Reichle et al. (1991) argued that communication intervention should be ecologically based; that is, the intervention should be functional not only in terms of the skills being taught, but also in terms of the context of instruction. It is rare for only one communicative function to be relevant to a given context. Rarely, for example, does one just happen to sit down and make repeated requests for objects or repeatedly name objects. Instead, most routines usually provide a few opportunities for a variety of communicative functions. During lunch, for instance, it is likely that the child will have need and opportunity to communicate a variety of functions (e.g., request more, request help, greet peers, maintain a conversation, and respond to questions). It would therefore seem to make sense to target multiple communication functions during intervention sessions that are embedded into a variety of functional routines. Implementing this aspect of a functional curriculum requires practitioners who can be flexible in how they structure intervention.

Flexibly Structured Teaching Arrangements

Contemporary ABA-based approaches to communication intervention are characterized by flexibly structured teaching arrangements (Ogletree, 2007). Teaching opportunities can be structured along a continuum of naturalness. At one end of this continuum, intervention sessions appear more clinical and structured. Training at this end of the continuum is characterized by the use of one-to-one training sessions during which the child receives numerous discrete-training trials on one, or perhaps a few, specific communication responses (Charlop-Christy et al., 2008; Duker et al., 2004. For example, intervention might occur in daily 20-min sessions during which the trainer could present 50–60 discrete-training trials. These trials are usually presented in rapid succession with the child allowed to consume or access the reinforcer during the brief (e.g., 30 s) intertrial interval. In this approach, each discrete trial typically consists of three components: (a) presentation of a discriminative stimulus (e.g., holding up an object and asking, "What is this?"), (b) waiting for, or prompting, a correct response, and (c) delivery of reinforcement contingent upon a correct response.

A study by Sigafoos, Drasgow, Halle, et al. (2004) illustrates the application of this type of more structured approach for teaching communication to individuals with autism. The study participants were an adolescent male (Jason, 16 years old) and a young a woman (Megan, 20 years old), both of whom had autism, severe intellectual disability, and no speech. Although the study addressed several aims and research questions, the one most relevant for the present discussion was whether Jason and Megan could learn to make requests using a speech-generating device. A correct request was defined as pressing a panel on the speech-generating device to produce the recorded message: "I want more." Preferred edibles were delivered as reinforcement for each correct request. If a correct request did not occur within 10 s of the start of the trial, the trainer used the least amount of physical guidance (i.e., a graduated guidance prompting procedure) necessary to prompt correct use of the speech-generating device. Training was conducted in structured one-to-one sessions. Within each 5-min session, the trainer provided six discrete-training trials by offering preferred edibles. The results showed that both participants learned to request preferred edibles using the speech-generating device. In fact, both participants acquired this new communication skill within 8–10 teaching sessions. This finding is consistent with many other studies that have adopted highly structured discrete-trial training formats for teaching communication skills to children with ASD (Duker et al., 2004).

At the other end of the continuum, communication intervention is characterized by a more naturalistic or incidental teaching approach (Charlop-Christy et al., 2008; Koegel, O'Dell, & Koegel, 1987). With this approach, teaching opportunities are embedded within the flow of a natural routine. For example, prior to bedtime, a parent might undertake communication intervention within the context of a book reading activity. To initiate the activity, the child might first receive an opportunity to request which book to read. After that, additional opportunities might be embedded within the activity to teach various picture naming (i.e., tact) responses ("What animal is that?", "What color is that?").

A study by Sigafoos and Littlewood (1999) illustrates the application of this type of more naturalistic approach for teaching communication to children with autism. The participant of this study was a young boy (aged 4.7 years) with autism who had no speech. The aim of the intervention was to teach the use of a gesture-mode requesting response. Specifically the child was taught to request preferred play activities by producing the manual sign for "More." Training occurred on the playground of his early intervention center during the regular recess time. During each recess period, the child received several embedded opportunities to make a request. Opportunities were created by momentarily interrupting the child's ongoing play. For example, the trainer would momentarily interrupt the child from getting on the slide or crawling through the tire tunnel. During this pause, a correct request would enable the activity to continue. If a correct request did not occur within 10 s, the child was prompted to produce the correct sign and then the activity continued. Prompting involved using the least amount of physical guidance necessary to assist the child in forming the sign. With this prompting procedure in place, correct requesting increased to a high level after approximately 100 instructional opportunities. This high level of correct requesting was maintained with a new teacher and also generalized to an earlier point in the routine (i.e., when he was interrupted while on his way to the playground).

The results showed that a functional communication skill could be taught in a more naturalistic context. This finding is consistent with the results of numerous other studies that have successfully taught a range of communication skills to children with ASD using naturalistic teaching arrangements (Charlop-Christy et al., 2008).

In line with this continuum model, communication outcomes for children with ASD may be enhanced when practitioners have the skills to vary the structure and naturalness of intervention to suit the child, context, and stage of intervention. When aiming for the rapid acquisition of a new communication skill, for example, there may be benefit in adopting a more structured discrete-trial approach. This approach may help to ensure that the child receives a sufficient number of learning opportunities to promote rapid acquisition of the response. Following acquisition, more naturalistic and incidental approaches should be incorporated into the intervention program as these will likely help to promote generalization and maintenance.

It would be a mistake to view discrete-trial training and more naturalistic approaches as sequential or mutually incompatible teaching arrangements. Sigafoos, Arthur-Kelly, and Butterfield (2006) argued that it is often beneficial to combine discrete-trial training within natural routines. For example, multiple opportunities to teach requests for food and drink could be embedded into the natural flow of breakfast, lunch, and dinner. This combination of discrete-trial training and naturalistic teaching arrangements is consistent with one aspect of the flexible and more contemporary approach to communication intervention described by Ogletree (2007).

Another aspect of flexibility in teaching is to remain alert to teachable moments by following the child's lead. Drasgow, Halle, and Sigafoos (1999) argued that teaching should only occur when there is some indication that the child is motivated to communicate. For example, a child may indicate motivation to reject by moving away from an activity or object. This scenario represents a naturally arising opportunity to run a discrete training trial in which the child is taught to use a more sophisticated form of communicative rejecting. At another time the child might indicate a desire for social interaction by approaching peers. This initiation on the part of the child signals an opportunity to teach more effective peer group entry strategies. Effective strategies include making an appropriate greeting response and initiating a conversation. Practitioners can often embed a large number of discrete training trials into a range of everyday activities by capitalizing on such naturally arising opportunities.

Evidence–Based Practice

Evidence-based practice is defined as "... the integration of the best available research evidence with educational/clinical expertise and relevant stakeholder perspectives to facilitate decisions for assessment and intervention that are deemed effective and efficient for a given stakeholder" (Schlosser & Raghavendra, 2004, p. 3). There has been a growing movement for practitioners to adopt this definition of evidence-based practice in communication assessment and intervention (Schlosser & Sigafoos, 2007). The EBP process is organized along the following steps: (a) ask a well-built question, (b) search for research evidence, (c) appraise the evidence, (d) apply the evidence, and (e) evaluate the effectiveness of the application (Schlosser & Raghavendra, 2004; Straus, 2007). To do so effectively will therefore require practitioners to (a) assess and incorporate stakeholder perspectives into their communication assessments and interventions, (b) identify and select the most relevant and effective empirically validated procedures and adapt these procedures to suit the unique characteristics of individual children, and (c) gain and apply the requisite educational or clinical expertise to effectively apply and evaluate assessment and treatment procedures.

Stakeholder Perspectives

Evidence-based practice places considerable emphasis on ensuring that stakeholder perspectives are incorporated into the design and implementation of assessment and intervention. Stakeholders in this context include any and all individuals whose perspectives may have a bearing on the feasibility of implementing an assessment or intervention concerning a given child (Schlosser, 2003). Here, the construct of evidence-based practice meshes well with the tradition of social validation in ABA-related approaches (Wolf, 1978). Thus, behavior analysts should find this aspect of

evidence-based practice a natural extension of what is often done already. For example, in the social validation literature, the following four groups of stakeholders have been identified which have been applied to evidence-based decision-making as well (Schlosser, 1999; Schlosser & Raghavendra, 2004): (a) direct stakeholders (i.e., the recipient of the intervention or assessment); (b) indirect stakeholders (e.g., family members of the child); (c) immediate community stakeholders (e.g., peers in the classroom); and (d) extended community stakeholders (e.g., the cashier in the local fast food restaurant who may not know the child). These groupings can facilitate the selection of relevant stakeholders relative to a particular child and decision.

The emphasis on incorporating stakeholders' perspectives is of critical importance in the practice of communication intervention because these key stakeholders will be the child's most frequent communicative partners (King, Batorowicz, & Shepherd, 2008). In addition, it is considered best practice to empower these stakeholders so that they can become directly involved in collaborating with professionals to implement the intervention (Lovaas, 2003). A high level of stakeholder commitment to the intervention is often critical to ensuring successful treatment outcomes and maintaining treatment gains.

Wolf (1978) argued that it is important to assess the social validity of ABA treatments to ensure that the interventions address socially important behaviors. He further argued that social validity should be assessed at three levels: (a) whether intervention goals are perceived as significant, (b) whether the intervention procedures are perceived as appropriate and acceptable, and (c) whether the results of the intervention have been perceived as meaningful.

In practice, however, stakeholder perceptions have often been assessed on a post hoc basis at the end of the intervention (Schlosser, 2003). While this evaluative information can be useful in providing summative data on the social validity and acceptability of the intervention, it provides little help in incorporating stakeholder perspectives into the design of intervention. Evidence-based practice, in contrast, emphasizes the value of incorporating stakeholder perspectives from the very beginning stages of the intervention planning process. To this end, stakeholder perspectives should be sought during the initial referral/intake process. Stakeholder perspectives at this stage can assist in identifying what skills to teach, what procedures to use, and how and where to use these procedures. In terms of the EBP process, it is therefore important that relevant stakeholders are involved from the first step, which involves asking a well-built question (Schlosser, Koul, & Costello, 2007), rather than only when it comes to applying the appraised evidence.

Also, the selection of appropriate target behaviors and negotiating stakeholder involvement in the teaching process are especially critical to the initial design of communication intervention programs for children with ASD. Decisions that need to be made include the mode(s) of communication that the child will be taught to use and the initial communicative functions/skills to target for acquisition. Duker, van Driel, and van de Bercken (2002) developed a useful tool for gaining stakeholder perspectives in these two critical areas. The unique aspect of this instrument is that it provides opportunities for stakeholders to consider the full range of speech and nonspeech communication modes (speech, gestures, manual sign, picture communication) and a range of communicative functions based on Skinner's (1957) functional classification of verbal behavior (i.e., mands, tacts, echoics).

Use of Empirically Supported Procedures

Evidence-based practice dictates that practitioners should make use of procedures that have been well established, or empirically supported, for their intended purpose. Well established in this context refers to procedures that have been subject to at least three rigorous and independent scientific evaluations and have proven to be consistently effective. With respect to ABA-based communication intervention, the generic strategies described in this chapter can all be considered well established. These procedures also appear sufficiently robust in the sense that they often remain highly effective when applied or packaged in various ways. The robust nature of these procedures enables individualization and flexibility in the provision of ABA-based communication intervention to children with ASD. The fact that ABA-based treatments can be effectively applied in a variety of flexible ways has enabled researchers to package these various applications into more comprehensive training programs, such as The Picture Exchange Communication System

(PECS), Pivotal Response Training, and Applied Verbal Behavior (see LeBlanc et al., 2006 and Matson et al., 2008 for reviews). There are many examples where generic ABA techniques have been packaged into programs that are well established for teaching communication to children with ASD (see Sigafoos, 1997 for a review).

There are of course always new and often more effective procedures being developed and evaluated. Practitioners will therefore need to be able to identify and appraise this emerging evidence. This can be a daunting task for busy educators and clinicians who may have had limited training in research methodology. The good news is that not all practitioners have to engage in all five steps of the EBP process for each well-built question. According to Straus (2007), the extent to which the practitioner will need to apply all steps will vary with (a) the nature of the encountered problem, the time constraints, and the level of expertise with each of the EBP steps. In the "doing" mode, Strauss suggests that the practitioner implements all steps. In the "using" mode, the critical appraisal step is eliminated. While this is a critical step because not all evidence is created equal (Schlosser, Wendt, & Sigafoos, 2007), a practitioner can often rely on evidence that has already been appraised. Haynes (2006) and Straus (2007) argue that busy practitioners should first seek out summaries (i.e., appraisals of systematic reviews and studies) before seeking out the reviews and studies themselves. The National Standards Project represents another source that the practitioner operating in the "doing" mode may consult (Wilczynski, Christian, & The National Autism Center, 2008). Finally, in the "replicating" mode, the practitioner not only drops the appraisal step, but also the search for evidence. Instead, the practitioner can rely on already completed searches for the same or similar well-built questions.

Flexible use of well-established techniques is a major component of evidence-based practice in communication intervention for children with ASD. Yet, there is more to this aspect of evidence-based practice than merely identifying and implementing appropriate empirically supported procedures. Sigafoos, Arthur, and O'Reilly (2003) described three factors that practitioners should consider in the selection of empirically supported procedures for use in evidence-based communication interventions. First, practitioners must select empirically supported procedures that are suited to the child's unique attributes and characteristics (e.g., the nature and types of communication impairment, associated conditions, preferences). Second, practitioners must collect and make use of learner-generated performance data to determine if the intervention is having the desired effects. Even the best procedures do not always work for every child. By collecting data on the child's performance during intervention (e.g., speed of acquisition, percentage of correct responses, error patterns), the practitioner will be able to determine if the procedure is having the desired effect. If not, steps can be taken to modify the procedure in an effort to improve treatment outcomes. Third, in order to make effective procedural modifications, practitioners require an understanding of the fundamental principles or mechanisms that underlie empirically validated procedures (Kazdin, 2007). Generic teaching strategies based on prompting and reinforcement, for example, are effective only to the extent that the basic principles of prompt fading and reinforcement have been adequately considered and incorporated into the intervention. Treatments often fail because practitioners lack the knowledge and expertise that would enable them to modify empirically supported procedures to suit the unique needs of the child and context (Linscheid, 1999).

Educational and Clinical Expertise

The third component of evidence-based practice is educational and clinical expertise in providing an assessment or intervention. In practice, this means that practitioners must have skills to implement empirically supported procedures with a high degree of treatment fidelity. Treatment fidelity refers to the extent to which the procedures are in fact implemented as intended (Schlosser, 2002). Treatments are more likely to be effective when they are consistently implemented as per the treatment protocol. Adhering to treatment protocols is also critical in the evaluation of treatment efficacy. If procedures are not implemented as intended and the treatment fails, it will be unclear why. Such a scenario could indicate that the procedure itself was ineffective or inappropriate or, rather, that it was not implemented correctly.

One hallmark of ABA-based procedures is that they are objectively described (see Table 6.3). The quality of the objective description will depend to some extent on the clarity and level of detail provided by the researcher. This is tested when practitioners attempt to implement the procedure based on a reading of the objective description. The mark of a good description is that a skilled practitioner will in fact be able to implement correctly on the basis of the objective description alone. Practitioners with less expertise, in contrast, may need to practice the procedure while receiving feedback from a mentor.

Summary

ASD is associated with a wide range of communication deficits and excesses that can negatively affect the child's quality of life. Communication intervention is therefore a major priority for children with ASD. Because communicative functioning can affect other areas of development, intervention to address communication impairment is best seen as part of the child's larger and more comprehensive treatment program.

Communication intervention based on the science of ABA is an integral part of the comprehensive treatment of children with ASD. As with other areas of adaptive behavior functioning, ABA-based procedures have proven consistently effective in addressing the communication needs of children with ASD. Indeed, research within the discipline of ABA has led to a number of highly effective procedures and programs for teaching a range of communicative skills to children with ASD.

Contemporary ABA-based approaches to communication intervention are characterized by the use of multiple modes of communication, functional curriculum, and flexible teaching arrangements. An emerging trend is the integration of ABA-based procedures with the principles of evidence-based practice. The emerging trend seeks to integrate the use of empirically supported procedures with stakeholder perspective and one's own clinical expertise to enhance the social validity and efficacy of intervention. Forty years of applied intervention research in ABA has provided an intervention technology that has proven to be consistently effective in enhancing communication in children with ASD. Practitioners who integrate this technology with the perspectives of stakeholders and their own clinical expertise may be more successful in addressing this major area of need for children with ASD.

References

American Psychiatric Association (2000). *Diagnostic and statistical manual of mental disorders* (4th ed., text revision). Washington, DC: Author.

Anderson, D. K., Lord, C., Sisi, S., DiLavore, P. S., Shulman, C., Thurm, A., et al. (2007). Patterns of growth in verbal abilities among children with autism spectrum disorder. *Journal of Consulting and Clinical Psychology, 75,* 594–604.

Baer, D. M., Wolf, M. M., & Risley, T. R. (1968). Some current dimensions of applied behavior analysis. *Journal of Applied Behavior Analysis, 1,* 91–97.

Baer, D. M., Wolf, M. M., & Risley, T. R. (1987). Some still current dimensions of applied behavior analysis. *Journal of Applied Behavior Analysis, 20,* 313–327.

Bates, E., Camaioni, L., & Volterra, V. (1975). The acquisition of performatives prior to speech. *Merrill-Palmer Quarterly, 21,* 205–226.

Bender, L., Goldschmidt, L., & Siva Sankar, D. V. (1962). Treatment of autistic schizophrenic children with LSD-25 and UML-491. *Recent Advances in Biological Psychiatry, 4,* 170–177.

Beukelman, D. R., & Mirenda, P. (2005). *Augmentative and alternative communication: Supporting children and adults with complex communication needs* (3rd ed.). Baltimore: Paul H. Brookes Publishing Co.

Bott, C., Farmer, R., & Rhode, J. (1997). Behavior problems associated with lack of speech in people with learning disabilities. *Journal of Intellectual Disability Research, 41,* 3–7.

Carmen, L. M. (1986). Acquisition, maintenance, and generalization of productive intraverbal behavior through transfer of stimulus control procedures. *Applied Research in Mental Retardation, 7,* 1–20.

Carpenter, R. L., Mastergeorge, A. M., & Coggins, T. E. (1983). The acquisition of communicative intentions in infants eight to fifteen months of age. *Language and Speech, 26,* 101–116.

Carr, E. G. (1982). Sign language. In R. Koegel, A. Rincover & A. Egel (Eds.), *Educating and understanding autistic children* (pp. 142–157). San Diego: College-Hill Press.

Carr, E. G., & Durand, V. M. (1985). Reducing behavior problems through functional communication training. *Journal of Applied Behavior Analysis, 18,* 111–126.

Charlop-Christy, M. H., Malmberg, D. B., Rocha, M. L., & Schreibman, L. (2008). Treating autistic spectrum disorder. In R. J. Morris & T. R. Kratochwill (Eds.), *The practice of child therapy* (4th ed., pp. 299–335). New York: Lawrence Erlbaum.

Chung, M. C., Jenner, L., Chamberlain, L., & Corbett, J. (1995). One year follow up pilot study on communication skill and challenging behavior. *European Journal of Psychiatry, 9,* 83–95.

Drasgow, E., Halle, J., & Sigafoos, J. (1999). Teaching communication to learners with severe disabilities: Motivation, response competition, and generalization. *Australasian Journal of Special Education, 23,* 47–63.

Duker, P., Didden, R., & Sigafoos, J. (2004). *One-to-one training: Instructional procedures for learners with developmental disabilities.* Austin, TX: Pro-Ed.

Duker, P. C., van Driel, S., & van de Bercken, J. (2002). Communication profiles of individuals with Down's syndrome, Angelman syndrome and pervasive developmental disorder. *Journal of Intellectual Disability Research, 46,* 35–40.

Durand, V. M. (1993). Problem behavior as communication. *Behaviour Change, 10,* 197–207.

Durand, V. M., & Merges, E. (2001). Functional communication training: A contemporary behavior analytic intervention for problem behaviors. *Focus on Autism and Other Developmental Disabilities, 16,* 110–119.

Evans, P. L. C., & Spittle, J. A. (1981). The development and use of a Premack symbol system in improving the communication skills of two children with learning difficulties. *Educational Psychology, 1,* 87–99.

Foxx, R. M., Schreck, K. A., Garito, J., Smith, A., & Weisenberger, S. (2004). Replacing the echolalia of children with autism with functional use of verbal labeling. *Journal of Developmental and Physical Disabilities, 16,* 307–320.

Freedman, A. M., Ebin, E. A., & Wilson, E. A. (1962). Autistic schizophrenic children: An experiment in the use of D-Lysergic Acid Diethylamide (LSD-25). *Archives of General Psychiatry, 6,* 35–45.

Fuller, P. R. (1949). Operant conditioning of a vegetative human organism. *American Journal of Psychology, 62,* 587–590.

Guess, D., Sailor, W., & Baer, D. M. (1974). To teach language to retarded children. In R. L. Schiefelbusch & L. L. Lloyd (Eds.), *Language perspectives: Acquisition, retardation, and intervention* (pp. 529–563). Baltimore: University Park Press.

Halle, J. W. (1987). Teaching language in the natural environment: An analysis of spontaneity. *Journal of the Association for Persons with Severe Handicaps, 12,* 28–37.

Hamilton, B. L., & Snell, M. E. (1993). Using the milieu approach to increase spontaneous communication book use across environments by an adolescent with autism. *Augmentative and Alternative Communication, 9,* 259–272.

Harwood, K., Warren, S., & Yoder, P. (2002). The importance of responsivity in developing contingent exchanges with beginning communicators. In J. Reichle, D. R. Beukelman & J. C. Light (Eds.), *Exemplary practices for beginning communicators* (pp. 59–95). Baltimore: Paul H. Brookes Publishing Co.

Haynes, R. B. (2006). Of studies, syntheses, synopses, summaries, and systems: the "5S" evolution of information services for evidence-based health care decisions. *ACP Journal Club, 145*(3), A8–A9.

Iwata, B., Pace, G., Dorsey, M., Zarcone, J., Vollmer, T., Smith, R., et al. (1994). The functions of self-injurious behavior: An experimental-epidemiological analysis. *Journal of Applied Behavior Analysis, 27,* 215–240.

Kaiser, A. P., & Grim, J. C. (2006). Teaching functional communication skills. In M. E. Snell & F. Brown (Eds.), *Instruction of students with severe disabilities* (6th ed., pp. 447–488). Upper Saddle River, NJ: Pearson.

Kanner, L. (1943). Autistic disturbances of affective contact. *Nervous Child, 2,* 217–250.

Kazdin, A. E. (2007). Mediators and mechanisms of change in psychotherapy research. *Annual Review of Clinical Psychology, 3,* 1–26.

Keen, D., Sigafoos, J., & Woodyatt, G. (2001). Replacing prelinguistic behaviors with functional communication. *Journal of Autism and Developmental Disorders, 31,* 385–398.

Kelley, M. E., Shillingsburg, M. A., Castro, M. J., Addison, L. R., & LeRue, R. H., Jr. (2007). Further evaluation of emerging speech in children with developmental disabilities: Training verbal behavior. *Journal of Applied Behavior Analysis, 40,* 431–445.

Kent, L. (1974). *Language acquisition program for the retarded or multiply impaired.* Champaign, IL: Research Press.

King, G., Batorowicz, B., & Shepherd, T. A. (2008). Expertise in research-informed clinical decision making: Working effectively with families of children with little or no functional speech. *Evidence-Based Communication Assessment and Intervention, 2,* 106–116.

Koegel, R. L., O'Dell, M. C., & Koegel, L. K. (1987). A natural language teaching paradigm for nonverbal autistic children. *Journal of Autism and Developmental Disorders, 17,* 187–200.

Lancioni, G. E., O'Reilly, M. F., Cuvo, A. J., Singh, N. N., Sigafoos, J., & Didden, R. (2007). PECS and VOCAs to enable students with developmental disabilities to make requests: An overview of the literature. *Research in Developmental Disabilities, 28,* 468–488.

Landa, R. (2007). Early communication development and intervention for children with autism. *Mental Retardation and Developmental Disabilities Research Reviews, 13,* 16–25.

LeBlanc, L. A., Esch, J., Sidener, T. M., & Firth, A. M. (2006). Behavioral language interventions for children with autism: Comparing applied verbal behavior and naturalistic teaching approaches. *Analysis of Verbal Behavior, 22,* 49–60.

Linscheid, T. R. (1999). Commentary: Response to empirically supported treatments for feeding problems. *Journal of Pediatric Psychology, 24,* 215–216.

Loncke, F. T., Campbell, J., England, A. M., & Haley, T. (2006). Multimodality: A basis for augmentative and alternative communication – psycholinguistic, cognitive, and clinical/educational aspects. *Disability and Rehabilitation, 28,* 169–174.

Lovaas, O. I. (1977). *The autistic child: Language development through behavior modification.* New York: Irvington.

Lovaas, O. I. (1987). Behavioral treatment and normal educational and intellectual functioning in young autistic children. *Journal of Consulting and Clinical Psychology, 55,* 3–9.

Lovaas, O. I. (2003). *Teaching individuals with developmental delays: Basic intervention techniques.* Austin, TX: Pro-Ed.

Lovaas, O. I., Berberich, J. P., Perloff, B. F., & Schaeffer, B. (1966). Acquisition of imitative speech by schizophrenic children. *Science, 151,* 705–707.

Machalicek, W., O'Reilly, M. F., Beretvas, N., Sigafoos, J., Lancioni, G., Sorrells, A., et al. (2008). A review of school-based instructional interventions for students with autism spectrum disorders. *Research in Autism Spectrum Disorders, 2,* 395–416.

Matson, J. L., Terlonge, C., & Minshawi, N. F. (2008). Children with intellectual disabilities. In R. J. Morris & T. R. Kratochwill (Eds.), *The practice of child therapy* (4th ed., pp. 337–361). New York: Lawrence Erlbaum.

Matson, J. L., & Wilkins, J. (2007). A critical review of assessment targets and methods for social skills excesses and deficits for children with autism spectrum disorders. *Research in Autism Spectrum Disorders, 1,* 28–37.

McEachin, J. J., Smith, T., & Lovaas, O. I. (1993). Long-term outcome for children with autism who received early intensive behavioral treatment. *American Journal on Mental Retardation, 97,* 359–391.

Miguel, C. F., Carr, J. E., & Michael, J. (2002). The effects of a stimulus-stimulus pairing procedure on the vocal behavior of children diagnosed with autism. *The Analysis of Verbal Behavior, 18,* 3–13.

Millar, D. C., Light, J. C., & Schlosser, R. W. (2006). The impact of augmentative and alternative communication intervention on the speech production of individuals with developmental disabilities: A research review. *Journal of Speech, Language, and Hearing Research, 49,* 248–264.

Mirenda, P. (2003). Toward functional augmentative and alternative communication for students with autism: Manual signs, graphic symbols, and voice output communication aids. *Language, Speech, and Hearing Services in Schools, 34,* 203–216.

National Institute of Child Health and Human Development. (2007). Autism Spectrum Disorders (ASDs). Retrieved July 25, 2008 from http://www.nichd.nih.gov/health/topics/asd.cfm

National Research Council. (2001). *Educating children with autism.* Washington, DC: National Academy Press.

O'Reilly, M., Sigafoos, J., Lancioni, G. E., Green, V. A., Olive, M., & Cannella, H. (2007). Applied behaviour analysis. In A. Carr, G. O'Reilly, P. N. Walsh & J. McEvoy (Eds.), *The handbook of intellectual disability and clinical psychology practice* (pp. 253–280). London: Routledge.

Ogletree, B. T. (2007). What makes communication intervention successful with children with autism spectrum disorders? *Focus on Autism and Other Developmental Disabilities, 22,* 190–192.

Osterling, J., Dawson, G., & McPartland, J. (2001). Autism. In C. E. Walker & M. C. Roberts (Eds.), *Handbook of clinical child psychology* (3rd ed., pp. 432–452). New York: Wiley.

Potter, B., & Brown, D. L. (1997). A review of studies examining the nature of selection-based and topography-based verbal behavior. *Analysis of Verbal Behavior, 14,* 85–104.

Reichle, J., York, J., & Sigafoos, J. (1991). *Implementing augmentative and alternative communication: Strategies for learners with severe disabilities.* Baltimore: Paul H. Brookes Publishing Co.

Richmond, M. G. (2006). Functional communication training: A review of the literature related to children with autism. *Education and Training in Developmental Disabilities, 41,* 213–224.

Rotholz, D., Berkowitz, S., & Burberry, J. (1989). Functionality of two modes of communication in the community by students with developmental disabilities: A comparison of signing and communication books. *Journal of the Association for Persons with Severe Handicaps, 14,* 227–233.

Sallows, G. O., & Graupner, T. D. (2005). Intensive behavioral treatment for children with autism. Four-year outcome and predictors. *American Journal on Mental Retardation, 110,* 417–438.

Schlosser, R. W. (1999). Social validation of interventions in augmentative and alternative communication. *Augmentative and Alternative Communication, 15,* 234–247.

Schlosser, R. W. (2002). On the importance of being earnest about treatment integrity. *Augmentative and Alternative Communication, 18,* 36–44.

Schlosser, R. W. (2003). *The efficacy of augmentative and alternative communication: Toward evidence-based practice.* San Diego: Academic Press.

Schlosser, R. W., Koul, R., & Costello, J. (2007). Asking well-built questions for evidence-based practice in augmentative and alternative communication. *Journal of Communication Disorders, 40,* 225–238.

Schlosser, R. W., & Raghavendra, P. (2004). Evidence-based practice in augmentative and alternative communication. *Augmentative and Alternative Communication, 20,* 1–21.

Schlosser, R. W., & Sigafoos, J. (2006). Augmentative and alternative communication interventions for persons with developmental disabilities: Narrative review of comparative single-subject experimental studies. *Research in Developmental Disabilities, 27,* 1–29.

Schlosser, R. W., & Sigafoos, J. (2007). Editorial: Moving evidence-based practice forward. *Evidence-Based Communication Assessment and Intervention, 1,* 1–3.

Schlosser, R. W., & Wendt, O. (2008). Effects of augmentative and alternative communication intervention on speech production in children with autism: A systematic review. *American Journal of Speech-Language Pathology, 17,* 212–230.

Schlosser, R. W., Wendt, O., & Sigafoos, J. (2007). Not all systematic reviews are created equal: Considerations for appraisal. *Evidence-Based Communication Assessment and Intervention, 1,* 138–150.

Shafer, E. (1993). Teaching topography-based and selection-based verbal behavior to developmentally disabled individuals: Some considerations. *Analysis of Verbal Behavior, 11,* 117–133.

Sigafoos, J. (1997). A review of communication intervention programs for people with developmental disabilities. *Behaviour Change, 14,* 125–138.

Sigafoos, J. (2000). Communication development and aberrant behavior in children with developmental disabilities. *Education and Training in Mental Retardation and Developmental Disabilities, 35,* 168–176.

Sigafoos, J., Arthur-Kelly, M., & Butterfield, N. (2006). *Enhancing everyday communication for children with disabilities.* Baltimore: Paul H. Brookes Publishing Co.

Sigafoos, J., Arthur, M., & O'Reilly, M. (2003). *Challenging behavior and developmental disability.* Baltimore: Paul H. Brookes Publishing Co.

Sigafoos, J., Drasgow, E., Halle, J. W., O'Reilly, M., Seely-York, S., Edrisinha, C., et al. (2004). Teaching VOCA use as a communicative repair strategy. *Journal of Autism and Developmental Disorders, 34,* 411–422.

Sigafoos, J., Drasgow, E., Reichle, J., O'Reilly, M., Green, V. A., & Tait, K. (2004). Tutorial: Teaching communicative rejecting to children with severe disabilities. *American Journal of Speech-Language Pathology, 13,* 31–42.

Sigafoos, J., Green, V. A., Payne, R., Son, S. H., O'Reilly, M., & Lancioni, G. E. (2009). A further comparison of picture exchange and speech-generating: Acquisition, preference, and collateral effects on social interaction. *Augmentative and Alternative Communication , 25,* 99–109.

Sigafoos, J., & Littlewood, R. (1999). Communication intervention on the playground: A case study on teaching requesting to a young child with autism. *International Journal of Disability, Development, and Education, 46,* 421–429.

Sigafoos, J., O'Reilly, M., Ganz, J., Lancioni, G., & Schlosser, R. (2005). Supporting self-determination in AAC interventions by assessing preference for communication devices. *Technology & Disability, 17,* 143–153.

Sigafoos, J., O'Reilly, M., Schlosser, R. W., & Lancioni, G. E. (2007). Communication intervention. In P. Sturmey & A. Fitzer (Eds.), *Autism spectrum disorders: Applied behavior analysis, evidence, and practice* (pp. 151–185). Austin, TX: Pro-Ed.

Sigafoos, J., Reichle, J., Doss, S., Hall, K., & Pettitt, L. (1990). "Spontaneous" transfer of stimulus control from tact to mand contingencies. *Research in Developmental Disabilities, 11,* 165–176.

Sigafoos, J., Schlosser, R. W., Green, V. A., O'Reilly, M. F., & Lancioni, G. E. (2008). Communication and social skills assessment. In J. L. Matson (Ed.), *Clinical assessment and intervention for autism spectrum disorders* (pp. 165–192). Burlington, MA: Academic Press.

Skinner, B. F. (1957). *Verbal behavior.* Englewood Cliffs, NJ: Prentice Hall.

Snell, M. E., Chen, L. Y., & Hoover, K. (2006). Teaching augmentative and alternative communication to students with severe disabilities: A review of intervention research 1997–2003. *Research and Practice for Persons with Severe Disabilities, 31,* 203–214.

Son, S. H., Sigafoos, J., O'Reilly, M., & Lancioni, G. E. (2006). Comparing two types of augmentative and alternative communication systems for children with autism. *Pediatric Rehabilitation, 9,* 389–395.

Soto, G., Belfiore, P. J., Schlosser, R. W., & Haynes, C. (1993). Teaching specific requests: A comparative analysis of skill acquisition and preference using two augmentative and alternative communication aids. *Education and Training in Mental Retardation, 28,* 169–178.

Straus, S. E. (2007). Evidence-based health care: Challenges and limitations. *Evidence-Based Communication Assessment and Intervention, 1,* 48–51.

Sundberg, M. L. (1980). *Developing a verbal repertoire using sign language and Skinner's analysis of verbal behavior.* Unpublished doctoral dissertation, Western Michigan University, Kalamazoo.

Sundberg, M. L., & Michael, J. (2001). The benefits of Skinner's analysis of verbal behavior for children with autism. *Behavior Modification, 25,* 698–724.

Sundberg, M. L., Michael, J., Partington, J. W., & Sundberg, C. A. (1996). The role of automatic reinforcement in early language acquisition. *The Analysis of Verbal Behavior, 13,* 21–37.

Tager-Flusberg, H., Paul, R., & Lord, C. (2005). Language and communication in autism. In F. Volkmar, R. Paul, A. Klin & D. Cohen (Eds.), *Handbook of autism and pervasive developmental disorders* (pp. 335–364). Indianapolis, IN: Wiley.

Tincani, M. (2004). Comparing the picture exchange communication system and sign language training for children with autism. *Focus on Autism and Other Developmental Disabilities, 19,* 152–163.

Vignes, T. (2007). A comparison of topography-based and selection-based verbal behavior in typically developed children and developmentally disabled persons with autism. *Analysis of Verbal Behavior, 23,* 113–122.

Wacker, D. P., Berg, W. K., Harding, J. W., Barretto, A., Rankin, B., & Ganzer, J. (2005). Treatment effectiveness, stimulus generalization, and acceptability to parents of functional communication training. *Educational Psychology, 25,* 233–256.

Wilczynski, S. M., Christian, L., & The National Autism Center. (2008). The National Standards Project: Promoting evidence-based practice in Autism Spectrum Disorders. In J. K. Luiselli, D. C. Russo, W. P. Christian & S. M. Wilczynski (Eds.), *Effective practices for children with autism: Educational and behavioral support interventions that work* (pp. 37–60). Oxford, NY: Oxford University Press.

Wolery, M., & Gast, D. L. (1984). Effective and efficient procedures for the transfer of stimulus control. *Topics in Early Childhood Special Education, 4*, 52–77.

Wolf, M. M. (1978). Social validity: The case for subjective measurement or how applied behavior analysis is finding its heart. *Journal of Applied Behavior Analysis, 11*, 203–214.

Woods, T. S. (1984). Generality in the verbal tacting of autistic children as a function of the "naturalness" in antecedent control. *Journal of Behavior Therapy and Experimental Psychiatry, 15*, 27–32.

World Health Organization. (2007). *International Statistical Classification of Diseases and Related Health Problems, 10th Revision (ICD-10)*. Retrieved July 23, 2008 from http://www.who.int/classifications/apps/icd/icd10online

Yoon, S., & Bennett, G. M. (2000). Effects of a stimulus-stimulus pairing procedure on conditioning vocal sounds as reinforcers. *The Analysis of Verbal Behavior, 17*, 75–88.

Chapter 7
Social Skills and Autism: Understanding and Addressing the Deficits

Mary Jane Weiss, Robert H. LaRue, and Andrea Newcomer

Social behavior is a core deficit area of autism spectrum disorders (ASD). Therefore, considerable literature in the ABA field has been developed to address this problem area. Specific behaviors treated and ABA techniques used will be the focus of the chapter. A critical appraisal of current status and future directions will also be provided.

Introduction

Autism is a severe developmental disorder marked by three core diagnostic features. These core features include impairments in reciprocal social interaction, delays in early language and communication, and the presence of restrictive, repetitive, and stereotyped behaviors. (American Psychiatric Association, 2000).

Autism was first identified and described by Leo Kanner (1943). Kanner noted the relative lack of affective engagement and communication with other people that has since become the primary characteristic of autism. A huge empirical literature has emerged, documenting the significant social challenges experienced by learners with autism (e.g., Attwood, 1998; Frith, 1989; Sigman & Capps, 1997). Symptoms of these social deficits include, poor eye contact, failure to develop peer relationships appropriate to their developmental level, abnormal voice and speech intonation, impairment in the use of multiple nonverbal behaviors

M.J. Weiss (✉)
Douglass Developmental Disabilities Center, Rutgers, The State University of New Jersey, 25 Gibbons Circle, New Brunswick, NJ, 08901-8528, USA
e-mail: weissnj@rci.rutgers.edu

(such as eye-to-eye gaze, facial expression, body postures, and social gestures), and failure to spontaneously seek to share enjoyment, interests, or achievements with other people (e.g., by a lack of showing, bringing, or pointing out objects of interest) (American Psychiatric Association, 2000). Learners with autism also do not orient to naturally occurring social stimuli to the same extent as non-autistic learners do (Dawson, Meltzoff, Osterling, Rinaldi, & Brown, 1998). Another complication is that the quantity, duration, and quality of social exchanges vary as a function of age, degree of impairment, and the setting/context (Matson & Swiezy, 1994).

While the social deficits of autism are often described, the nature or etiology of this specific deficit remains poorly understood.

Origin of Deficit: Theory of Mind

The concept of Theory of Mind was first proposed in basic research involving chimpanzees (Premack & Woodruff, 1978). The Theory of Mind, in a general sense, refers to the ability to take the perspective of others to understand and predict behavior. Researchers have suggested that the development of the Theory of Mind begins within the first year of life. These initial steps in the development of Theory of Mind include gaze following, joint attention, drawing the attention of others with pointing, understanding if objects are animate or inanimate, and awareness of others as intentional agents (Barresi & Moore, 1996; Falck-Ytter, Gredebäck, & von Hofsten, 2006; Tremoulet & Feldman, 2000).

Researchers have suggested that the development of Theory of Mind is an area of weakness for individuals across the autism spectrum. Researchers have indicated that learners with autism have specific difficulties with tasks requiring the understanding of another person's beliefs (Baron-Cohen, Leslie, & Frith, 1985; Moore, 2002). Theorists have suggested that the Theory of Mind provides an explanation for the communication and social challenges that define autism spectrum disorders. The Theory of Mind requires the ability to use joint attention and gaze following, which are commonly documented deficits in autism (Baron-Cohen, 1989; Dawson et al., 2004; Loveland & Landry, 1986). Understanding the animate/inanimate nature of objects is also a common deficit in learners with autism (Blake, Turner, Smoski, Pozdol, & Stone, 2003; Rutherford, Pennington, & Rogers, 2006).

The Physiology of Social Deficits

A number of brain areas are involved in social behavior. Brain areas involved in social behavior include the medial prefrontal cortex (mPFC), anterior cingulate cortex (ACC), inferior frontal gyrus, superior temporal sulcus (STS), the amygdala and anterior insula. In addition, researchers have suggested that social impairments may also be related to vagal nerve dysfunction (Porges, 1995). Studies have shown that damage to these areas creates disruptions in social behavior in humans as well as other mammals.

Amygdala–Fusiform System

Many researchers have theorized that learners with autism have functional abnormalities in some of the social areas of the brain. Specific sites implicated in the social abnormalities in autism include the amygdala and the fusiform face area (or fusiform gyrus). Researchers have suggested that the development of face perception and social cognitive skills are supported by the amygdala–fusiform system, and that deficits in this network are instrumental in the development of autism (Schultz, 2005). Although not part of current diagnostic criteria for autism, a considerable amount of evidence indicates that learners with autism ASD have marked deficits in face perception (Derulle, Rondan, Gepner, & Tardif, 2004; Grelotti, Gauthier, & Schultz, 2002; Klin et al., 1999). Researchers suggest that the ability to recognize faces is a critical component to successful functioning within a social group.

Vagal Nerve Dysfunction

Researchers have hypothesized that some of the symptoms of autism may be related to dysfunction in vagal nerve activity, which has been linked to a number of psychiatric disorders (Porges, 1995, 1997). Relatively little research has investigated this phenomenon and information related to this may help to inform the intervention process for learners with autism.

The vagus nerve is a cranial nerve that fulfills multiple roles throughout the body. One role is the support of homeostatic function in the body (e.g., regulation of digestion, respiration, heart rate). Another role of the vagus nerve is that it regulates the body's response to environmental challenges, which affects social behavior. In higher mammals, a branch of the vagus nerve (myelinated vagus) regulates social communication, calming, and had the ability to inhibit sympathetic-adrenal influences when necessary (can prevent fight-or-flight arousal). Recent research has indicated that individuals with psychiatric disorders often have dysfunction in the branch of the vagus that regulates these functions. Specifically, individuals with the inability to regulate the function of the vagus nerve (referred to as having "low vagal tone") are susceptible to a variety of behavior and social problems, such as, fearful emotionality, off-task behavior (Blair & Peters, 2004), negative emotional affect, behavior problems, social skills deficits (Calkins & Keane, 2004), peer coping, and impaired self-regulation (e.g., Porges, 1995, 1997), anxiety (e.g., Thayer, Friedman, & Borkovec, 1996), hostility (Sloan et al., 1994), and disorders of impulse control (Beauchaine, 2001).

The Challenges of Learning and Teaching Social Skills

In addition to speculation on the causes and origins of the social deficits associated with autism, there has been great interest in how such skills might be effectively improved. In general, it is an area in which gains have been modest and the development of innovative clinical approaches has been limited.

Social skills, which are centrally important to the success of individuals on the autism spectrum, are among the most elusive targets to teach. One impediment to teaching such skills is that there may not be much intrinsic interest on the part of consumers with autism spectrum disorders (ASD) in learning these skills. Many people with ASD lack social interest and fail to comprehend social nuances. Additionally, they often exhibit little social initiation, as well as reduced social responsiveness.

Furthermore, it is often difficult to identify teaching methods for such skills. Most social skills are multi-element skills that require the individual to engage in several different and distinct tasks. Furthermore, most of the skills in the social realm involve an element of judgment (i.e., is it appropriate to engage in this behavior at this time?) Such complexities make it difficult to teach such skills. How can we operationalize social judgment? How can we prepare learners for the endless possibilities that exist in the natural environment?

Basic Components of Social Skills

Social skill deficits include deficits in social initiation, social responses, and social comprehension (which may simply be circumstances which require complex or multi-component initiations and responses). All of these central areas impede social integration and limit how the individual interacts with others in their environments.

Social initiations include greeting others, asking questions of others, commenting to others, and asking to join ongoing activities. In general, social initiations are weaker as a response class than social responses. Social responses include responding to the social overtures of others such as greetings, questions, and offers to join activities. Applied Behavior Analysis (ABA) has been shown to be extremely effective in building social initiations and social responses.

Qualitative Aspects of Social Behaviors

There are qualitative aspects to social initiations and responses that affect the functional utility of the social skills learned. Social initiations and responses emitted may lack clarity (e.g., a child who waits near the water table as a mand to join). They may also be blatantly inappropriate (e.g., a child who initiates a game of chase by pulling another child's hair). They may lack independence, and require facilitation from an adult. Such assistance may be subtle (e.g., encouragement) or intrusive (e.g., scripting).

Another qualitative aspect of social skills is latency to respond. For a social response to be functional, it must occur within an acceptable timeframe. If there is a delay of 5 or 10 s after a child is greeted and before they respond, many social opportunities are lost. Many peers will simply leave the social interaction when they do not receive a timely response. They may also infer that their friend is not interested in or able to respond to them, thereby reducing the likelihood of future initiations.

Social Comprehension

Social comprehension is used to describe the complicated social responses and initiations that are part of navigating the social world. It includes understanding social rules, engaging in behaviors that are expected in given contexts, and interpreting social nuances. Social comprehension skills are elusive for making meaningful progress and are difficult to define and teach.

There are a number of commercially available curricula to target the development of such skills that have well-formulated lessons for a variety of skills (e.g., Baker, 2003a, 2003b; McGinnis & Goldstein, 1990; Richardson, 1996; Taylor & Jasper, 2001). Many of these curricula are written by behavior analysts, and outline methodical teaching strategies and the collection of data to guide decisions. They are extremely useful clinical resources indeed for the identification of and instruction in social skills.

Often, a variety of approaches are used together, in a packaged approach, to address such issues. Such packages may combine both empirically validated and non empirically validated techniques. Commonly used components of such packages include video modeling, social stories, rule cards, and role plays.

Video Modeling

Several studies have shown that *video modeling* can be an effective tool for teaching learners with autism. Video modeling has been shown to be useful for teaching the imitation of peers (Haring, Kennedy, Adams, &

Pitts-Conway, 1987), learning sign language (Watkins, Sprafkin, & Krolikowski, 1993), developing play skills (Charlop-Christy, Le, & Freeman, 2000), and building conversation skills (Charlop & Milstein, 1989; Sherer et al., 2001). Because so much research supports its utility in teaching skills, video modeling is being used increasingly clinically to build a variety of skills, including functional academic skills, community-relevant skills, conversational exchanges, and play skills (e. g., Snell & Brown, 2000; Taylor, 2001; Weiss & Harris, 2001).

Many students with ASD are strong visual learners, and often enjoy watching videos. Many learners with autism may attend better to a model presented in a video clip than they would to a live model demonstrating a skill. Clinically, video modeling is often done with an adult demonstrating the skill first. By using an adult model, it is easier to ensure that the salient aspects of the target behavior will be highlighted. Alternately, older peer tutors or mature peers can be used as models. These choices have obvious advantages, because of their similarities to the target students.

Video modeling usually involves having learners observe a video clip of the desired actions and then prompting procedures are used to help the learner engage in the behaviors. Initially, there may be simultaneous imitation of what is being watched (doing the actions along with the model on tape), followed by delayed imitation of what was observed (watching the clip and then engaging in the play). Rote responding can be a significant concern, so it is essential to program variability into the video modeling protocol.

Another extension of video instruction is to use videotape as a source of feedback to the learners on their performance during play activities. Reinforcement and corrective feedback can be provided, and better strategies for targeted areas of weakness can be modeled and rehearsed (e.g., Taylor, 2001). This might have special relevance for learners who have demonstrated difficulty in comprehending social nuances, such as sticking to the topic in a conversation.

Several guidelines for the use of video with learners have been given (e. g., Krantz, MacDuff, Wadstrom, & McClannahan, 1991). Suggestions include assessing learners for appropriate prerequisite skills; removing extraneous stimuli from the videotape; attending to the history of the learner with the persons presenting the video or modeling on video; and considering cognitive level as a possible factor affecting relevance.

Social Stories

As mentioned previously, learners with autism often have difficulty understanding expectations in social situations. Over the past decade, social stories have become increasingly popular as an intervention strategy for learners with ASD (Barry & Burlew, 2004; Sansosti, Powell-Smith, & Kincaid, 2004). Social stories are brief descriptions of expectations that are explained in the context of a "story" created on an individual basis to describe a specific scenario the learner will encounter. Typically, the story is written from the perspective of the learner, in a meaningful format for people with ASD (Gray, 2000). A social story is created specifically for the student it is intended to help. Practitioners can create stories that are supplemented with pictorial cues or photos in addition to textual information (Reynhout & Carter, 2006). The use of stories to explain social rules and contingencies has been shown to be beneficial for learners with autism.

Gray (2000) outlined suggestions for developing effective social stories. Specifically, Gray outlined the types of sentences to be used in social stories. There are currently seven recognized sentence types used to create social stories (Barry & Burlew, 2004; Crozier & Tincani, 2007; Reynhout & Carter, 2006):

- *Descriptive:* Sentences that provide factual information.
- *Perspective:* Sentences that provide insight regarding the thoughts, feelings, and behaviors of others.
- *Affirmative:* Sentences that are used to reassure the learner.
- *Directive:* Sentences that tell the learner what behaviors are expected.
- *Control:* Sentences that use analogies to explain situations.
- *Cooperative:* Sentences that tell the learners who can assist them in different situations.
- *Consequence:* Sentences that tell what will happen as a result of the actions.

Gray (1995, 2000) offers two options for how to construct social stories using the different types of sentences: the *basic* social story ratio and the *complete* social story ratio. In the *basic* social story ratio, Gray suggests using 2–5 descriptive, perspective, and/or affirmative sentences for each directive sentence. The *complete* social story ratio includes the addition of control and cooperative sentences. For each control or cooperative sentence, 2–5 descriptive, perspective, affirmative, and/or directive sentences are recommended. The objective of the social story is to describe rather than direct. The assumption is that changes in behavior may be a result of a greater understanding of expectations and events in their environment (The Gray Center, 2008). Social stories reported in the literature are primarily composed of descriptive, directive, consequence, and perspective sentences (Reynhout & Carter, 2006). Social stories can be used to both increase and decrease behavior. For example, social stories can be used to explain the actions required to deposit a check at the bank or to explain the contingencies required to access a desired reinforcer (e.g., to access a trip to the park, they must not engage in any aggressive behavior). Social stories are often used for multi-element situations (which change on a frequent basis), fear situations, and to reduce challenging behaviors.

While the use of social stories is common in clinical practice, the number of carefully controlled investigations is relatively small. Most clinical guidelines for using social stories have not been empirically validated and require more comprehensive investigation.

Barry and Burlew (2004) used a multiple baseline across two participants to show the effects of social story instruction on independent choice making and appropriate play. The authors reported that the level of prompting required for choice making decreased for both participants and the duration of appropriate play increased. However, the study did not control for other treatments in place in the classroom at the time of intervention.

Thiemann and Goldstein (2001) used social stories in conjunction with text cards, visual cues, and video feedback to increase the social behavior of five learners with autism. The targeted social behaviors included contingent responses, securing attention, commenting, and requesting. The effect of social stories was evaluated using a multiple baseline design across skills. Intervention occurred in a small group setting with two typical peers along with the child with autism. Social stories helped developing the social behavior of the learners with autism. Two learners demonstrated generalization to new social skills. However, the authors reported that these effects may have been due, in part, to the overlap between the skills. While these results are encouraging, the authors reported that there was a general lack of maintenance across skills and learners.

Often, social stories are used in combination with other treatments, as part of a packaged social skills intervention (Reynhout & Carter, 2006; Rogers, 2000). In fact, when part of packaged interventions, some gains have been noted (Sansosti & Powell-Smith, 2008; Swaggart et al., 1995). However, multiple treatments limit the extent to which treatment effects can be attributed to social stories.

When studies employ more than one treatment method (Barry & Burlew, 2004; Burke, Kuhn, & Peterson, 2004; Thiemann & Goldstein, 2001), the degree to which social stories are responsible for that effect is unclear. Delano and Snell (2006) set out to build upon the research of Thiemann and Goldstein by using the same social skills, but isolating social stories as the only treatment. During intervention, skills increased for all three learners; however, as the influence of the stories faded, so did the treatment effects. Two learners showed generalization of skills to their general education classroom. Treatment effects were higher than baseline, but failed to maintain at intervention levels.

The tendency for social stories to be implemented concurrently with other interventions is a serious challenge to understanding their potential efficacy. Another major challenge in the use of social stories, both from a clinical and a research standpoint, is the paucity of available information on the essential elements of their use. Development of the stories is highly variable, presentation to the student is highly idiosyncratic, and staff-training procedures have not been addressed. There are few guidelines for how to use the social story and when to curtail its usage. Two commonly used, but empirically unsupported, strategies to fade the use of a social story are to reduce the number of times the story is read each week and systematically removing sentences from the story, specifically the directive ones. There has been no controlled study looking at length of intervention phase.

The literature describes a variety of strategies to implement the social story. They include having the teacher or parent read to the child (Crozier & Tincani, 2007), having the child read (Thiemann & Goldstein, 2001), listening to or watching the story on a computer or TV (More, 2008; Sansosti & Powell-Smith, 2008), and listening to the story embedded in a song (Brownell, 2002).

Implementation is variable in nearly every aspect of use. Crozier and Tincani (2007) developed a treatment integrity checklist to evaluate how well the intervention of social stories was implemented. The critical components of the treatment were:sitting across from the learner placing the book on the table in front of the learner reading the book with the learner encouraging the learner to look and point at the story telling the learner it's time to do the activity directing the learner to the activity

This tool allows for some assessment of whether the instructor is following a specified protocol for the introduction and review of the story. As such, it represents progress in the operational definition of how to incorporate social stories into a student's educational program.

There has also been some interest in evaluating exactly how social stories might be used to reduce challenging behaviors. Swaggart et al. (1995) and Burke et al. (2004) used social stories to explain a behavioral contingency that had been put in place (i.e., response-cost, positive reinforcement) to reduce behavior disturbances. Both studies demonstrated decreases in problem behavior and Burke et al. showed maintenance of effects at three-month follow-up.

In general, however, at the present time, the wide use of social stories is perplexing, given the limited data available regarding their efficacy. Nevertheless, they remain a very popular tool for intervention. Parents and teachers alike report liking social stories (Burke et al., 2004; Dodd, Hupp, Jewell, & Krohn, 2008), and often will follow recommendations to create and review social stories. It may be that social stories enhance parent and teacher attention to targeted behaviors, which may make it more likely that desirable behaviors are prompted and reinforced. There also appears to be a discrepancy between the perceived effects of treatment and the future use of the social stories. Dodd et al. reported that the two parents in their study were unsure if the social stories had an effect on the target behaviors, but planned to continue using them and even create new stories for other skills. Investment may come from face-validity or natural quality of approach for parents (e.g., all parents read to kids). Similarly, Crozier and Tincani (2007) reported that teachers liked using social stories and found their outcomes to be favorable, but did not continue to use the stories beyond the scope of the research study. The authors suspect that the time consuming nature of reading a social story before an activity may have not made it feasible for teachers with large groups of students. To maintain the behavior, the stories would need to be a part of the lesson planning and become integrated into the classroom routine.

Even in studies that have shown promising treatment effects using social stories, there is a lack of knowledge about the critical components. By developing more effective methods for evaluating social stories, improvements in creating and implementing them can be made. It is possible that their effectiveness may be a result of other elements of the packaged interventions. In general, it is clinically wise to use social stories in combination with direct behavior change procedures.

Rule Cards

Another visual support strategy for social skills intervention is the rule card or a similar approach known as the *Power Card Strategy* (Gagnon, 2001). The Power Card is a small card that the learner carries that summarizes a strategy to use when a particular scenario arises. The card, typically the size of a business card or note card, is individualized for the learner by having a picture of a preferred interest. Learners with autism often have limited interests, but find these interests tend to be highly reinforcing. The behavior or skill is encouraged through its connection to the special interest (Keeling, Smith Miles, Gagnon, & Simpson, 2003).

Keeling et al. (2003) used the Power Card Strategy to decrease the whines and screams of a 10-year-old student with autism. The student typically engaged in these behaviors when placed in game situations. A multiple baseline design was implemented across three game activities. On the first day of intervention a longer Power Card Script was read, in which the child's favorite cartoon character modeled appropriate responses for both winning and losing games. Prior to all other intervention sessions, the shorter Power Card was read, which listed three strategies for winning and three for losing, which came from the longer script. The Power Card was effective in decreasing whines and screams and the intervention generalized to the third activity, which never used the Power Card. The student began to use the strategies on the card in new settings with peers and even told a classmate what he could say after he had lost. A limitation of the study was that data were only presented for problem behavior, not targeted behavior.

A closely related intervention is the script-fading procedure. For example, Krantz and McClannahan (1998) embedded textual prompts in the activity picture schedules of preschoolers with autism. The schedule showed what to play with and the textual prompt was for a short directive statement for the student to make to the teacher. The number of social initiations increased for all the children, as did the number of unscripted interactions. The textual prompts were faded out and the number of interactions maintained and generalized to new activities. This study adds to the literature by describing an intervention that worked for children with minimal reading skills. In a similar study Stevenson, Krantz, and McClannahan (2000) used an audio taped script to increase the social interactions of four students, ages 10–15. Once scripts were faded, all participants were able to produce high levels of unscripted responses and results were maintained. The authors cite generalization as an area that needs more research.

Summary of Strategies to Build Social Comprehension

Social skills are complicated to define, teach, and evaluate. Often, they are targeted in a wide variety of ways, and are addressed through a package of instructional strategies. Some of the commonly used approaches include social stories, rule cards, and video modeling. Social stories, while probably the most widely utilized of these approaches, has a paucity of data supporting its effectiveness. While there have been some reports of success, it is not clear whether social stories themselves are responsible for the effects. In fact, it is likely that other, more direct behavior change procedures used in combination with social stories were responsible for those effects. Component analyses would help to isolate the unique contribution of social stories. In addition, research is needed on the critical elements of social stories as an intervention approach. Video modeling and social scripting have good empirical support. From a clinical perspective, variability in scripts and models must be included as part of effective intervention. Rule cards are an interesting clinical direction, particularly when combined with role-plays or other behavioral rehearsal techniques.

New Directions

There have been some other approaches to social skills training that may have clinical utility for learners on the autism spectrum. In some cases, these approaches may have been demonstrated as effective with other populations of learners. In other cases, they may be theoretically compelling. We will discuss interventions to increase perspective taking, problem solving, and joint attention.

Perspective Taking

Perspective taking generally refers to the ability to understand the thoughts and feeling (or perspective) of others. While these skills emerge during the preschool years for typically developing children, children with autism often have significant impairments in their ability to understand the perspectives of others. The ability to understand the perspectives of others is of particular importance as it is closely related to other critical social skills, including turn-taking, empathy, sharing, conversation skills, and initiations (LeBlanc et al., 2003).

Theory of Mind (ToM) is an abstract theory encompassing many skills and mental capacities. One is said to have a ToM when they can infer and understand others' desires, beliefs, and feelings (Ozonoff & Miller, 1995). Research on ToM often uses measures of appearance reality, false belief, and representational change to operationally define perspective taking and ToM (Charlop-Christy & Daneshvar, 2003; Taylor & Carlson, 1997). For example, tests evaluate the person's ability to distinguish between what something may appear to be and what it truly is. Similarly, tests may evaluate the person's ability to accurately label what people believe about a situation, particularly when they have different or incomplete information.

Literature on teaching perspective taking skills is very limited. Two studies have used video modeling to teach perspective taking (Charlop-Christy & Daneshvar, 2003; LeBlanc et al., 2003). In these studies, children with autism ranging in age from 6 to 13 years were taught to answer questions by watching videos of others answering the questions correctly.

Charlop-Christy and Daneshvar (2003) used three false-belief tasks, referred to in the literature as, the Sally-Anne task, the M&M's task, and the hide-and-seek task. Training was provided on each of the tasks until the child was able to show generalization of the skill on a similar example. All three participants were able to learn the tasks and correctly answer questions on similar tasks. Only two participants were able to pass the posttest (an untrained Sally-Anne task) at the conclusion of the training. This study provides evidence that video modeling and multiple exemplar training may be useful components to social skills training packages.

LeBlanc et al. (2003) used a similar method with the addition of reinforcers delivered for correct answers. They had similar results to Charlop-Christy and Daneshvar, including two out of three of their participants passing the untrained Sally-Anne task at the end.

Anecdotally, Charlop-Christy and Daneshvar report that the participant who did not pass the post-test also had the most trouble answering questions about what he had seen in the video (memory questions) and he was the least social and the least verbal of the three participants. The non-passing participant in the LeBlanc et al. study, was the oldest participant at 13 years (the other participants were both 7 years old). There is some evidence of a correlation between performance on perspective-taking tasks and age equivalent scores on the Daily Living scale of the Vineland Adaptive Behavior Scales (Rehfeldt, Dillen, Ziomek, & Kowalchuk, 2007).

Perspective taking interventions are theoretically compelling, as they target the central social deficit of autism (described in the ToM literature). There is great potential clinical utility in this area. However, much research is needed in understanding how to best teach such skills, and more importantly, in how to teach them in ways that transfer to natural social circumstances.

Problem Solving

Another compelling social deficit associated with autism is difficulty in identifying and managing social conflicts of various kinds. The term "problem solving" refers to the ability to use available information to come up with strategies to solve problems (Agran, Blanhard, Wehmeyer, & Hughes, 2002). Learners with autism often exhibit a lack of problem-solving abilities, selecting the wrong strategy in a scenario, or do not know when to switch from one strategy to another

(Gagnon, 2001). When solutions are generated, there are often problems that arise when the solutions are not socially appropriate (Channon, Charman, Heap, Crawford, & Rios, 2001).

There is general agreement among practitioners that problem-solving skills are imperative for successful outcomes in school and community settings. However, this is an area that continues to be limited by a lack of information about what to teach and how to teach it. As a result, teachers are often simply not providing the necessary opportunities for students to improve in this area (Agran et al., 2002).

Some research suggests that one component of successful problem solving, may be autobiographical memory. Goddard, Howlin, Dritschel, and Patel (2007) compared the autobiographical memory and problem-solving abilities of adults with Asperger Syndrome to neurotypical adults. They found that those with Asperger Syndrome were less likely than their neurotypical counterparts to come up with detailed and effective solutions to social problems. In addition, the researchers reported significantly longer latencies to recall memories and a fewer number of memories recalled overall in the Asperger group.

As we have reviewed, solving problems is an important part of successful navigation in school. In addition, it is central to navigating the social world. Many students with other types of presenting problems, such as ADHD, have benefited substantially from problem-solving approaches. Problem-solving training usually involves helping learners to identify problems and select appropriate solutions. Children with ASD often have difficulties with deciphering the ambiguity of social problems, and with evaluating options for a course of action. They may be impulsive or fail to see the range of options. Problem-solving training (e. g., Shure, 2001a, 2001b, 2004) can help students with ASD to identify problems, generate alternative solutions, evaluate the effectiveness of different potential courses of action, and choose the best option. This can be done as a class-wide intervention or as an individual approach.

A variation of problem solving is the social autopsy (Bieber, 1994). This approach helps to identify cause-and-effect relationships between one's behavior and the reactions of others. This clinical approach involves discussing the situation after the event and creating a plan to prevent further instances (Dunn, 2006).

Problem solving and perspective taking interventions are both designed to address some of the more complicated social deficits associated with autism spectrum disorders. These are central deficits, which impede social problem solving and the development of relationships.

Joint Attention

Children are often initially referred for a diagnosis of autism spectrum disorder when they fail to acquire language at a rate similar to their typically developing peers. However, another common deficit in observed in learners with autism at this early juncture is a lack of joint attention. Joint attention skills typically develop before a child's first words. Recently, the topic of joint attention has come into sharp focus in the literature because it may have important implications for both early diagnosis and intervention (Bruinsma, Koegel, & Koegel, 2004). The term *joint attention* can be difficult to define because it encompasses a variety of phenomena (i.e., gaze following, social referencing, protoimperative gestures, protodeclarative gestures, and monitoring) and is closely related to many others. In addition to the many operational definitions used in the literature, there is usually a more implicit meaning associated with the term. Descriptions of joint attention often include terms like, "sharing attention" or "knowing what another is looking at and experiencing".

Joint attention is frequently described as a coordinated shift in attention between an object or event and another person, which occurs in a social context. The term is used to refer to both recruiting (or initiating) attention and responding to the bids of others. For instance, a child recruiting attention may point to a toy while saying, "look," or reach for a toy while turning to an adult for help. Other examples would include a child responding to bids for attention from others, turning to look when the child hears their name called, or looking back and forth from a toy being held out to the person holding it. Children with autism typically exhibit significant deficits in joint attention.

Whalen and Schreibman (2003) distinguished between two main types of recruiting attention: protoimperative and protodeclarative. While both types of attention recruitment may be similar in topography, they differ in function. According to Whalen and Schreibman protoimperative gestures and vocalizations are those used to request access to an object. Protodeclarative gestures and vocalizations are used to recruit attention for sharing or mutual attending to an object.

Recently, Mundy et al. (2007) elaborated on the different types of joint attention as well. The authors described the concepts of protoimperative and protodeclarative gestures and vocalizations as initiating behavior regulation/requests (IBR) and initiating joint attention (IJA), respectively. In addition, Mundy et al. described the response to joint attention (RJA) and response to behavior requests (RBR) to characterize the responding to others' bids for joint attention.

Importance of Joint Attention

Joint attention is considered an important skill because of its possible relation to several domains of development. The development of joint attention has been linked to language development, adaptive social-emotional behavioral development (Sheinkopf, Mundy, Claussen, & Willoughby, 2004), and frontal lobe function (Mundy & Crawson, 1997). Joint attention may be central to understanding language outcomes later in childhood. Morales et al. (2000) found that response to joint attention was directly related to vocabulary development in learners between -6 and 24 months. In a review of the literature, Bruinsma et al. (2004) found that time spent engaging in joint attention behaviors was positively related to the child's later vocabulary size.

Teaching Joint Attention

There is growing evidence to support that joint attention can indeed be taught for those who do not naturally acquire it. In a study conducted by Kasari, Freeman, and Paparella (2006), children were assigned to one of three experimental groups: a joint attention intervention group, a symbolic play intervention group, and a control group. Treatment procedures were held constant in the joint attention and symbolic play groups, primarily consisting of discrete trial training, shaping, and milieu teaching techniques. The groups differed along the treatment goals, either teaching joint attention skills or symbolic play. Sessions were conducted daily for 30 min over the course of 5–6 weeks. Improvements in joint attention and joint engagement were found for both treatment groups as compared to the control group. These improvements were also shown to generalize from the interventionist to the child's caregiver. Based on these results, the recommendation was that early intervention programs should address not only *what* is being taught, but also *how* they are targeting skills for intervention. This study also shows the relatively short amount of time it takes children to learn and generalize theses skills.

In a similar study by Kasari, Paparella, Freeman, and Jahromi (2008), the authors compared the effects of different interventions (joint attention intervention, symbolic play intervention) on expressive language in 3- and 4-year-old learners with autism. They found expressive language gains for both the joint attention and symbolic play intervention groups relative to the control group. In addition to the initial improvements, treatment effects grew stronger over time (12-month follow-up compared to control group). This suggests significant benefits of including joint attention training and symbolic play training when designing interventions for young children with autism.

Joint attention interventions are compelling for similar reasons to those reviewed for teaching perspective taking skills. If we can target these core deficits with our interventions, the magnitude of socially significant change may be much greater. As with perspective taking, much work remains to be done in identifying how to teach such skills and how to generalize such skills to natural interactions and contexts.

Peers: Building Social Bridges to Other Children

Many individuals with autism spectrum disorders struggle to achieve social reciprocity (Rutter, 1985; Rutter, Mahwood, & Howlin, 1992), which impedes their ability to make and strengthen connections with others. Developing such reciprocity with peers is a pivotal skill for developing friendships (e.g., Dunn & Maguire, 1992), and is an important goal in working with individuals with ASD.

The majority of research that has been done in social skills has been done with young children with autism. Researchers initially focused on teaching social reciprocity between young children with autism

and adults (e.g., Strain, Shores, & Kerr, 1976; Strain & Timm, 1974). While this approach provided predictability (in the adults' behaviors), it also sometimes fostered dependence on adults. In fact, some studies showed that when adult support was reduced, social behaviors declined (e.g., Odom, Hoyson, Jamieson, & Strain, 1985).

It has also been argued that the presence of and interaction with adults alters the social environment. It can be intrusive, it may be artificial, and it likely reduces the naturalistic quality of child to child interactions (McGee, Almeida, Sulzer-Azaroff, & Feldman, 1992; Kliewer, 1995). When adult support is used, it is important that such support be weaned as quickly as possible to reduce the artificiality and dependence on adults (e.g., Odom, Chandler, Ostrosky, McConnell, & Reaney, 1992).

Peers as Agents of Change

The use of peers as the agents of social change has several distinct advantages. Their involvement, from the onset of training, substantially increases the likelihood of generalization to other peers. The risk of dependence on adults is also reduced. In addition, the degree of artificiality is reduced, as the interactions much more closely parallel the real-life situations that the children encounter on a daily basis in their social environments. It may also be that the use of peers builds learning opportunities, as peers are readily available in the natural environment.

When peers are used as agents of integration, there are several common approaches that have been historically used. The three most common methods include: proximity, prompt/reinforce, and peer initiation (e.g., Lord & Magill, 1989; Odom & Strain, 1984). In the first approach, children with autism and typically developing children are simply placed together in close physical proximity. The typically developing children are known to be socially competent with well-developed language skills, and they serve as effective models for social interaction. In the *proximity* model, peers are generally not instructed in any special way (although there may be a socially rich curriculum). The theory/philosophy is that *exposure* to typically developing peers will have social benefits.

In the *prompt/reinforce* model, peers are trained to prompt and to reinforce the children with autism. In this way, they serve as additional trainers in the environment, and they use techniques similar to those employed by the child's teachers. They may prompt/remind children with autism to attend, to listen again to instructions, or to answer them in a specific way. They might offer them praise statements or other rewards for appropriate or compliant behavior. In this approach, these interactions are supported by teaching staff, who help to orchestrate such interactions and who coach the peers in effectively helping their friends.

Peer initiation training focuses on developing peer skills in initiating to and in persisting with children with autism. Specifically, peers are systematically taught how to initiate a child with autism, with individualized strategies that facilitate response for that child. They may be taught to secure their attention with an attention cue or to use visual aids in delivering instructions. In addition, they are taught to repeat their efforts when they are unsuccessful. In other words, they are taught not to give up, but to try again when their overtures are not successful.

Proximity techniques require little facilitation, and are commonly used in inclusive environments (e.g., Johnson & Johnson, 1984; Rynders & Schleien, 1991; Rynders et al., 1993; Schleien, Mustonen, & Rynders, 1995). Although all of the methods are associated with positive results, both the prompt/reinforcement and the peer initiation training models are more effective than the proximity model. However, the prompt/reinforcement and peer initiation models are less naturalistic than the proximity model (e.g., Lord & Hopkins, 1986; Roeyers, 1996). This probably limits the degree to which such training reflects the environments that learners may ultimately join. (Most environments will not have trained peers.) Thus, generalization of the effects is questionable.

It does seem fairly clear that proximity alone is insufficient for producing reliable change. It appears that children with autism need more salient cues than simple demonstration to produce changes in their social behavior (Weiss & Harris, 2001). Carr and Darcy (1990) illustrated this when they taught children to play follow the leader with peer modeling and prompting. Peers who modeled and physically prompted the children with autism to imitate them were successful. It was not sufficient to simply have the child with autism observe their peers.

Other Methods

Some researchers have suggested that it may also be helpful for peers to interact with children with autism in specific ways. For example, while much research has focused on helping peers to ask questions, it may be useful to teach them to make comments. Goldstein, Kaczmarek, Pennington, and Shafer (1992) taught peers to make comments to children with autism and found a significant improvement in social behaviors. A speculative explanation is that comments may facilitate interaction precisely because they do not demand a specific response from the child with autism.

Peer buddy systems have also been shown to be useful. Laushey and Heflin (2000) used a peer buddy program for kindergarteners in which a daily buddy was assigned to children with autism. The buddy was told to stay with, play with, and talk to his/her buddy. Social interactions increased substantially as a result of this approach. Targeted skills included asking for an object, responding to the question asked, getting attention, waiting for a turn, and looking at a conversational partner. Children with autism responded to multiple peers, and generalization to a new classroom environment was also documented. These generalization benefits are notable, given the necessity of transfer to natural environments and contexts.

Self-monitoring by peers involved in training also has some potential benefits. Sainato, Goldstein, and Strain (1992) taught peers to use self-evaluation strategies in assessing how well they had interacted with children with autism. Specifically, the peers assessed how well they got a child's attention, initiated a play activity, or responded to a child.

Pivotal response training (PRT) has also been very promising in facilitating interactions between children with autism and their peers. PRT is focused on increasing pivotal behaviors that are central to wide areas of functioning (Koegel & Koegel, 1995). PRT has been shown to produce generalized behavioral changes and to address other challenging issues such as motivation and responsiveness to multiple cues. Pierce and Schreibman (1995, 1997) taught peers to user PRT through a combination of modeling, role plays, and didactic instruction. Results indicated that there were increases in interactions, initiations, joint attention, and engagement. The generalization benefits and the increases in socio-communicative behaviors such as joint attention are very impressive, given how difficult it can be to achieve generalized effects and to build complex multi-element socio-communicative behaviors.

Benefits to Participants

Much data have been published about the benefits of integration to children with autism spectrum disorders, as well as to their typically developing peers (Kamps et al., 1992; Kamps, Barbetta, Leonard, & Delquadri, 1994). In general, students improve in social initiations, social responding, sustaining social interactions, taking turns, sharing items, and offering help. It has also been shown that structured integration experiences have a broad and positive generalized effect on acceptance of individuals with disabilities by their typically developing peers (Kamps et al., 1994).

It has been further suggested that such integration programs might benefit peers in global ways, similar to the benefits often reported about siblings of children with autism (e.g., Feiges & Weiss, 2004; Harris & Glasberg, 2003). It may be that exposure to disability and assisting someone with a disability may increase tolerance, understanding, and empathy, and may even foster a desire to help others.

Summary of Historical Peer Training Approaches

Social deficits in autism are substantial and pervasive. It is a serious challenge to teach these skills effectively and efficiently, and in ways which promote independence in natural settings. The use of peers as agents of change in this area is compelling, as it (potentially) substantially reduces dependence on adults, increases the natural quality of the teaching environment, and capitalizes on naturally occurring teaching opportunities.

When peers are used as agents of change, it is best to provide some training to increase the effectiveness of their efforts. Training in prompting and reinforcing children with autism, as well as in persisting when unsuccessful in interactions, increases the success of peer integration efforts. In addition, positive effects have also been demonstrated with peer buddy systems, peer pivotal response training, and self-management training of peers.

Peers as Agents of Change: Current Trends

In recent years, there has been more focused interest in the development of relationships between children with autism and their typically developing peers. Parents of children with autism report that they often do not have friends, despite their participation in an inclusive environment (Orsmond, Wyngaarden Krauss, & Malick Seltzer, 2004). Many students on the spectrum also report problems in social functioning (Knott, Dunlop, & Mackay, 2006). As children with autism age, it seems that they experience intensified feelings of loneliness (Bauminger & Kasari, 2000; Chamberlain, Kasari, & Rotheram-Fuller, 2007), possibly reflecting a more nuanced understanding of social integration and relationships over time. In recent years, mapping of social networks has shed some light on how students with autism are assimilated and integrated into the larger social environment. Researchers examine variables such as the reciprocity of friendship connections.

In addition, they have sought more specific information about how to best address the social deficits exhibited with peers, given that the gains of most training approaches are modest (Bellini, Peters, Benner, & Hopf, 2007; Rao, Beidel, & Murray, 2008; White, Keonig, & Scahill, 2007). In general, approaches that include peers directly in training efforts are much more successful than those that do not include them (Kasari, 2008). Both peer training programs and combination approaches (targeting both peer skills and instruction to children with autism) are more effective than only teaching the child with autism. Unanswered questions include how generalization can best be fostered, how individualization can be incorporated to address child-specific issues, and what the most important elements of intervention are.

Generality and Social Validity

In peer training and in all areas of social skill instruction and intervention, clinicians and researchers are concerned with the generalization of learned skills to the natural environment and with the social relevance of the skills learned. This is all the more important in the realm of social skills training, where anything short of transfer to the natural environment is meaningless.

Assessment of social skills mastery must include adaptation to the natural environment. When skills are taught in analogue or formal ways, the transfer to naturally occurring interactions and contexts is essential.

Summary

Individuals with ASD have significant social deficits. Their social difficulties include problems in responding to others and in making social overtures. In addition, there are problems in the quality of social initiations and responses that individuals with ASD make. Often, they are unclear, inappropriate, prompted, or delayed. Such poor quality responses result in less social success. In addition, many social skills are complex, multi-element skills. In addition to requiring multiple sub-skills, there is also the need for social judgment in when and how to socially interact. This has made it all the more difficult to operationally define social skills.

A variety of techniques are commonly used for teaching social skills to individuals with ASD. Some of those techniques are not empirically validated or have been used primarily with other populations. Often, they are used as part of a package of interventions designed to address a specific deficit or issue. For example, social stories or rule cards may be used in combination with a variety of other procedures. They may be useful additional components to a package of behavioral teaching interventions. Such package interventions may assist the clinician in teaching these multi-element skills. Additionally, they may provide more practice/learning opportunities and increase the degree to which training prepares learners for the range of possible experiences in the social world. As in the case with all interventions, direct behavior-change procedures should always be used to affect behavior. In addition, data on the effectiveness of all strategies used with individual learners should be collected, and should be used to determine which elements of intervention should continue to be used with the learner.

New directions for social skill intervention include addressing the deficits of problem solving, perspective taking, and joint attention. More research is needed to identify critical elements of these targeted interventions, as well as to identify strategies for enhancing the generalization of learned skills to real-life social exchanges.

References

Agran, M., Blanhard, C., Wehmeyer, M. L., & Hughes, C. (2002). Increasing the problem-solving skills of students with developmental disabilities participating in special education. *Remedial and Special Education, 23*, 279–288.

American Psychiatric Association. (2000). *Diagnostic and statistical manual of mental disorders, Fourth Edition, Text Revision.* (DSM-IV-TR). Washington, DC: American Psychiatric Association.

Attwood, T. (1998). *Asperger's syndrome: A guide for parents and professionals.* Philadelphia: Jessica Kingsley.

Baker, J. E. (2003a). *Social skills picture book: Teaching play, emotion, and communication to children with autism.* Arlington, TX: Future Horizons.

Baker, J. E. (2003b). *Social skills training.* Shawnee Mission, KS: Autism Asperger Publishing Company.

Baron-Cohen, S. (1989). Joint-attention deficits in autism: Towards a cognitive analysis. *Development and Psychopathology, 1*, 185–189.

Baron-Cohen, S., Leslie, A. M., & Frith, U. (1985). Does the autistic child have a 'theory of mind'? *Cognition, 21*(1), 37–46.

Barresi, J., & Moore, C. (1996). Intentional relations and social understanding. *Behavioral and Brain Sciences, 19*, 107–122.

Barry, L. M., & Burlew, S. B. (2004). Using social stories to teach choice and play skills to children with autism. *Focus on Autism and Other Developmental Disabilities, 19*, 45–51.

Bauminger, N., & Kasari, C. (2000). Loneliness and friendship in high-functioning children with a autism. *Child Development, 71*, 447–456.

Beauchaine, T. P. (2001). Vagal tone, development, and Gray's motivational theory: Toward an integrated model of autonomic nervous system functioning in psychopathology. *Development and Psychopathology, 13*, 183–214.

Bellini, S., Peters, J. K., Benner, L., & Hopf, A. (2007). A meta analysis of school based social skills interventions for children with autism spectrum disorders. *Remedial and Special Education, 28*, 153–162.

Bieber, J. (1994). *Learning disabilities and social skills with Richard Lavoie: Last one picked...First one picked on.* Washington, DC: Public Broadcasting Service.

Blair, C., & Peters, R. (2004). Physiological and neurocognitive correlates of adaptive behavior in preschool among children in Head Start. *Developmental Neuropsychology, 24*(1), 479–497.

Blake, R., Turner, L. M., Smoski, M. J., Pozdol, S. L., & Stone, W. L. (2003). Visual recognition of biological motion is impaired in children with autism. *Psychological Science, 14*(2), 151–157.

Brownell, M. D. (2002). Musically adapted social stories to modify behaviors in students with autism: Four case studies. *Journal of Music Therapy, 39*, 117–144.

Bruinsma, Y., Koegel, R. L., & Koegel, L. K. (2004). Joint attention and children with autism: A review of the literature. *Mental Retardation and Developmental Disorders, 10*, 169–175.

Burke, R. V., Kuhn, B. R., & Peterson, J. L. (2004). Brief report: A storybook ending to children's bedtime problems – The use of a rewarding social story to reduce bedtime resistance and frequent night waking. *Journal of Pediatric Psychology, 29*, 389–396.

Calkins, S. D., & Keane, S. P. (2004). Cardiac vagal regulation across preschool: Stability, continuity, and relations to adjustment. *Developmental Psychobiology, 45*, 101–112.

Carr, E. G., & Darcy, M. (1990). Setting generality of peer modeling in children with autism. *Journal of Autism and Developmental Disorders, 20*, 49–59.

Chamberlain, B., Kasari, C., & Rotheram-Fuller, E. (2007). Involvement or isolation: The social networks of children with autism in regular classrooms. *Journal of Autism and Developmental Disorders, 37*, 230–242.

Channon, S., Charman, T., Heap, J., Crawford, S., & Rios, P. (2001). Real-life-type problem-solving in Asperger's syndrome. *Journal of Autism and Developmental Disorders, 31*, 461–469.

Charlop-Christy, M. H., & Daneshvar, S. (2003). Using video modeling to teach perspective taking to children with autism. *Journal of Positive Behavior Interventions, 5*(1), 12–21.

Charlop-Christy, M. H., & Milstein, J. P. (1989). Teaching autistic children conversational speech using video modeling. *Journal of Applied Behavior Analysis, 22*, 275–285.

Charlop-Christy, M. H., Le, L., & Freeman, K. A. (2000). A comparison of video modeling with in vivo modeling for teaching children with autism. *Journal of Autism and Developmental Disorders, 30*, 537–552.

Crozier, S., & Tincani, M. (2007). Effects of social stories on prosocial behavior of preschool children with autism spectrum disorders. *Journal of Autism and Developmental Disorders, 37*, 1803–1814.

Dawson, G., Meltzoff, A. N., Osterling, J., Rinaldi, J., & Brown, E. (1998). Children with autism fail to orient to naturally occurring social stimuli. *Journal of Autism and Developmental Disorders, 28*(6), 479–485.

Dawson, G., Toth, K., Abbott, R., Osterling, J., Munson, J., Estes, A., et al. (2004). Early social attention impairments in autism: Social orienting, joint attention, and attention to distress. *Developmental Psychology, 40*(2), 271–283.

Delano, M., & Snell, M. E. (2006). The effects of Social Stories on the social engagement of children with autism. *Journal of Positive Behavior Intervention, 8*, 29–42.

Deruelle, C., Rondan, C., Gepner, B., & Tardif, C. (2004). Spatial frequency and face processing in children with autism and Asperger syndrome. *Journal of Autism and Developmental Disorders, 34*(2), 199–210.

Dodd, S., Hupp, S. D. A., Jewell, J. D., & Krohn, E. (2008). Using parents and siblings during a social story intervention for two children diagnosed with PDD-NOS. *Journal of Developmental and Physical Disabilities, 20*, 217–229.

Dunn, M. (2006). *S. O. S.: Social Skills in Our Schools: A social skills program for children with pervasive developmental disorders, including high functioning autism and Asperger syndrome and their typical peers.* Shawnee Mission, KS: Autism Asperger Publishing Company.

Dunn, J., & Maguire, S. (1992). Sibling and peer relationships in childhood. *Journal of Child Psychiatry and Psychology, 33*, 67–105.

Falck-Ytter, T., Gredebäck, G., & von Hofsten, C. (2006). Infants predict other people's action goals. *Nature Neuroscience, 9*(7), 878–879.

Feiges, L. S., & Weiss, M. J. (2004). *Sibling stories: Reflections on life with a brother or sister on the autism spectrum.* Shawnee Mission, KS: Autism Asperger Publishing Company.

Frith, U. (1989). *Autism: Explaining the enigma.* Oxford: Blackwell.

Gagnon, E. (2001). *Power cards: Using special interests to motivate children and youth with Asperger syndrome and autism.* Kansas City, KS: Autism Asperger Publishing Company.

Goddard, L., Howlin, P., Dritschel, B., & Patel, T. (2007). Autobiographical memory and social problem-solving in Asperger syndrome. *Journal of Autism and Developmental Disorders, 37*, 291–300.

Goldstein, H., Kaczmarek, L., Pennington, R., & Shafer, K. (1992). Peer-mediated intervention: Attending to commenting on, and acknowledging the behavior of preschoolers with autism. *Journal of Autism and Developmental Disorders, 25*, 289–305.

Gray, C. A. (1995). Teaching children with autism to 'read' social situations. In K. A. Quill (Ed.), *Teaching children with autism; strategies to enhance communication and socialization* (pp. 219–242). Albany, NY: Delmar.

Gray, C. (2000). How to write a social story. *The new social story handbook* (illustrated edition). Arlington, TX: Future Horizons.

Grelotti, D. J., Gauthier, I., & Schultz, R. T. (2002). Social interest and the development of cortical face specialization: What autism teaches us about face processing. *Developmental Psychobiology, 40*(3), 213–225.

Haring, T., Kennedy, C., Adams, M., & Pitts-Conway, V. (1987). Teaching generalization of purchasing skills across community settings to autistic youth using videotape modeling. *Journal of Applied Behavior Analysis, 20*, 89–96.

Harris, S. L., & Glasberg, B. A. (2003). *Siblings of children with autism: A guide for families.* Bethesda, MD: Woodbine House.

Johnson, D. W., & Johnson, R. T. (1984). Classroom structure and attitudes toward handicapped students in mainstream settings: A theoretical model and research evidence. In R. L. Jones (Ed.), *Attitudes and attitude change in special education: Theory and practice* (pp. 118–142). Reston, VA: Council for Exceptional Children.

Kamps, D. M., Barbetta, P. M., Leonard, B. R., & Delquadri, J. C. (1994). Classwide peer tutoring: An integration strategy to improve reading skills and promote peer interactions among students with autism and general education peers. *Journal of Applied Behavior Analysis, 27*, 49–61.

Kamps, D. M., Leonard, B. R., Vernon, S., Dugan, E. P., Delquadri, J. C., Gershon, B., et al. (1992). Teaching social skills to students with autism to increase peer interactions in an integrated first-grade classroom. *Journal of Applied Behavior Analysis, 25*, 281–288.

Kanner, L. (1943). Autistic disturbances of affective contact. *Nervous Child, 2*, 217–250. Reprint (1968). *Acta Paedopsychiatrica, 35*(4), 100–136.

Kasari, C. (2008). *Peer relationships, friendships, and loneliness at school for children with ASD.* Presentation at Organization for Autism Research Annual Research Convocation, Atlanta, GA.

Kasari, C., Freeman, S., & Paparella, T. (2006). Joint attention and symbolic play in young children with autism: A randomized controlled intervention study. *Journal of Child Psychology and Psychiatry, 47*(6), 611–620.

Kasari, C., Paparella, T., Freeman, S., & Jahromi, L. B. (2008). Language outcome in autism: Randomized comparison of joint attention and play interventions. *Journal of Consulting and Clinical Psychology, 76*(1), 125–137.

Keeling, K., Smith Miles, B., Gagnon, E., & Simpson, R. L. (2003). Using the power card strategy to teach sportsmanship skills to a child with autism. *Focus on Autism and Other Developmental Disabilities, 18,* 105–111.

Kliewer, C. (1995). Young children's communication and literacy: A qualitative study of language in the inclusive preschool. *Mental Retardation, 33,* 143–152.

Klin, A., Sparrow, S. S., de Bildt, A., Cicchetti, D. V., Cohen, D. J., & Volkmar, F. R. (1999). A normed study of face recognition in autism and related disorders. *Journal of Autism and Developmental Disorders, 29*(6), 499–508.

Knott, F., Dunlop, A., & Mackay, T. (2006). Living with ASD: How do children and their parents assess their difficulties with social interaction and understanding? *Autism, 10*(6), 609–617.

Koegel, L. K., & Koegel, L. K. (1995). *Teaching children with autism: Strategies for initiating interactions and improving learning opportunities.* Baltimore, MD: Brookes.

Krantz, P. J., & McClannahan, L. E. (1998). Social interaction skills for children with autism: A script-fading procedure for beginning readers. *Journal of Applied Behavior Analysis, 31,* 191–202.

Krantz, P. J., MacDuff, G. S., Wadstrom, O., & McClannahan, L. E. (1991). Using video with developmentally disabled learners. In P. W. Dowrick (Ed.), *Practical guide to video in the behavioral sciences* (pp. 256–266). New York, NY: Wiley.

Laushey, K. M., & Heflin, J. (2000). Enhancing social skills of kindergarten children with autism through the training of multiple peers as tutors. *Journal of Autism and Developmental Disorders, 30,* 183–193.

LeBlanc, L. A., Coates, A. M., Daneshvar, S., Charlop-Christy, M. H., Morris, C., & Lancaster, B. M. (2003). Using video modeling and reinforcement to teach perspective-taking skills to children with autism. *Journal of Applied Behavior Analysis, 36,* 253–257.

Lord, C., & Hopkins, J. M. (1986). The social behavior of autistic children with younger and same age nonhandicapped peers. *Journal of Autism and Developmental Disorders, 16,* 249–262.

Lord, C., & Magill, J. (1989). Methodological and theoretical issues in studying peer directed behavior and autism. In G. Dawson (Ed.), *Autism: Nature, diagnosis, and treatment* (pp. 326–345). New York: Guilford.

Loveland, K. A., & Landry, S. H. (1986). Joint attention and language in autism and developmental language delay. *Journal of Autism and Developmental Disorders, 16*(3), 335–349.

Matson, J. L., & Swiezy, N. B. (1994). Social skills training with autistic children. In J. L. Matson (Ed.), *Autism in children and adults: Etiology, assessment and intervention.* Sycamore, IL: Sycamore Publishing Company.

McGee, G. C., Almeida, M. C., Sulzer-Azaroff, B., & Feldman, R. S. (1992). Prompting reciprocal interaction via peer incidental teaching. *Journal of Applied Behavior Analysis, 25,* 117–126.

McGinnis, E., & Goldstein, A. P. (1990). *Skillstreaming.* Champaign, IL: Research Press.

Moore, S. (2002). *Asperger syndrome and the elementary school experience.* Shawnee Mission, KS: Autism Asperger Publishing Company.

Morales, M., Mundy, P., Delgado, C. E. F., Yale, M., Messinger, D., Neal, R., et al. (2000). Responding to joint attention across the 6- through 24-month age period and early language acquisition. *Journal of Applied Developmental Psychology, 21*(3), 283–298.

More, C. (2008). Digital stories targeting social skills for children with disabilities: Multidimensional learning. *Intervention in School and Clinic, 43,* 168–177.

Mundy, P., & Crawson, M. (1997). Joint attention and early social communication implications for research on intervention with autism. *Journal of Autism and Developmental Disorders, 27,* 653–676.

Mundy, P., Block, J., Vaughan Van Hecke, A., Delgadoa, C., Venezia Parlade, M., & Pomares, Y. (2007). Individual differences and the development of infant joint attention. *Child Development, 78*(3), 938–954.

Odom, S. L., Chandler, K., Ostrosky, M., McConnell, M. R., & Reaney, S. (1992). Fading teacher prompts from peer-initiation interventions for young children with disabilities. *Journal of Applied Behavior Analysis, 25,* 307–317.

Odom, S. L., Hoyson, S., Jamieson, B., & Strain, P. S. (1985). Increasing handicapped preschoolers social interactions: Cross-setting and component analysis. *Journal of Applied Behavior Analysis, 18,* 3–16.

Odom, S. L., & Strain, P. S. (1984). Peer mediated approaches to prompting children's social interactions: A review. *American Journal of Orthopsychiatry, 54,* 544–557.

Orsmond, G. I., Wyngaarden Krauss, M., & Malick Seltzer, M. M. (2004). Peer relationships and social and recreational activities among adolescents and adults with autism. *Journal of Autism and Developmental Disorders, 34,* 245–256.

Ozonoff, S., & Miller, J. N. (1995). Teaching theory of mind: A new approach to social skills training for individuals with autism. *Journal of Autism and Developmental Disorders, 25*(4), 415–433.

Pierce, K., & Schreibman, L. (1995). Increasing complex social behaviors in children with autism: Effects of peer-implemented pivotal response training. *Journal of Applied Behavior Analysis, 28,* 285–295.

Pierce, K., & Schreibman, L. (1997). Multiple peer use of pivotal response training to increase social behaviors of classmates with autism: Results from trained and untrained peers. *Journal of Applied Behavior Analysis, 30,* 157–160.

Porges, S. W. (1995). Orienting in a defensive world: Mammalian modifications of our evolutionary heritage. A polyvagal theory. *Psychophysiology, 32,* 301–318.

Porges, S. W. (1997). Emotion: An evolutionary by-product of the neural regulation of the autonomic nervous system. *Annals of the New York Academy of Sciences, 807,* 62–77.

Premack, D. G., & Woodruff, G. (1978). Does the chimpanzee have a theory of mind? *Behavioral and Brain Sciences, 1,* 515–526.

Rao, P. A., Beidel, D. C., & Murray, M. J. (2008). Social skills interventions for children with Asperger's syndrome or high-functioning autism: A review and recommendations. *Journal of Autism and Developmental Disorders, 38*(2), 353–361.

Rehfeldt, R. A., Dillen, J. E., Ziomek, M. M., & Kowalchuk, R. K. (2007). Assessing relational learning deficits in perspective-taking in children with high-functioning autism spectrum disorder. *Psychological Record, 57*(1), 23–48.

Reynhout, G., & Carter, M. (2006). Social stories for children with disabilities. *Journal of Autism and Developmental Disorders, 36,* 445–469.

Richardson, R. C. (1996). *Connecting with others: Lessons for teaching social and emotional competence.* Champaign, IL: Research Press.

Roeyers, H. (1996). The influence of nonhandicapped peers on the social interactions of children with a pervasive developmental disorder. *Journal of Autism and Developmental Disorders, 26*, 303–320.

Rogers, S. J. (2000). Interventions that facilitate socialization in children with autism. *Journal of Autism and Developmental Disorders, 30*(5), 399–409.

Rutherford, M. D., Pennington, B. F., & Rogers, S. J. (2006). The perception of animacy in young children with autism. *Journal of Autism and Developmental Disorders, 36*(8), 983–992.

Rutter, M. (1985). Infantile autism. In D. Shaffer, A. Ernhardt & L. Greenhill (Eds.), *A clinician's guide to child psychiatry* (pp. 48–78). New York: Free Press.

Rutter, M., Mahwood, L., & Howlin, P. (1992). Language delay and social development. In P. Fletcher & D. Hale (Eds.), *Specific speech and language disorders in children*. London: Whurr.

Rynders, J., & Schleien, S. (1991). *Together successfully: Creating recreational and educational programs that integrate people with and without disabilities*. Arlington, TX: Association for Retarded Citizens of the United States.

Rynders, J., Schleien, S., Meyer, L., Vandercook, T., Mustonen, T., Colond, J., et al. (1993). Improving integration outcomes for children with and without severe disabilities through cooperatively structured recreation activities: A synthesis of research. *Journal of Special Education, 26*, 386–407.

Sainato, D. M., Goldstein, H., & Strain, P. S. (1992). Effects of self-evaluation on preschool children's use of social interaction strategies with their classmates with autism. *Journal of Applied Behavior Analysis, 25*, 127–141.

Sansosti, F. J., & Powell-Smith, K. A. (2008). Using computer-presented social stories and video models to increase the social communication skills of children with high-functioning autism spectrum disorders. *Journal of Positive Behavior Interventions, 10*, 162–178.

Sansosti, F. J., Powell-Smith, K. A., & Kincaid, D. (2004). A research synthesis of social story interventions for children with autism spectrum disorders. *Focus on Autism and Developmental Disorders, 19*, 194–204.

Schleien, S. J., Mustonen, T., & Rynders, J. E. (1995). Participation of children with autism and nondisabled peers in a cooperatively structured community art program. *Journal of Autism and Developmental Disorders, 25*, 397–413.

Schultz, R. T. (2005). Developmental deficits in social perception in autism: The role of the amygdala and fusiform face area. *International Journal of Developmental Neuroscience, 23*, 125–141.

Sheinkopf, S. J., Mundy, P., Claussen, A. H., & Willoughby, J. (2004). Infant joint attention skill and preschool behavioral outcomes in at-risk children. *Development and Psychopathology, 16*, 273–291.

Sherer, M., Pierce, K. L., Parades, S., Kisacky, K. L., Ingersoll, B., & Schreibman, L. (2001). Enhancing conversation skills in children with autism via video technology: Which is better, "self" or "other" as a model. *Behavior Modification, 25*, 140–158.

Shure, M. B. (2001a). *I can problem solve (kindergarten and primary grades)*. Champaign, IL: Research Press.

Shure, M. B. (2001b). *I can problem solve (intermediate elementary grades)*. Champaign, IL: Research Press.

Shure, M. B. (2004). *I can problem solve (preschool)*. Champaign, IL: Research Press.

Sigman, M., & Capps, L. (1997). *Children with autism: A developmental perspective*. Cambridge, MA: Harvard University Press.

Sloan, R. P., Shapiro, P. A., Bigger, J. T., Bagiella, M., Steinman, R. C., & Gorman, J. M. (1994). Cardiac autonomic control and hostility in healthy subjects. *American Journal of Cardiology, 74*, 298–300.

Snell, M. E., & Brown, F. (2000). *Instruction of students with severe handicaps*. Upper Saddle River, NJ: Prentice Hall.

Snell, M. E., & Janney, R. (2000). *Social relationships and peer support*. Baltimore, MD: Brookes.

Stevenson, C. L., Krantz, P. J., & McClannahan, L. E. (2000). Social interaction skills for children with autism: A script-fading procedure for nonreaders. *Behavioral Interventions, 15*(1), 1–20.

Strain, P. S., Shores, R. E., & Kerr, M. M. (1976). An experimental analysis of "spillover" effects on the social interactions of behaviorally handicapped preschool children. *Journal of Applied Behavior Analysis, 9*, 31–40.

Strain, P. S., & Timm, M. A. (1974). An experimental analysis of social interaction between a behaviorally disordered preschool child and her classroom peers. *Journal of Applied Behavior Analysis, 7*, 583–590.

Swaggart, B. L., Gagnon, E., Bock, S. J., Earles, T. L., Quinn, C., Myles, B. S., et al. (1995). Using social stories to teach social and behavioral skills to children with autism. *Focus on Autistic Behavior, 10*, 1–16.

Taylor, B. A. (2001). Teaching peer social skills to children with autism. In C. Maurice, G. Green & R. Foxx (Eds.), *Making a difference: Behavioral intervention for autism* (pp. 83–96). Austin, TX: Pro-Ed.

Taylor, M., & Carlson, S. M. (1997). The relation between individual differences in fantasy and theory of mind. *Child Development, 68*(3), 436–455.

Taylor, B. A., & Jasper, S. (2001). Teaching programs to increase peer interaction. In C. Maurice, G. Green & R. Foxx (Eds.), *Making a difference: Behavioral intervention for autism* (pp. 97–162). Austin, TX: Pro-Ed.

Thayer, J. F., Friedman, B. H., & Borkovec, T. D. (1996). Autonomic characteristics of generalized anxiety disorder and worry. *Biological Psychiatry, 39*, 255–266.

The Gray Center. (2008). *What is a social story?* http://www.thegraycenter.org.

Thiemann, K. S., & Goldstein, H. (2001). Social stories, written text cues, and video feedback: Effects on social communication of children with autism. *Journal of Applied Behavior Analysis, 34*, 425–446.

Tremoulet, P. D., & Feldman, J. (2000). Perception of animacy from the motion of a single object. *Perception, 29*, 943–951.

Watkins, L. T., Sprafkin, J. N., & Krolikowski, D. M. (1993). Using videotaped lessons to facilitate the development of manual sign skills in students with mental retardation. *Augmentative and Alternative Communication, 9*, 177–183.

Weiss, M. J., & Harris, S. L. (2001). *Reaching out, joining in: Teaching social skills to young children with autism*. Bethesda, MD: Woodbine House.

Whalen, C., & Schreibman, L. (2003). Joint attention training for children using behavior modification procedures. *Journal of Child Psychiatry, 44*, 456–468.

White, S. W., Keonig, K., & Scahill, L. (2007). Social skills development in children with autism spectrum disorders: A review of the intervention research. *Journal of Autism and Developmental Disorders, 37*(10), 1858–1868.

Chapter 8
Rituals and Stereotypies

Jeffrey H. Tiger, Karen A. Toussaint, and Megan L. Kliebert

This group of behaviors constitutes third core feature of ASD. ABA is the most effective means of addressing the problems. The specific problems and research based interventions will be addressed.

What Are Stereotypies and Rituals?

The presence of restricted or repetitive interests, activities, and behaviors represents the third core behavioral symptom leading to a diagnosis of an autism spectrum disorder (ASD) based upon the DSM-IV and ICD-10. The term "repetitive behavior" commonly includes simple motor movements (e.g., hand flapping, body rocking, facial posturing), repetitive vocalizations (e.g., repeating sounds or phrases emitted by another person or object), ritualistic behaviors (e.g., shutting all the doors in a house, lining up objects), and a general insistence on sameness (e.g., signs of distress associated with deviations from typical schedules). The simple presence of repetitive behaviors is not unique to individuals with autism; such behaviors are commonly present in individuals with mental retardation, schizophrenia, obsessive compulsive disorder, Tourette's disorder, and even among young, typically developing children. The frequency and severity of repetitive behaviors tends to be greater and more debilitating among individuals diagnosed with autism (McDougle et al., 1995; Smith & Van Houten, 1996).

Repetitive behaviors may emerge even among very young children with autism; the most common of which are motor and vocal stereotypies. Richler, Bishop, Kleinke, and Lord (2007) found that the repetitive use of objects, unusual sensory interests, complex mannerisms, and hand/finger mannerisms were reported in more than 50% of children with autism as early as age 2. Further, these authors reported that unusual preoccupations and abnormal/idiosyncratic responses to sensory stimuli were reported in over 33% of children with autism at age 2. Both prevalence estimates were significantly different from matched populations of children of typical development or those diagnosed with other developmental disabilities. In addition, parents of children with autism rated the occurrence of these repetitive behaviors to be of greater severity in terms of their disruption of everyday functioning than did parents of matched non-ASD peers.

In describing the phenomenology of stereotypy in 224 children with autism, Campbell et al. (1990) reported that 25% engaged in some form of object stereotypy, 16% engaged in hand flapping, 15% engaged in body rocking, 12% engaged in head tilting, 28% engaged in a stereotypy related to another lower extremity, and 18% engaged in a stereotypy related to another upper extremity. In addition it has been reported that repetitive self-injurious behavior (SIB) occurs between 6% (Bartak & Rutter, 1976) and 30% (Schroeder, Schroeder, Smith, & Dalldorf, 1978) of individuals with autism.

The simple occurrence of stereotypy and other repetitive behaviors, with the exception of SIB, alone are not necessarily problematic but become problematic when they limit the extent to which individuals successfully interact with their environment. Specifically, the occurrence of stereotypy is negatively related to the acquisition of academic and social skills (Dunlap, Dyer, & Koegel, 1983; Epstein, Doke, Sajwaj, Sorrell, & Rimmer, 1974; Koegel & Covert, 1972;

J.H. Tiger (✉)
Department of Psychology, Louisiana State University,
Baton Rouge, LA, 70803, USA
e-mail: jtiger@lsu.edu

J.L. Matson (ed.), *Applied Behavior Analysis for Children with Autism Spectrum Disorders*,
DOI 10.1007/978-1-4419-0088-3_8, © Springer Science+Business Media, LLC 2009

Koegel, Firestone, Kramme, & Dunlap, 1974; Lovaas, Litrownik, & Mann, 1971; Morrison & Rosales-Ruiz, 1997; Risley, 1968). That is, when children engage in stereotypy, they do so to an extent that competes with their interacting with other individuals, participating in learning activities, and contacting other reinforcement contingencies in their environment resulting in a failure to develop novel skills.

Given the problems associated with the occurrence of stereotypy, a thorough understanding of the conditions responsible for the development of stereotypy and the development of treatments to eliminate or minimize the occurrence of stereotypy have remained important areas of research for applied scientists, and in particular for behavior analysts. This chapter will serve to highlight research that has contributed to our understanding and treatment of this problem behavior.

Why Do Children with Autism Engage in Stereotypies and Rituals?

Although physiology certainly plays a contributory role in the development of stereotypy, behavior-analytic research has focused considerably more attention on the environmental influences that result in stereotypy's development and maintenance. Early investigations with institutionalized populations found the occurrence of stereotypy to be inversely related to the presence of other materials and the amount of social interaction in their environment (Berkson & Mason, 1963, 1965; Davenport & Berkson, 1963) indicating that environmental influences did play an important role. However, it was not until the development of the functional analysis model of behavioral assessment (Iwata et al., 1982/1994; Hanley, Iwata, & McCord, 2003) that the role of environmental consequences in the maintenance of stereotypy and other repetitive problem behaviors could be understood. Unlike the methods of observing correlations between environmental events and repetitive problem behavior, this methodology involved systematically introducing and removing specified antecedent and consequent events surrounding problem behavior through a series of test and control conditions, and thus was capable of demonstrating functional relationships between specific variables and the occurrence and non-occurrence of problem behavior (see Hanley et al., 2003 for a thorough

review of these procedures). That is, this methodology was effective at identifying and isolating the specific reinforcers that maintain problem behavior, be they social (i.e., consequences delivered by another person such as attention, access to leisure items or food, or escape from non-preferred environments) or non-social (i.e., consequences that are produced directly by behavior such as visual, auditory, tactile, or vestibular stimulation, pain attenuation, or sensory attenuation; Vollmer, 1994).

Rapp and Vollmer (2005) recently conducted a review of the literature relevant to the outcomes of functional analyses of stereotypic behaviors and reported that stereotypy was most commonly maintained by non-social sources of reinforcement. That is, behaviors such as hand mouthing, hand flapping, and body rocking are rarely maintained by the delivery of attention, tangible items, or escape from non-preferred events, but rather by the direct sensory consequences of the behavior. This contrasts with other forms of problem behavior such as self-injury and aggression, which are more commonly sensitive to social reinforcers (Iwata, Pace, Dorsey et al., 1994).

Although the vast majority of cases of stereotypy are maintained by automatic sources of reinforcement, there have been a few reported instances in which stereotypy has been maintained by social reinforcers as well, so this possibility should not be discounted (Goh et al., 1995; Kennedy, Meyer, Knowles, & Shukla, 2000). These cases highlight the importance of conducting functional analyses prior to developing treatments for stereotypic behaviors as opposed to making an a priori assumption that the behaviors are maintained by sensory consequences. Treatments based upon an assumption of automatic reinforcement will be ineffective in the subset of cases maintained by social reinforcers (Iwata, Pace, Cowdery, & Miltenberger, 1994), and thus we recommend conducting functional analysis prior to initiating treatments for stereotypy in every case. If social reinforcers are found to maintain stereotypy, we recommend implementing interventions that eliminate the social consequence following stereotypy and deliver it either on a fixed-time schedule or following some more desirable communicative response (Carr et al., 2000; Tiger, Hanley, & Bruzek, 2008). For the remainder of this chapter we will focus on the development of function-based interventions for stereotypy maintained by automatic sources of reinforcement. In particular we will focus upon four broad categories of intervention: eliminating or attenuating the sensory consequences of stereotypy, the development of alternative skill repertoires, reinforcement for the non-occurrence of stereotypy, and punishment of stereotypy.

Developing Interventions for Stereotypy and Other Repetitive Behaviors

Eliminating or Attenuating the Sensory Consequences of Stereotypy

The term function-based treatment refers to interventions that are designed to eliminate the reinforcer that maintains problem behavior (i.e., involve arranging extinction). For instance, a function-based treatment for problem behavior maintained by attention would be any intervention that involved not delivering attention following problem behavior. Behavior maintained by automatic reinforcement presents a particular treatment challenge in that the reinforcer is often inaccessible to a caregiver and may not be possible to withhold entirely. That is, it is relatively easy for a parent to avoid providing their attention following a problem behavior, but more difficult for a parent to withhold the stimulation generated by their child's body rocking.

Rincover, Cook, Peoples, and Packard (1979) provided one of the earliest systematic demonstrations of the use of sensory extinction to reduce stereotypic behaviors with four children diagnosed with autism who engaged in high rates of stereotypic behaviors (hand flapping, object spinning, picking, and finger flapping). Initially, the authors formed hypotheses regarding the potential sensory reinforcers which may have maintained these behaviors, such as the sound of the spinning object and the visual stimulation of finger flapping. Next the authors attenuated the sensory consequences of engaging in each behavior (e.g., carpeting the table upon which objects were typically spun resulted in a muffled sound and turning off the lights or blindfolding individuals eliminated visual stimulation). These sensory extinction procedures were found to reduce the occurrence of stereotypy for each of the four participants.

In a similar regard, Aiken and Salzberg (1984) eliminated the sensory consequences of loud vocalizations,

hand clapping, and dropping items by playing white noise through head phones with two participants. The use of such procedures is eloquent in their experimental demonstration of the effects of sensory extinction, but highly impractical in terms of implementation (i.e., it would be questionable to recommend blindfolding individuals continuously to eliminate hand flapping or to have them continuously experience ambient white noise).

An alternative technique for implementing sensory extinction has been the use of protective equipment to attenuate the sensory consequences of stereotypy. Dorsey, Iwata, Reid, and Davis (1982) demonstrated the effectiveness of protective equipment as an extinction procedure for the automatically reinforced self-injurious head hitting, head banging, and hand biting of three individuals with mental retardation. The sensory consequences of these behaviors were disrupted by having the participants wear a football helmet and padded gloves to minimize the stimulation experienced from hitting and resulted in substantial reductions in these self-injurious behaviors. Similarly, Mazaleski, Iwata, Rodgers, Vollmer, and Zarcone (1994) reduced the stereotypic hand mouthing of two individuals with profound mental retardation by placing oven mitts over their hands, which disrupted sensation both to the fingers and to the mouth. The use of protective equipment may be somewhat more practical to implement than the previously described extinction procedures, but the restriction of stereotypy through protective equipment may be associated with decreased opportunities for appropriate behavior (e.g., it can be difficult to manipulate items with padded gloves or mittens) and may be associated with muscle atrophy, bone demineralization, and shortening of tendons if the equipment restricts movement (Fisher, Piazza, Bowman, Hanley, & Adelinis, 1997).

A third technique for implementing sensory extinction has been referred to as response blocking or response interruption (Lerman & Iwata, 1996; McCord, Grosser, Iwata, & Powers, 2005; Reid, Parsons, Phillips, & Green, 1993; Smith, Russo, & Le, 1999) Reid et al. implemented this technique with two individuals with profound mental retardation who engaged in stereotypic hand mouthing. This procedure involved the therapist placing their hand in front of the participant's mouth, preventing attempts at the response from reaching completion. This form of extinction procedures does not require specialized equipment, but it does require the continuous monitoring of the individual and thus may be very costly in terms of the manpower required to implement the procedure with integrity. Very few investigations have evaluated the effects of imperfect implementation of this procedure with some evidence that repetitive behavior can worsen (i.e., occur at higher rates) if blocking is implemented intermittently (Lerman & Iwata).

Given that it is likely that blocking will not be implemented with perfect integrity (i.e., there will be periods of time in which caregivers will not be able to implement blocking, such as when driving) it may be desirable to develop stimulus control over the occurrence of the stereotypic response (Falcomata, Roane, & Pabico, 2007; Piazza, Hanley, & Fisher, 1996; Rollings & Baumeister, 1981). For instance, Piazza et al. described the use of a stimulus control procedure to reduce the covert cigarette pica (i.e., ingestion of cigarettes) of a young man with autism. Pica was initially reduced by providing access to non-contingent food and disrupting the occurrence of pica with a mild reprimand ("No butts"). Periods in which the interruption procedure would be implemented were then paired with a purple card, and periods in which the interruption procedure would not be implemented were paired with a yellow card. The purple card gained control over pica in that no attempts to ingest cigarette butts were made when the purple card was present. This purple card was then introduced into novel settings and continued to suppress the occurrence of pica, even when the blocking procedure would no longer be implemented. Although pica is a behavior that is never appropriate to allow, similar procedures could prove useful with other non-life threatening forms of behavior.

Extinction procedures implemented in isolation suffer from a number clinical limitations in addition to the practical ones already discussed. For one, withholding access to a particular form of reinforcement will result in a deprivation state from that reinforcer and may then evoke additional stereotypic behavior under this deprivation state (Rapp, 2006). For instance, if extinction is implemented during an instructional period which is then followed by a meal, it is possible that the disruption of stereotypy during the instructional period will create a deprivation state for the sensory consequences of stereotypy, and higher than normal levels of stereotypy may then be observed during the meal period.

Blocking of one form of stereotypy may also increase the occurrence of other forms of stereotypy or more problematic behaviors such as property destruction and aggression (Fellner, Laroche, & Sulzer-Azaroff, 1984; Fisher, Lindauer, Alterson, & Thompson, 1998; Rapp, Vollmer, St. Peter, Dozier, & Cotnoir, 2004). Fisher et al. reported two cases of individuals with mental retardation who engaged in property destruction and stereotypic toy play (i.e., tapping in one case and string play in another). When tapping was restricted, one participant broke household items (e.g., lamps) and then engaged in stereotypic tapping with the fragments. Similarly, when the second participant's string play was restricted, she would shred cloth materials (e.g., draperies and clothing) and then engage in string play with the shreds. These more severe destructive behaviors were minimized when more appropriate materials, similar to the fragments and shreds, that could be manipulated were provided.

Developing Alternative Skill Repertoires

Due to both the practical and clinical limitations of implementing extinction for automatically reinforced repetitive behaviors, such procedures are rarely implemented in isolation; rather, alternative and augmentative treatment approaches have become more common in the research literature and practice. One such approach is to promote engagement in activities that are incompatible with stereotypy. In some instances, this is as simple as providing access to leisure items. Berkson and Mason (1965) first reported that the simple presence of leisure materials was associated with decreased rates of stereotypic behavior among institutionalized individuals with developmental disabilities and simply handing materials to individuals may be sufficient in some cases to eliminate the occurrence of stereotypy. This procedure of providing access to novel materials has been described by a number of names including non-contingent reinforcement (NCR) and environmental enrichment (Favell, McGimsey, & Schell, 1982; Goh et al., 1995; Horner, 1980; Rapp, 2007; Ringdahl, Vollmer, Marcus, & Roane, 1997; Roane, Kelly, & Fisher, 2003; Sidener, Carr, & Firth, 2005; Vollmer, Marcus, & LeBlanc, 1994).

The success of environmental enrichment programs is predicated on the extent to which clients engage with the provided materials in lieu of stereotypic behavior, which is not guaranteed. An important consideration is to include high quality and high preference activities or materials. Vollmer et al. (1994) reported a comparison between treatment environments enriched with either preferred or non-preferred leisure items with a young boy with severe developmental disabilities who engaged in automatically maintained SIB. Appropriate toy play was high and SIB was low when and only when high preference materials were incorporated into the enriched environment.

Preferences among individuals with autism and other developmental disabilities are idiosyncratic in that the events, activities, and materials that serve as powerful reinforcers for one individual may be completely ineffective as reinforcers for another individual. Thus, the identification of each individual's preferences will contribute to the effectiveness of any reinforcement-based intervention. Caregiver interview is commonly the first step in determining preferred items. Fisher, Piazza, Bowman, and Amari (1996) provided a useful interview tool termed the Reinforcer Assessment for Individuals with Severe Disabilities, or RAISD, in which caregivers are provided examples of potential reinforcers experienced through different sensory modalities (e.g., visual, auditory, tactile, vestibular, olfactory, and gustatory), are asked to nominate materials or events that are likely to be enjoyable for the individual, and then to rank their perceptions of the individuals' preferences for these potential reinforcers in order. Caregiver report is a useful first step in identifying high preference items, but has been shown to have limited agreement with more systematic approaches to assessing individuals' preferences (Cote, Thompson, Hanley, & McKerchar, 2007; Green, Reid, White, Halford, Brittain, & Gardner, 1988). Direct preference assessments are recommended for identifying a hierarchy of preferences following the nomination procedure.

During a direct preference assessment, a potential reinforcer is presented to an individual to determine if he/she will then approach and manipulate the item (or consume it in the case of edible items). Items may be presented singly (Pace, Ivancic, Edwards, Iwata, & Page, 1985), in pairs (Fisher et al., 1992), or in multiple stimulus arrays (DeLeon & Iwata, 1996). The percentage of trials each item is approached is then rank ordered relative to each item resulting in a preference hierarchy. Stimuli ranked as highly preferred by these

procedures have been found to be more effective when delivered as reinforcers than those stimuli ranked as less preferred.

In addition to ensuring that materials are highly preferred, some have suggested attempting to identify materials that specifically produce stimulation similar to that generated by the repetitive behaviors. For instance, Piazza et al. (1998) compared the effects of two treatments on the occurrence of pica (i.e., the ingestion of inedible objects). The authors hypothesized that pica maintained by automatic reinforcement is most likely reinforced by stimulation to the mouth. Their treatment procedures involved providing free access to items that also provided oral stimulation, termed matched stimuli (e.g., food items, teething rings) or other items that were identified as highly preferred, but did not provide oral stimulation (e.g., swings, fans, mirrors). Matched-stimulation items resulted in substantial reductions in pica relative to those that were preferred but did not provide similar forms of stimulation (for a similar evaluation see Piazza, Adelinis, Hanley, Goh, & Delia, 2000).

In order to efficiently identify specific matched and non-matched stimuli to compete with the occurrence of problem behavior, some have recommend conducting a brief competing items assessment (Fisher, DeLeon, Rodriguez-Catter, & Keeney, 2004; Fisher, O'Conner, Kurtz, DeLeon, & Gotjen, 2000; Piazza et al., 1998; Shore, Iwata, DeLeon, Kahng, & Smith, 1997) in which the durations of item engagement and problem behavior are measured in the presence of each item individually during brief sessions (e.g., 5 min). Those items that fail to compete with stereotypy during a brief assessment can be eliminated from further consideration and those that effectively compete with stereotypy may be included in further intervention programming. Ideally, multiple potential competing items will be identified and incorporated into enriched environments to minimize satiation effects (Lindberg, Iwata, Roscoe, Worsdell, & Hanley, 2003).

Despite the inclusion of high-quality competing sources of reinforcement, some individuals will continue to engage in high rates of stereotypy and low-rates of item engagement (e.g., Favell et al., 1982). There are a number of potential explanations for this finding. Individuals may simply not have a history of reinforcement for interacting with particular items. Thus it is a useful starting point to include periodic prompts to engage with materials (Hanley, Iwata,

Thompson, & Lindberg, 2000; Lerman, Kelley, Vorndran, & Van Camp, 2003). For instance, Lerman et al. reported a case of a young girl with autism who engaged in head and tooth tapping. During one of their analyses, a treatment condition was introduced in which tapping was blocked and a variety of high preference leisure items were delivered. However, item interaction remained low until the experimenters prompted item interaction by physically guiding the participant to manipulate the items every 20 s if she was not doing so independently.

Other individuals may not have the skill repertoire necessary to extract reinforcement from the provided items. Additional skill training or modification of the environment will be necessary to improve the effectiveness of enriched environments. For instance, Vollmer et al. (1994) reported two cases in which an enriched environment was arranged with preferred items that required activation to operate (e.g., sound-making toys). This treatment was initially ineffective because the toys were difficult to operate. Stereotypy was reduced only when the therapists activated the preferred materials for the participants following a simple reaching response. To achieve a greater degree of independence, one of the sound-making toys was connected to a large microswitch that could be operated independently by their participant and low levels of stereotypy were maintained.

It is worth considering the effort required to engage in a newly taught skill relative to stereotypy. It may be possible, in at least some instances, to decrease the effort required to engage in a more socially appropriate behavior such that it is more likely to compete with stereotypy. Piazza, Hanley, Blakely-Smith, and Kinsman (2000) described the case of a boy with profound mental retardation and cortical blindness who engaged in pica and hand mouthing. Their initial treatment condition involved providing access to toys that were more appropriate for mouthing; however, this treatment occasioned high levels of pica and hand mouthing because the participant would frequently drop his toys and not be able to locate them. The effort associated with relocating his toys was then minimized by attaching each item to a vest he wore via strings, and he was taught to use the strings to retrieve the toys. This manipulation resulted in consistently low levels of pica and hand mouthing and high levels of more appropriate object mouthing.

It may also be possible to increase the effort associated with stereotypy, and thereby decrease its occurrence. Increasing the response effort of stereotypy has generally been accomplished by adding physical resistance to the limb or limbs associated with stereotypy without completely immobilizing the limb. For instance, Hanley, Piazza, Keeney, Blakely-Smith, and Worsdell (1998) increased the effort associated with stereotypic head hitting by placing wrist weights on the participants arms, resulting in a 92% reduction in head hitting relative to baseline conditions without the weights. Further, these wrist weights did not compete with other adaptive behaviors that were measured (specifically self-feeding and pacifier-to-mouth play) and were associated with the development of novel communicative behavior.

Zhou, Goff, and Iwata (2000) provided an additional demonstration of the effects of increasing the response effort required to engage in stereotypy with four adults with profound mental retardation who engaged in hand mouthing. The effort associated with hand mouthing was increased by placing the participants in soft flexible sleeves that increased resistance for bending at the elbow, but still allowed hand mouthing to occur. Similar to the results of Hanley et al. (1998), these authors found that increasing the effort associated with stereotypy decreased the occurrence of this behavior and increased the occurrence of other appropriate object manipulation.

For some individuals, it may be necessary to arrange differential reinforcement contingencies to promote and strengthen object manipulation. For instance, the stereotypy of one participant in Rapp et al. (2004) remained high and no object manipulation was observed during an environmental enrichment condition. However, when each instance of object manipulation resulted in a 2-s drink from a bottle of juice, object manipulation increased well above levels of stereotypy. The effectiveness of a differential-reinforcement based treatment relies on the identification of a reinforcer that may be delivered repeatedly and whose value will remain greater than that of stereotypy.

The sensory consequences of stereotypy are likely to serve as an extremely potent reinforcer, with potentially greater value than the edibles or leisure items commonly delivered as reinforcers within a differential-reinforcement based treatment or during skill acquisition programming (Charlop, Kurtz, & Kasey, 1990). In other words, in many cases it may be extremely difficult, if not impossible, to identify an alternative reinforcer to compete with the occurrence of stereotypy. As a result, some researcher have suggested that rather than attempting to eliminate these behaviors all together, it may be possible to utilize the reinforcing value of stereotypy to enhance desirable behaviors with children with autism (Hanley et al., 2000; Hung, 1978; Wolery, Kirk, & Gast, 1985).

Delivering access to stereotypy as a reinforcer involves restricting access to stereotypy, commonly via response blocking, and allowing access to stereotypy following the occurrence of some desirable behavior. Hung (1978) restricted access to stereotypy for two withdrawn adolescents with autism enrolled in a summer camp and delivered tokens exchangeable for access to brief periods in which to engage in stereotypy contingent upon appropriate utterances. Appropriate vocalizations increased for both participants. Similarly, Wolery et al. (1985) increased the academic participation of two children with autism by delivering contingent access to stereotypy. This approach may be particularly beneficial in the treatment of stereotypy in that it strengthens a desirable response and eliminates stereotypy during important instructional or socially-interactive periods, but allows stereotypy to occur during periods controlled by a caregiver. It is worth noting however that there is a limited research base upon which to make specific recommendations regarding the parameters of this strategy. It is not clear for how long stereotypy should be restricted, what quantity or duration of the desirable response should be required to be emitted, nor what duration of access to stereotypy should be provided contingent upon each desirable response. These variables represent an important direction for continued research.

Reinforcement for the Non-occurrence of Stereotypy

Differential reinforcement of the non-occurrence of stereotypy (DRO) involves providing high quality reinforcers contingent upon periods of time in which an individual abstains from stereotypy (Cowdery, Iwata, & Pace, 1990; Fellner et al., 1984; Foxx & Azrin, 1973; Repp, Deitz, & Speir, 1974; Taylor, Hoch, & Weissman, 2005). Cowdery et al. provided one example of a DRO procedure with a 9-year-old boy who engaged in severe, stereotypic self-scratching and

self-rubbing. This procedure involved delivering pennies (conditioned reinforcers) that were exchangeable for a variety of back-up reinforcers (e.g., TV, snacks, video games, other play materials) contingent upon periods of time in which the participant abstained from self-scratching. Initially this DRO interval was set for 2 min and was gradually expanded to 30 min as the treatment proved successful.

Similar to NCR, the first step in arranging a DRO-based intervention is to identify highly preferred stimuli that may be delivered as reinforcers. After these have been identified, the next step is to determine initial durations of the DRO interval (i.e., how long need the individual abstain from stereotypy prior to delivering reinforcement). If the DRO interval is set too short (i.e., reinforcement is delivered frequently) it is likely that satiation will set in, and the treatment will lose its effectiveness. If the DRO interval is set too long, it is possible that such an omission criteria will not be met, and thus behavior will not contact the reinforcement contingency. For these reasons, DRO intervals are best set idiosyncratically, based upon each individual's presenting level of problem behavior. Vollmer, Iwata, Zarcone, Smith, and Mazaleski (1993) described a process for setting their DRO intervals by first collecting baseline data on the occurrence of stereotypy and from this data calculating the mean inter-response interval (IRI), or the time between each response cluster. That is, if an individual engaged in problem behavior at a rate of 6 per min, there would be a mean of 10-s between each response, and thus their initial DRO interval would be set to 10-s. Interestingly, Vollmer et al., continued to adjust their DRO equivalent to the previous sessions' IRI's such that the DRO interval continued to adjust upward as their procedure was effective at lowering stereotypy. Adjusting DRO intervals over time will decrease the overall number of reinforcers delivered, and thus minimize long-term reinforcer satiation.

It is also important to decide whether DRO intervals will reset immediately following the occurrence of problem behavior. During a resetting DRO, each instance of problem behavior will immediately restart the DRO interval (e.g., another 10-s would need to elapse without problem behavior); thus there is a constant response-reinforcer interval (Vollmer & Iwata, 1992). During a non-resetting DRO, reinforcement is programmed to occur at specific time intervals, and the occurrence of problem behavior prior to the elapse of that time interval simply causes the omission of that reinforcer. In this regard, the response-reinforcer interval may vary depending upon the time during which problem behavior occurs. We are not aware of any comparative studies to suggest that either resetting or non-resetting DRO intervals are superior, but both have been independently shown to be effective (Repp, Deitz, & Deitz, 1976; Repp et al., 1974).

One of the challenges associated with implementing either resetting or non-resetting DRO procedures is that they require the constant monitoring of the occurrence or non-occurrence of problem behavior in order to determine if reinforcement should be delivered, and thus may not be practically implemented in many typical care settings. Momentary DRO procedures may provide an alternative that may be substantially easier to implement with fidelity. For instance, after determining the self injury of three individuals with profound mental retardation was maintained by social sources of reinforcement, Lindberg, Iwata, Kahng, and DeLeon (1999) described the use of a momentary DRO procedure in which rather than observing problem behavior for the entire duration of an interval, a therapist noted the occurrence or non-occurrence of problem behavior at the instant an interval ended and delivered reinforcement only if behavior was not occurring at that instant. Despite the fact that numerous problem behaviors could occur without postponing the delivery of reinforcement, this momentary procedure was equally effective as a DRO procedure with continuous observation. This finding may be limited to cases of socially-maintained problem behavior as these procedures were implemented with extinction in place (i.e., self-injury in these cases no-longer resulted in the delivery of reinforcement). The role of the "total omission" contingency when problem behavior continues to produce reinforcement, is unclear, as is the case in treating stereotypy, and thus remains an important area for future research.

Punishment

Despite the most extraordinary efforts of the most trained clinicians, some cases will still remain in which a reinforcer of sufficient strength to compete with stereotypy cannot be identified and extinction procedures cannot be successfully implemented. In these cases, a practitioner is limited to two options. The first is to cease the treatment of stereotypy. The negative impact of stereotypy and the challenges it imposes upon the life of the individual should be weighed against the cost of continued intervention. Clinicians should implement punishment-based procedures in cases in which the occurrence of stereotypy is debilitating or detracts from the individual's quality of life (Van Houten et al., 1988).

The early stereotypy treatment literature is replete with examples of the use of highly intrusive forms of punishment such as electric shock (Baumeister & Forehand, 1972; Risley, 1968), slapping (Foxx & Azrin, 1973; Koegel et al., 1974), aversive tastes (Foxx & Azrin, 1973; Friman, Cook, & Finney, 1984), aversive odors (Clarke & Thomason, 1983), and water misting (Friman et al., 1984). However, more recent research has also shown the effectiveness of more benign forms of punishment such as verbal reprimands (Baumeister & Forehand, 1972; Foxx & Azrin, 1973), overcorrection (Doke & Epstein, 1975; Epstein et al., 1974; Foxx & Azrin, 1973; Harris & Wolchik, 1979; Maag, Rutherford, Wolchik, & Parks, 1986; Ollendick, Matson, & Martin, 1978) time-out and response-cost procedures (Falcomata, Roane, Hovanetz, Kettering, & Kenney, 2004; Pendergrass, 1972).

When implemented, punishments should be selected which are both sufficiently aversive as to reduce stereotypy but also socially acceptable to the caregivers responsible for implementing the treatment. The punishments should be delivered immediately following each instance of stereotypy at a sufficient intensity to suppress the behavior (see Lerman & Vorndran, 2002 for more comprehensive coverage). Additional sources of reinforcement (e.g., DRO or enriched environments) should continue to be provided to enhance the effectiveness of the punishment (Thompson, Iwata, Conners, & Roscoe, 1999).

Conclusions and Recommendations

Stereotypy, rituals, and other repetitive behaviors are one of the core behavioral symptoms leading to a diagnosis of autism. Although the topography of these behaviors varies from individual to individual, these behaviors often share the same functional properties in that they tend to be maintained by automatic sources of reinforcement, with important exceptions. There have been demonstrations and replications of a number of operant-based interventions in the behavior analytic literature that involve eliminating or attenuating the sensory consequences of the behavior, providing matched or competing forms of stimulation to substitute for the sensory consequences of stereotypy, delivering alternative forms of reinforcement for appropriate behavior or for the non-occurrence of stereotypy, and arranging punishments to follow the occurrence of stereotypy. There is limited evidence that it may be possible to allow access to stereotypy to occur during certain periods (either scheduled times for following some desirable behavior) rather than eliminate the behavior entirely; however, more research is needed to elaborate upon the integral parameters of such an approach.

References

Aiken, J. M., & Salzberg, C. L. (1984). The effects of a sensory extinction procedure on stereotypic sounds of two autistic children. *Journal of Autism and Developmental Disorders, 14*, 291–299.

Bartak, L., & Rutter, M. (1976). Differences between mentally retarded and normally intelligent autistic children. *Journal of Autism and Child Schizophrenia, 6*, 109–120.

Baumeister, A. A., & Forehand, R. (1972). Effects of contingent shock and verbal command on body rocking of retardates. *Journal of Clinical Psychology, 28*, 586–590.

Berkson, G., & Mason, W. A. (1963). Stereotyped movements of mental defectives: III. Situation effects. *American Journal of Mental Deficiency, 68*, 409–412.

Berkson, G., & Mason, W. A. (1965). Stereotyped movements of mental defectives. IV. The effects of toys and the character of the acts. *American Journal of Mental Deficiency, 70*, 511–524.

Campbell, M., Locascio, J. J., Choroco, M. C., Spencer, E. K., Malone, R. P., Kafantaris, V., et al. (1990). Stereotypies and Tardive Dyskinesia: Abnormal movements in autistic children. *Psychopharmacology Bulletin, 26*, 260–266.

Carr, J. E., Coriarty, S., Wilder, D. A., Gaunt, B. T., Dozier, C. L., Britton, L. N., et al. (2000). A review of "noncontingent" reinforcement as treatment for aberrant behavior of individuals with developmental disabilities. *Research in Developmental Disabilities, 21*, 377–391.

Charlop, M. H., Kurtz, P. F., & Casey, F. G. (1990). Using aberrant behaviors as reinforcers for autistic children. *Journal of Applied Behavior Analysis, 23*, 163–181.

Clarke, J. C., & Thomason, S. (1983). The use of an aversive smell to eliminate autistic self-stimulatory behavior. *Child and Family Behavior Therapy, 5*(3), 51–61.

Cote, C. A., Thompson, R. H., Hanley, G. P., & McKerchar, P. M. (2007). Teacher report and direct assessment of preferences for identifying reinforcers for young children. *Journal of Applied Behavior Analysis, 40*, 157–166.

Cowdery, G. E., Iwata, B. A., & Pace, G. M. (1990). Effects and side effects of DRO as treatment for self-injurious behavior. *Journal of Applied Behavior Analysis, 23*, 497–506.

Davenport, R. K., Jr., & Berkson, G. (1963). Stereotyped movements of mental defectives: II. Effects of novel objects. *American Journal of Mental Deficiency, 67*, 879–882.

DeLeon, I. G., & Iwata, B. A. (1996). Evaluation of a multiple-stimulus presentation format for assessing reinforcer preferences. *Journal of Applied Behavior Analysis, 29*(4), 519–533.

Doke, L. A., & Epstein, L. H. (1975). Oral overcorrection: Side effects and extended applications. *Journal of Experimental Child Psychology, 20*, 496–511.

Dorsey, M. F., Iwata, B. A., Reid, D. H., & Davis, P. A. (1982). Protective equipment: Continuous and contingent application in the treatment of self-injurious behavior. *Journal of Applied Behavior Analysis, 15*, 217–230.

Dunlap, G., Dyer, K., & Koegel, R. L. (1983). Autistic self-stimulation and intertrial interval duration. *American Journal of Mental Deficiency, 88*, 194–202.

Epstein, L. H., Doke, L. A., Sajwaj, T. E., Sorrell, S., & Rimmer, B. (1974). Generality and the side effects of overcorrection. *Journal of Applied Behavior Analysis, 7*, 385–390.

Falcomata, T. S., Roane, H. S., Hovanetz, A. N., Kettering, T. L., & Kenney, K. M. (2004). An evaluation of response cost in the treatment of inappropriate vocalizations maintained by automatic reinforcement. *Journal of Applied Behavior Analysis, 37*, 83–87.

Falcomata, T. S., Roane, H. S., & Pabico, R. R. (2007). Unintentional stimulus control during the treatment of pica displayed by a young man with autism. *Research in Autism Spectrum Disorders, 1*, 350–359.

Favell, J. E., McGimsey, J. F., & Schell, R. M. (1982). Treatment of self-injury by providing alternate sensory activities. *Analysis and Interventions in Developmental Disabilities, 2*, 83–104.

Fellner, D. J., LaRoche, M., & Sulzer-Azaroff, B. (1984). The effects of adding interruption to differential reinforcement on targeted and novel self-stimulatory behaviors. *Journal of Behavior Therapy and Experimental Psychiatry, 15*, 315–321.

Fisher, W. W., DeLeon, I. G., Rodriguez-Catter, V., & Keeney, K. M. (2004). Enhancing the effects of extinction of attention-maintained behavior through noncontingent delivery of attention or stimuli identified via a competing items assessment. *Journal of Applied Behavior Analysis, 37*, 171–184.

Fisher, W. W., Lindauer, S. E., Alterson, C. J., & Thompson, R. H. (1998). Assessment and treatment of destructive behavior maintained by stereotypic object manipulation. *Journal of Applied Behavior Analysis, 31*, 513–527.

Fisher, W. W., O'Conner, J. T., Kurtz, P. F., DeLeon, I. G., & Gotjen, D. L. (2000). The effects of noncontingent delivery of high- and low-preference stimuli on attention-maintained destructive behavior. *Journal of Applied Behavior Analysis, 33*, 79–83.

Fisher, W. W., Piazza, C. C., Bowman, L. G., & Amari, A. (1996). Integrating caregiver report with a systematic choice assessment to enhance reinforcer identification. *American Journal on Mental Retardation, 101*, 15–25.

Fisher, W., Piazza, C. C., Bowman, L. G., Hagopian, L. P., Owens, J. C., & Slevin, I. (1992). A comparison of two approaches for identifying reinforcers for persones with severe and profound disabilities. *Journal of Applied Behavior Analysis, 25*(2), 491–498.

Fisher, W. W., Piazza, C. C., Bowman, L. G., Hanley, G. P., & Adelinis, J. D. (1997). Direct and collateral effects of restraints and restraint fading. *Journal of Applied Behavior Analysis, 30*, 105–120.

Foxx, R. M., & Azrin, N. H. (1973). The elimination of autistic self-stimulatory behavior by overcorrection. *Journal of Applied Behavior Analysis, 6*, 1–14.

Friman, P. C., Cook, J. W., & Finney, J. W. (1984). Effects of punishment procedures on the self-stimulatory behavior of an autistic child. *Analysis and Interventions in Developmental Disabilities, 4*, 39–46.

Goh, H., Iwata, B. A., Shore, B. A., DeLeon, I. G., Lerman, D. C., Ulrich, S. M., et al. (1995). An analysis of the reinforcing properties of hand mouthing. *Journal of Applied Behavior Analysis, 28*, 269–283.

Green, C. W., Reid, D. H., White, L. K., Halford, R. C., Brittain, D. P., & Gardner, S. M. (1988). Identifying reinforcers for persons with profound handicaps: Staff opinion versus systematic assessment of preferences. *Journal of Applied Behavior Analysis, 21*, 31–43.

Hanley, G. P., Iwata, B. A., & McCord, B. E. (2003). Functional analysis of problem behavior: A review. *Journal of Applied Behavior Analysis, 36*, 147–185.

Hanley, G. P., Iwata, B. A., Thompson, R. H., & Lindberg, J. S. (2000). A component analysis of "stereotypy as reinforcement" for alternative behavior. *Journal of Applied Behavior Analysis, 33*, 285–297.

Hanley, G. P., Piazza, C. C., Keeney, K. M., Blakely-Smith, A., & Worsdell, A. S. (1998). Effects of wrist weights on self-injurious and adaptive behaviors. *Journal of Applied Behavior Analysis, 31*, 307–310.

Harris, S. L., & Wolchik, S. A. (1979). Suppression of self-stimulation: Three alternative strategies. *Journal of Applied Behavior Analysis, 12*, 185–198.

Horner, R. D. (1980). The effects of an environmental "enrichment" program on the behavior of institutionalized profoundly retarded children. *Journal of Applied Behavior Analysis, 13*, 473–491.

Hung, D. W. (1978). Using self-stimulation as reinforcement for autistic children. *Journal of Autism and Childhood Schizophrenia, 8*, 355–366.

Iwata, B. A., Dorsey, M. F., Slifer, K. J., Bauman, K. E., & Richman, G. S. (1994). Toward a functional analysis of self-injury. *Journal of Applied Behavior Analysis, 27*, 197–209. Reprinted from *Analysis and Intervention in Developmental Disabilities, 2*, 3–20, 1982.

Iwata, B. A., Pace, G. M., Cowdery, G. E., & Miltenberger, R. G. (1994). What makes extinction work: An analysis of procedural form and function. *Journal of Applied Behavior Analysis, 27*, 131–144.

Iwata, B. A., Pace, G. M., Dorsey, M. F., Zarcone, J. R., Vollmer, T. R., Smith, R. G., et al. (1994). The functions of self-injurious behavior: An experimental-epidemiological analysis. *Journal of Applied Behavior Analysis, 27*, 215–240.

Kennedy, C. H., Meyer, K. A., Knowles, T., & Shukla, S. (2000). Analyzing the multiple functions of stereotypical behavior for students with autism: Implications for assessment and treatment. *Journal of Applied Behavior Analysis, 33*, 559–571.

Koegel, R. L., & Covert, A. (1972). The relationship of self-stimulation to learning in autistic children. *Journal of Applied Behavior Analysis, 5*, 381–387.

Koegel, R. L., Firestone, P. B., Kramme, K. W., & Dunlap, G. (1974). Increasing spontaneous play by suppressing self-stimulation in autistic children. *Journal of Applied Behavior Analysis, 7*, 521–528.

Lerman, D. C., & Iwata, B. A. (1996). A methodology for distinguishing between extinction and punishment effects associated with response blocking. *Journal of Applied Behavior Analysis, 29*, 231–233.

Lerman, D. C., Kelley, M. E., Vorndran, C. M., & Van Camp, C. M. (2003). Collateral effects of response blocking during the treatment of stereotypic behavior. *Journal of Applied Behavior Analysis, 36*, 119–123.

Lerman, D. C., & Vorndran, C. M. (2002). On the status of knowledge for using punishment: Implications for treating behavior disorders. *Journal of Applied Behavior Analysis, 35*, 431–464.

Lindberg, J. S., Iwata, B. A., Kahng, S., & DeLeon, I. G. (1999). DRO contingencies: An analysis of variable-momentary schedules. *Journal of Applied Behavior Analysis, 32*, 123–136.

Lindberg, J. S., Iwata, B. A., Roscoe, E. M., Worsdell, A. S., & Hanley, G. P. (2003). Treatment efficacy of noncontingent reinforcement during brief and extended application. *Journal of Applied Behavior Analysis, 36*, 1–19.

Lovaas, O. I., Litrownik, A., & Mann, R. (1971). Response latencies to auditory stimuli in autistic children engaged in self-stimulatory behavior. *Behavior Research and Therapy, 9*, 39–49.

Maag, J. W., Rutherford, R. B., Wolchik, S. A., & Parks, B. T. (1986). Brief report: Comparison of two short overcorrection procedures on the stereotypic behavior of autistic children. *Journal of Autism and Developmental Disorders, 16*, 83–87.

Mazaleski, J. L., Iwata, B. A., Rodgers, T. A., Vollmer, T. R., & Zarcone, J. R. (1994). Protective equipment as treatment for stereotypic hand mouthing: Sensory extinction or punishment effects? *Journal of Applied Behavior Analysis, 27*, 345–355.

McCord, B. E., Grosser, J. W., Iwata, B. A., & Powers, L. A. (2005). An analysis of response-blocking parameters in the prevention of pica. *Journal of Applied Behavior Analysis, 38*, 391–394.

McDougle, C. J., Kresch, L., Goodman, W. K., Naylor, S. T., Volkmar, F. R., Cohen, D. J., et al. (1995). A case-controlled study of repetitive thoughts and behavior in adults with autistic disorder and obsessive compulsive disorder. *American Journal of Psychiatry, 152*, 772–777.

Morrison, K., & Rosales-Ruiz, J. (1997). The effect of object preferences on task performance and stereotypy in a child with autism. *Research in Developmental Disabilities, 18*, 127–137.

Ollendick, T. H., Matson, J. L., & Martin, J. E. (1978). Effectiveness of hand overcorrection for topographically similar and dissimilar self-stimulatory behavior. *Journal of Experimental Child Psychology, 25*, 396–403.

Pace, G. M., Ivancic, M. T., Edwards, G. L., Iwata, B. A., & Page, T. J. (1985). Assessment of stimulus preference assessment and reinforcer value with profoundly retarded individuals. *Journal of Applied Behavior Analysis, 18*(3), 249–255.

Pendergrass, V. E. (1972). Timeout from positive reinforcement following persistent, high-rate behavior in retardates. *Journal of Applied Behavior Analysis, 5*, 85–91.

Piazza, C. C., Adelinis, J. D., Hanley, G. P., Goh, H., & Delia, M. D. (2000). An evaluation of the effects of matched stimuli on behaviors maintained by automatic reinforcement. *Journal of Applied Behavior Analysis, 33*, 13–27.

Piazza, C. C., Hanley, G. P., Blakely-Smith, A., & Kinsman, A. M. (2000). Effects of search skills training on the pica of a blind boy. *Journal of Developmental and Physical Disabilities, 12*, 35–41.

Piazza, C. C., Fisher, W. W., Hanley, G. P., LeBlanc, L. A., Worsdell, A. S., Lindauer, S. E., et al. (1998). Treatment of pica through multiple analyses of its reinforcing functions. *Journal of Applied Behavior Analysis, 31*, 165–189.

Piazza, C. C., Hanley, G. P., & Fisher, W. W. (1996). Functional analysis and treatment of cigarette pica. *Journal of Applied Behavior Analysis, 29*, 437–450.

Rapp, J. T. (2006). Toward an empirical method for identifying matched stimulation for automatically reinforced behavior: A preliminary investigation. *Journal of Applied Behavior Analysis, 39*, 137–140.

Rapp, J. T. (2007). Further evaluation of methods to identify matched stimulation. *Journal of Applied Behavior Analysis, 40*, 73–88.

Rapp, J. T., & Vollmer, T. R. (2005). Stereotypy I: A review of behavioral assessment and treatment. *Research in Developmental Disabilities, 26*, 527–547.

Rapp, J. T., Vollmer, T. R., St. Peter, C., Dozier, C. L., & Cotnoir, N. M. (2004). Analysis of response allocation in individuals with multiple forms of stereotyped behavior. *Journal of Applied Behavior Analysis, 37*, 481–501.

Reid, D. H., Parsons, M. B., Phillips, J. F., & Green, C. W. (1993). Reduction of self-injurious hand mouthing using response blocking. *Journal of Applied Behavior Analysis, 26*, 139–140.

Repp, A. C., Deitz, S. M., & Deitz, D. E. D. (1976). Reducing inappropriate behaviors in a classroom and in individual sessions through DRO schedules of reinforcement. *Mental Retardation, 14*, 11–15.

Repp, A. C., Deitz, S. M., & Speir, N. C. (1974). Reducing stereotypic responding of retarded persons by the differential reinforcement of other behavior. *American Journal of Mental Deficiency, 79*, 279–284.

Richler, J., Bishop, S. L., Kleinke, J. R., & Lord, C. (2007). Restricted and repetitive behavior disorders in young children with autism spectrum disorders. *Journal of Autism and Developmental Disorders, 37*, 73–85.

Rincover, A., Cook, R., Peoples, A., & Packard, D. (1979). Sensory extinction and sensory reinforcement principles for programming multiple adaptive behavior change. *Journal of Applied Behavior Analysis, 12*, 221–233.

Ringdahl, J. E., Vollmer, T. R., Marcus, B. A., & Roane, H. S. (1997). An analogue evaluation of environmental enrichment: The role of stimulus preference. *Journal of Applied Behavior Analysis, 30*, 203–216.

Risley, T. R. (1968). The effects and side effects of punishing the autistic behaviors of a deviant child. *Journal of Applied Behavior Analysis, 1*, 21–34.

Roane, H. S., Kelly, M. L., & Fisher, W. W. (2003). The effects of noncontingent access to food on the rate of object mouth-ing across three settings. *Journal of Applied Behavior Analysis, 36*, 579–582.

Rollings, J. P., & Baumeister, A. A. (1981). Stimulus control of stereotypic responding: Effects on target and collateral behavior. *American Journal of Mental Deficiency, 86*, 67–77.

Schroeder, A., Schroeder, C., Smith, B., & Dalldorf, J. (1978). Prevalence of self-injurious behavior in a large state facility for the retarded. *Journal of Autism and Child Schizophrenia, 8*, 261–269.

Shore, B. A., Iwata, B. A., DeLeon, I. G., Kahng, S. W., & Smith, R. G. (1997). An analysis of reinforcer substitutability using object manipulation and self-injury as competing responses. *Journal of Applied Behavior Analysis, 30*(1), 21–41.

Sidener, T. M., Carr, J. E., & Firth, A. M. (2005). Superimposition and withholding of edible consequences as treatment for automatically reinforced stereotypy. *Journal of Applied Behavior Analysis, 38*, 121–124.

Smith, E. A., & Van Houten, R. (1996). A comparison of the characteristics of self-stimulatory behaviors in "normal": Children and children with developmental delays. *Research in Developmental Disabilities, 17*, 253–268.

Smith, R. G., Russo, L., & Le, L. D. (1999). Distinguishing between extinction and punishment effects of response blocking: A replication. *Journal of Applied Behavior Analysis, 32*, 367–370.

Taylor, B. A., Hoch, H., & Weissman, M. (2005). The analysis and treatment of vocal stereotypy in a child with autism. *Behavioral Interventions, 20*, 239–253.

Thompson, R. H., Iwata, B. A., Conners, J., & Roscoe, E. M. (1999). Effects of reinforcement for alternative behavior during punishment of self-injury. *Journal of Applied Behavior Analysis, 32*, 317–328.

Tiger, J. H., Hanley, G. P., & Bruzek, J. (2008). Functional communication training: A review and practical guide. *Behavior Analysis in Practice, 1*, 16–23.

Van Houten, R., Axelrod, S., Bailey, J. S., Favell, J. E., Foxx, R. M., Iwata, B. A., et al. (1988). The right to effective behavioral treatment. *Journal of Applied Behavior Analysis, 21*, 381–384.

Vollmer, T. R. (1994). The concept of automatic reinforcement: Implications for behavioral research in developmental disabilities. *Research in Developmental Disabilities, 15*, 187–207.

Vollmer, T. R., & Iwata, B. A. (1992). Differential reinforcement as treatment for behavior disorders: Procedural and functional variations. *Research in Developmental Disabilities, 13*, 393–417.

Vollmer, T. R., Iwata, B. A., Zarcone, J. R., Smith, R. G., & Mazaleski, J. L. (1993). The role of attention in the treatment of attention-maintained self-injurious behavior: Noncontingent reinforcement and differential reinforcement of other behavior. *Journal of Applied Behavior Analysis, 26*, 9–21.

Vollmer, T. R., Marcus, B. A., & LeBlanc, L. A. (1994). Treatment of self-injury and hand mouthing following inconclusive functional analyses. *Journal of Applied Behavior Analysis, 27*, 331–344.

Wolery, M., Kirk, K., & Gast, D. L. (1985). Stereotypic behavior as a reinforcer: Effects and side effects. *Journal of Autism and Developmental Disorders, 15*, 149–161.

Zhou, L., Goff, G. A., & Iwata, B. A. (2000). Effects of increased response effort on self-injury and object manipulation as competing responses. *Journal of Applied Behavior Analysis, 33*, 29–40.

Chapter 9
Self–injury

Timothy R. Vollmer, Kimberly N. Sloman, and Andrew L. Samaha

One of the most dangerous and debilitating behavior problems in the entire field of developmental disabilities is self-injurious behavior. This set of target behaviors is also a frequent concern in ASD. A review of common targets for intervention and research supported treatment will be covered. Current status of the field and future directions will be discussed

Self–injury

One of the most perplexing and challenging forms of behavior in autism is self-injury. Self-injurious behavior (SIB) has been reported in clinical documentation and in the research literature to take various forms including self-hitting, head banging, self-pinching, self-scratching, eye-gouging, self-kicking, hair-pulling, self-biting, and many others. McDermott, Zhou, and Mann (2008) reported that children with autism are 7.6 times more likely to be treated for self-inflicted injuries than members of a typically developing control group. Of course not all individuals with autism display SIB, but the problem is significant in that population. For example Bodfish, Symons, Parker, and Lewis (2000) reported that in a sample of 32 individuals diagnosed with autism, 69% displayed some form of SIB. The prevalence statistics are widely varied in different studies, but all suggest that the problem is far greater in autism than in the general population (Dominick, Davis, Lainhart, Tager-Flusberg, & Folstein, 2007).

T.R. Vollmer (✉)
Department of Psychology, University of Florida, Gainesville, FL, 32611-2250 P.O. Box 112250, USA
e-mail: vollmera@ufl.edu

Although SIB is commonly described as highly repetitive behavior that can occur at frequencies of up to dozens of instances per minute (Iwata, Dorsey, Slifer, Bauman & Richman, 1994), the behavior also can be episodic insofar as it either occurs under highly specific stimulus contexts or in bursts after long periods without problematic behavior (e.g., O'Reilly, 1997). A majority of the evidence suggests that SIB is learned behavior that is often inadvertently reinforced (strengthened) by common social consequences to the behavior, such as attention from adults, access to preferred items or activities, or escape from instructional or undesired activities. Sometimes the behavior occurs because it produces stimulation by itself and, therefore, will persist in the absence of social reinforcement (a phenomenon known as "automatic reinforcement," Skinner, 1953; Vaughan & Michael, 1982).

In this chapter we will first describe the known "operant functions" of SIB. Second, we will describe behavioral assessment methods for SIB. Third, we will describe how the assessment information can be used to initiate behavioral treatments. Not all of the examples used will come directly from participants with autism, but the same or similar principles apply.

The Operant Functions of SIB

A majority of the evidence suggests that SIB is operant behavior. Operant behavior is controlled by its consequences. For example, a person can turn a doorknob and the door opens as a result; hence, turning the knob is operant behavior. Similarly, a child is engaging in operant behavior when she bangs her head against the wall because in the past someone gave her food to "calm her down.". Some indirect evidence exists to suggest that some SIB in the form of self-biting may be reflexive rather than operant. It is known that several species of animals, including humans, will bite down forcefully on whatever is available when presented with extremely loud or painful stimulation (Hutchinson, 1977). Thus, it is conceivable that some self-biting is in response to aversive noise or other noxious stimulation. Although a reflexive biting response should be considered in future SIB research, a vast majority of evidence supports operant functions of SIB. These functions will be discussed below as follows.

Some SIB is maintained by socially mediated positive reinforcement. *Socially mediated* means only that the reinforcement is delivered by another person. *Positive* means that some stimulation is *presented* as a consequence to behavior. *Reinforcement* means *to strengthen* (in the sense that behavior is more likely to occur under similar circumstances in the future). Of course few care providers would intentionally reinforce SIB, but many natural reactions from the social environment inadvertently produce a reinforcement effect. Socially mediated reinforcement can be attention in the form of reprimands, comfort statements, or physical proximity (Iwata, Pace, Dorsey, et al., 1994) or can be tangible items such as food, toys, or activities. It is a very common and perhaps even natural adult response to reprimand, comfort, or try to calm down an individual when severe behavior occurs (e.g., Thompson & Iwata, 2001) and probably the adult's behavior is, in turn, reinforced by the temporary cessation of SIB (Sloman et al., 2005).

Some SIB is maintained by socially mediated negative reinforcement. Again, *socially mediated* means that it is delivered by another person. *Negative* means that some stimulation is *removed, terminated, or avoided* as a consequence to behavior. *Reinforcement* again means *to strengthen* (increase the future likelihood of) the behavior. Thus, the distinction between socially mediated positive reinforcement and socially mediated negative reinforcement is that in the latter aversive stimulation is essentially "turned off" when SIB occurs. For example, a care provider might make a request to complete an academic or self self-care activity but then stop making requests when SIB occurs (e.g., "okay, we'll do that later"). As with positive reinforcement, such a reaction by a teacher, parent, or other care provider is not aimed to reinforce the behavior. Rather, the termination of instructions or demands is probably reinforced by the temporary cessation of SIB. The problem is that the SIB becomes more likely to occur in similar situations in the future.

Some SIB is not socially reinforced. In these cases, the stimulus products of the behavior can produce either automatic positive or automatic negative reinforcement. The term *automatic* means the reinforcement is not delivered by another person (Vaughan & Michael, 1982). Automatic positive reinforcement can occur if the behavior produces some kind of pleasing sensation. Automatic negative reinforcement can occur when the behavior terminates some aversive physical sensation, such as when self-scratching terminates an itching sensation or ear-hitting momentarily alleviates the pain produced by an ear infection.

In the next section we will describe how behavioral assessments are used to identify the operant function of behavior, or at least to generate hypotheses about the operant function of behavior.

Behavioral Assessment of SIB

Indirect Assessment

Indirect assessment refers to methods used to gather information about possible functions of behavior, without directly observing the behavior. During indirect assessments, informants are asked to provide descriptions of the behavior and information about common environmental events surrounding the target behavior. There are numerous indirect assessment formats available ranging from informal interviews to more structured interviews (e.g., O'Neill et al., 1997), questionnaires (e.g., Matson & Vollmer, 1995), and rating scales (e.g., Durand & Crimmins, 1988).

A majority of the structured formats attempt to identify possible sources of reinforcement for the target behavior including social positive reinforcement (e.g., the delivery of reprimands or comfort statements, access to preferred items), social negative reinforcement (e.g., escape from academic demands, escape from close proximity to others), and positive or negative automatic reinforcement (e.g., sensory stimulation, attenuation of painful physical or internal stimuli). Generally, informants are asked to rate the accuracy of statements describing relations between the response

and environmental events. For example, in the Functional
Analysis Screening Tool (FAST) (© The Florida
Center on Self-Injury, 2005), informants are asked to
provide a description of the topography, severity and
frequency of the behavior, times when the behavior is
most and least likely to occur, and "yes" or "no"
answers to a series of questions (e.g., "Does the problem behavior occur when the person is asked to perform a task or to participate in activities?"). Similarly,
in the Questions About Behavior Function (QABF)
assessment (Matson & Vollmer, 1995), informants are
asked to rate how often on a scale of 0–3 specific antecedent and consequent events occur. For example, the
informant would be asked to rate the statement, "He
engages in SIB to draw attention to himself" and higher
ratings for this statement may indicate that SIB is reinforced by access to attention.

Indirect assessments are an integral part of any
comprehensive behavioral assessment as they initiate a
dialog between the therapist and caregivers and provide a forum to collect preliminary information about
SIB. For example, indirect assessments can help determine objective descriptions of the target response
(operational definitions) as well as information about
the frequency and severity of the SIB. In addition,
these assessments provide information about common
antecedents (events that immediately precede) and
consequences (events that immediately follow as a
result of) behavior. Other benefits of indirect assessments are that they can be administered relatively
quickly (e.g., 15–20 min.), and they require little training to conduct. Furthermore, indirect assessments may
accommodate behavior that is not amenable to direct
assessment methods. This may include responses that
occur too infrequently to be reliably observed through
direct assessment methods, or responses that cannot be
allowed to occur due to the severity of behavior (e.g.,
head banging against sharp objects, eye gouging).
However, in most cases, it is recommended that indirect assessments should not be used as the sole means
to acquire information about SIB.

There are numerous documented limitations of
indirect assessments as a stand-alone assessment. First,
because they rely on verbal reports, which are often
delayed in time from the actual occurrence of behavior; information gathered through indirect assessments
may be unreliable. That is, informants may be unable
to accurately recall environmental events or may provide information irrelevant to the function of the

behavior. Structured interviews and checklists may
provide a means to direct the informant to relevant
environmental events. However, a second limitation of
these assessments is that the information gathered is
correlational. Therefore, it is possible that the informant accurately recalls surrounding environmental
events but that these events are not causally related to
behavior. For example, a teacher may accurately report
that she generally provides reprimands following
instances of head banging, yet reprimands are not
functionally related to the behavior (St. Peter et al.,
2005).

The reliability of several of the structured indirect
assessment methods has been evaluated by comparing
the outcomes across two or more informants or the
same informant over time. Research on the reliability
of indirect assessment methods has yielded mixed
results. Although some studies have reported high levels of interrater reliability (e.g., Durand & Crimmins,
1988), the majority has reported poor outcomes (e.g.,
Arndorfer, Miltenberger, Woster, Rortvedt, & Gaffaney,
1994; Sturmey, 1994; Zarcone et al. 1991), which calls
into question the utility of questionnaires and checklists as stand-alone assessments. However, some
researchers have argued that indirect assessments may
still be useful on an individual level and should be
evaluated on a case-by-case basis (Sturmey, 1994). In
addition, poor reliability between two observers may
be due to the fact that the behavior serves different
functions in the presence of different people or environments. Furthermore, if the two assessments are
temporally distant, poor reliability scores may be
caused by a change in behavioral function over time
(e.g., Lerman, Iwata, Smith, Zarcone, & Vollmer,
1994). Thus, the reliability of indirect assessments
may be improved by administering them in a small
time window to individuals in the same environment
who have similar exposure to the SIB.

Several studies have evaluated the validity of indirect assessments by comparing the outcomes to other
assessment methods such as descriptive and functional
analyses. Such validity studies have also yielded mixed
results. Several studies have used correlations between
the outcomes of indirect and direct assessment methods as indicators of validity (e.g., Arndorfer et al.,
1994; Durand & Crimmins, 1988). For example,
Arndorfer et al. compared the results from structured
interviews to functional analyses (Iwata, Dorsey, et al.,
1994) and found correspondence between the two

methods. Similarly, Durand and Crimmins found that the outcomes from the Motivation Assessment Scale (MAS) matched the outcomes from functional analyses (Carr & Durand, 1985) for all eight participants in the study. In contrast, several studies have reported poor validity, or a lack of correspondence between the outcomes of indirect and direct assessment methods (e.g., Crawford, Brockel, Schauss, & Miltenberger 1992, Paclawskyj et al., 2001). Considering these varied outcomes, future research may help to determine factors that can improve correspondence between various assessment formats and ultimately improve the validity of indirect assessments.

In summary, indirect assessments may provide a starting point to inform subsequent assessment components (e.g., descriptive and functional analyses) and may also provide an alternative when direct assessments cannot be conducted. However, due to the correlational nature of the information and problems inherent in verbal reports, outcomes of indirect assessments should be viewed with caution and supplemented with direct assessment measures when possible.

Descriptive Analysis

Descriptive analysis refers to the direct observation of behavior during natural contexts (Bijou, Peterson, & Ault, 1968). During descriptive analyses, data are collected on the frequency or duration of the target behavior and typically, surrounding antecedent and consequent events. However, no systematic manipulation of variables is made. Data gathered during descriptive analyses may provide necessary information for general assessment or treatment evaluation purposes such as operational definitions of behavior, baseline levels of responding, and correlated environmental events. Three of the most common descriptive analysis methods are the scatterplot, A-B-C assessment, and direct observation by a professional. The first two methods are commonly conducted by careproviders throughout the day using a paper and pencil method. The third method, direct observation, is commonly conducted by therapists or trained professionals during smaller time windows throughout the day using computerized or paper and pencil recording methods.

The scatterplot was first described as a method for behavioral assessment of SIB by Touchette,

MacDonald, and Langer (1985) and is comprised of a chart that is divided into intervals of time (e.g., 15 or 30 min) across successive days. One column of a scatterplot sheet typically represents 1 day of recording, whereas an entire scatterplot sheet generally represents several weeks of recording. Using the scatterplot, data are collected and recorded for the frequency of SIB during a set interval (i.e., box on the chart). If no instances of behavior are recorded, the box is left blank. If instances of behavior are recorded, the boxes are filled differentially depending on the frequency of the response (e.g., a hatch mark for one instance of behavior and a filled box for 2 or more instances of behavior). Scatterplots are easy to implement and require relatively little training to use. In addition, scatterplot analyses sometimes provide information about estimates of rates of behavior and temporal patterns of behavior over time. These patterns may be associated with specific environmental events that can be altered to decrease the occurrence of the behavior. For example, Touchette et al. charted scatterplots for three participants and found clear patterns for two participants (i.e., higher frequency of problem behavior during specific times of the day). In addition, Touchette et al. were able to use the information from the scatterplot to identify which environmental events were correlated with the time of day and, consequently, established effective treatments for the two participants.

Despite the fact that scatterplots are a widely used assessment and data collection tool in classrooms, residential facilities and inpatient settings, very little research has been conducted to validate use of the method. One exception is a study conducted by Kahng et al. (1998) in which scatterplot analyses were implemented for 15 participants. Results showed no clear temporal patterns of responding for any of the participants. Thus, scatterplots may fail to identify useful patterns or correlated environmental events for some individuals. There are several possible reasons for the lack of consistency between the Touchette et al. and Kahng et al. results. First, in Kahng et al., the interval length (30 min) may have been too large to capture differences in frequency in high rate problem behavior across the day. Second, the data recording techniques used in scatterplot analyses may be insensitive to changes in frequency of behavior. For example, in both studies, two or more instances of SIB were denoted by filling in the interval box. It is possible that a given individual engaged in SIB twice per interval during most of the day, and higher rates (e.g., ten times per interval) during other intervals. Yet, because the frequencies were denoted similarly, there would be no differentiation of responding on the scatterplot. Thus, when using scatterplots, it is important to construct individualized data collection procedures to better suit the frequency of problem behavior and the individual's schedule. A third possible reason for the disparity of results between Touchette et al. and Kahng et al. is that, in Kahng et al., some individual's daily schedules may have varied too greatly from day to day to observe clear temporal patterns. Therefore, scatterplots may be more effectively used for individuals who have consistent and structured schedules. However, more research is necessary to identify the extent of the utility of scatterplots in behavioral assessment.

During ABC assessments, careproviders (e.g., parents, teachers, etc.) use a data sheet to record each instance of SIB in one column and descriptions of events that immediately precede (antecedents) and follow (consequences) behavior in the surrounding columns. For example, "Antecedent: I asked Jenny to brush her hair; Behavior: SIB; Consequence: I put the brush away and held Jenny." Like scatterplot analyses, ABC assessments require very little training and are easy to implement. In addition, if completed consistently, ABC assessments provide actual baseline rates of SIB as well as information about possible reinforcers maintaining self-injury.

However, there are some potential disadvantages to ABC recording. First, if an open-ended narrative is used, caregivers are likely to record subjective and technically imprecise rather than objective environmental events. For example, "Antecedent: Jenny got frustrated; Behavior: SIB; Consequence: I tried to calm her down." In this example, getting frustrated is a presumed emotional state, and there is no reference to observable environmental events. Presumably some environmental event caused the "frustration," so it is ultimately not an objective causal variable associated with SIB. To address this shortcoming, some ABC data sheets provide a list of several different objectified antecedent and consequent events. A second disadvantage of ABC assessments is that environmental events are only recorded when SIB occurs. Therefore, it is impossible to evaluate the likelihood of certain environmental events are when SIB does not occur. For example, attention might occur with a high probability whether or not SIB occurs; and an ABC sheet might give the false impression that SIB produces the attention.

Direct observation by a professional involves real-time data collection of behavior and environmental events. Technological developments in recent years have greatly improved the scope of these assessments. During direct observation, therapists typically use hand held computer programs that allow for observation of numerous environmental events (e.g., delivery and removal of academic demands, delivery and removal of access to preferred tangible items) and target responses to be recorded simultaneously. The outcome is a stream of behavior and environmental events that can be analyzed to examine possible reinforcement contingencies or at least correlations between behavior and environmental events.

As one example of the direct observation approach, Lerman and Iwata (1993) conducted descriptive and functional analyses for six participants who engaged in SIB. They calculated conditional probabilities (i.e., the probability of an event given the occurrence of behavior) for a variety of antecedent and consequent events in order to identify possible reinforcement contingencies. For example, if both the conditional probability of instructional demands preceding SIB and the conditional probability of escape following SIB were high, the hypothesis would be that SIB was reinforced by escape from instructional demands. Vollmer, Borrero, Wright, Van Camp, and Lalli (2001) calculated an additional probability, the background probability of an event, and compared this to the conditional probability of the event given behavior. They conducted descriptive analyses for 11 participants and used the above aforementioned probabilities to determine possible positive (i.e., the background probability of an event is lower than the conditional probability of an event), neutral (i.e., the background and conditional probabilities are roughly equal), and negative (i.e., the background probability is higher than the conditional probability of an event). The notion was that possible positive contingencies are at least a sufficient condition for a reinforcement effect.

The major limitation of all descriptive analysis methods is that because environmental variables are not manipulated, information gathered through these assessments is correlational. Correlated events are not necessarily functionally related to behavior. St. Peter et al. (2005) conducted functional analyses for four participants and found that attention was not a reinforcer for problem behavior for any of the participants. However, St. Peter et al. then used descriptive analyses to examine relations between attention and problem behavior and found that the delivery of attention was highly correlated with problem behavior for all participants. Furthermore, several studies have compared the results from descriptive and functional analyses and found that often they do not correspond (e.g., Lerman & Iwata, 1993, Mace & Lalli, 1991). Thus, descriptive analyses are generally determined to be inappropriate as a sole means of identifying functional relations for problem behavior.

Despite limitations, descriptive analyses may provide useful information to inform functional analyses and treatments. For example, direct observation can improve operational definitions of behavior. In addition, direct observation provides information on the naturally occurring rates of behavior (i.e., a baseline), which can later be used to assess treatment effects. Both direct observation and ABC assessments may help to identify idiosyncratic events related to behavior (e.g., Borrero, Vollmer, & Borrero, 2004). Furthermore, direct observation may provide useful information when functional analyses cannot be conducted safely. Recently, descriptive analyses have been used to identify precursors to more severe forms of behavior (Borrero & Borrero, 2008). Precursor analyses may be particularly useful when the target problem behavior is determined to be too dangerous for a functional analysis, such as may be the case with the most severe forms of SIB (e.g., if a single response should not be allowed to occur).

Functional Analyses

A functional analysis generally refers to the manipulation of variables to determine cause and effect relationships. However, in the realm of applied behavior analysis, functional analysis now usually refers to a specific assessment procedure used to identify reinforcers maintaining problem behavior. During a functional analysis, potential reinforcing events are delivered after the occurrence of problem behavior to identify functional relations. Although the intentional delivery of potentially reinforcing events may seem counterintuitive, this approach is analogous to allergy testing during which patients are exposed to various allergens to determine an effective course of treatment. During functional analyses, participants are exposed to analogs of situations they commonly experience in everyday life in order to determine an effective course of treatment. Functional analysis offers advantages over indirect and descriptive methods because the information gathered is not correlational. Thus, functional analyses may prevent the implementation of ineffective treatments or treatments that are contraindicated (e.g., Iwata, Pace, Cowdery, & Miltenberger, 1994).

When conducting functional analyses of SIB, several considerations and safety precautions should be taken. First, it should be determined if the response is amenable to a functional analyses. For example, functional analyses should not be conducted if the SIB would cause immediate danger to the participant, such as the case of pica (ingestion of inedible objects) with sharp objects. In marginal cases, medical personnel should always be available for consultation related to session-termination criteria or suitability of a functional analysis in general from a medical perspective. Also, because clear functional analysis outcomes rely on at least moderate rates of behavior to assess relations between behavior and environmental events, functional analyses may be less useful for extremely low rate SIB. In these cases, other assessment formats or variations on the standard functional analysis procedure should be used.

The most commonly used functional analysis procedure was first described by Iwata, Dorsey, et al. (1994). Functional analyses were conducted for nine individuals who engaged in SIB. Clear functional analysis results were obtained for six of the nine participants. The general procedures involved alternating the presentation of three test conditions and one control condition repeatedly in a multielement experimental design until clear outcomes were obtained. The purpose of the control condition was to create a situation in which SIB was unlikely to occur. That is, the participant was given free access to preferred items, the therapist provided attention intermittently, and no demands were placed on the participant. Differentially higher rates in the test conditions relative to the control condition were used to indicate a reinforcement effect. The test conditions in Iwata et al. included social attention, demand, and alone. In many current applications, another condition typically called "tangible" is included when necessary. Next, general protocols for the common test conditions derived from Iwata et al. are described.

During the attention condition, the participant is given access to preferred items, while the therapist pretends to do work away from the participant. Contingent upon each instance of SIB, the therapist provides brief access to attention to the participant and then returns to his or her work. Differentially higher rates of SIB in the attention condition compared to the control condition indicate the behavior is reinforced by access to attention. Typically, the type of attention used in this condition is matched to the form of attention observed in the participant's natural environment. More specifically, if the participant's caregivers usually provide reprimands or comfort statements after the self-injury, those forms of attention would be used during the functional analysis. Other variations of the attention condition, sometimes called the divided or diverted attention condition, have been conducted in which the therapist's attention is directed toward another individual until an instance of SIB occurs.

A second type of social positive reinforcement condition, known as the tangible condition, has sometimes been included in functional analyses. Although some studies have shown that the delivery of tangible items does not commonly follow problem behavior (e.g., Thompson & Iwata, 2001), several studies have shown that at least a small percentage of SIB is maintained by access to preferred tangible items or activities (e.g., Iwata, Pace, Dorsey, et al., 1994). However, this condition is typically only included if other assessments (i.e., indirect assessments and/or descriptive analyses) show evidence of delivery of tangible items following problem behavior in the individual's natural environment. During this condition, the therapist interacts with the participant but restricts access to preferred items. Contingent upon each instance of SIB, the therapist provides brief access to the preferred items. Differentially higher rates of SIB in this condition relative to the control condition indicate that SIB is reinforced by access to preferred tangible items. A related test condition described in recent studies suggests that problem behavior may be occasioned by interruption of ongoing "free-operant" behavior and reinforced by access to the interrupted activity (e.g., Fisher, Adelinis, Thompson, Worsdell & Zarcone, 1998; Hagopian, Bruzek, Bowman, & Jennett, 2007). For example, instructing a child with autism to not engage in stereotypy, which is sometimes a preferred activity, may evoke SIB. To test such a possibility, the participant is allowed to engage in the preferred activity. The thera-

pist then interrupts the activity by providing statements such as "Don't do that!" Contingent upon each instance of SIB, the participant is allowed to resume the activity. Differentially higher rates of SIB in this condition relative to the control condition indicate that SIB is reinforced by access to the preferred activity.

The purpose of the escape condition is to test if behavior is maintained by socially mediated negative reinforcement in the form of escape from (usually) instructional demands. During this condition, access to preferred items is restricted and the therapist presents demands on a time-based schedule using a three-prompt instructional sequence. The therapist provides brief praise for compliance with the demands before resuming the instructional sequence. Contingent upon each instance of SIB, the therapist removes the instructional materials and provides a brief break from demands. Differentially higher rates of SIB in this condition relative to the control condition indicate that SIB is reinforced by escape from demands. Typically, the types of demands that are selected are matched to the demands usually experienced by the participant in his or her natural environment. A wide range of demands has been used including academic and vocational tasks, personal hygiene routines, household chores, and medical routines. In addition, a variation of this condition, known as the social escape condition, has been developed to evaluate whether problem behavior is reinforced by escape from close proximity to other individuals or social situations (e.g., Borrero et al., 2004).

The purpose of the alone or no consequence condition is to test if behavior is sensitive to nonsocially mediated or automatic reinforcement. More specifically, this condition is used to evaluate whether SIB persists in the absence of social consequences. During the alone condition, the participant is left alone in the room and observed through a one-way mirror. During the no consequence variation, the individual remains in the room with the therapist who provides no programmed consequences for SIB. Differentially higher rates of SIB in the alone or no consequence condition relative to the control condition indicate that SIB is automatically reinforced. Also, high rates across all of the test and control conditions may in some cases indicate that SIB is automatically reinforced because the automatic reinforcement is available during any condition.

The most commonly cited limitations of functional analyses are that they (a) require a specialized setting,

(b) are time consuming, and (c) are complicated to conduct. To ensure proper control of the relevant environmental variables, it is true that most functional analyses are conducted in highly controlled settings. However, functional analyses have also been conducted in a variety of settings including schools, residential, and inpatient facilities. They have been conducted in a traditional manner (i.e., in a separate isolated area) or as a part of the individual's ongoing daily activities (e.g., Sigafoos & Saggers, 1995). To accommodate time constraints, brief functional analyses have been developed (e.g., Cooper, Wacker, Sasso, Reimers & Donn, 1990; Cooper et al., 1992; Derby et al., 1992; Harding, Wacker, Cooper, Millard, & Jensen-Kovalan, 1994; Northup et al., 1991). Brief functional analyses generally involve one to two brief presentations of each test condition. In a large-scale analysis, Derby et al. 1992 found that these abbreviated assessments have produced clear outcomes for roughly half of the participants. Further, the evaluation of within-session response patterns can result in abbreviated sessions (Vollmer, Marcus, and Ringdahl, 1995). Finally, although conducting functional analyses does require some training, several studies have shown that teachers, staff members, and undergraduate psychology majors can be trained in a limited amount of time to conduct functional analyses, sometimes even just by reading instructions relating to session protocols (e.g., Moore & Fisher, 2007, Wallace, Doney, Mintz-Resudek, & Tarbox, 2004).

A more serious potential limitation of functional analyses is that they may be inappropriate for some forms of behavior. For example, functional analyses may be inappropriate for behavior that causes an immediate danger to the participant, or behavior that occurs too infrequently to reliably observe. Variations on the standard functional analysis method have been proposed to address these limitations. For severe and dangerous forms of behavior, some researchers have suggested assessing less severe forms of precursor behavior that reliably precedes SIB. For example, Smith and Churchill (2002) identified precursors for four individuals who engaged in SIB. They conducted functional analyses of both the precursor behavior and SIB and showed that the functions of the precursor behavior corresponded with the function of SIB. Other variations of functional analyses have been used to address the problem of low rate behavior by increasing the duration of the test conditions from 10–15 min to 45–60 min (Kahng, Abt, & Schonbachler, 2001).

A final potential limitation of functional analysis is that the results are sometimes difficult to interpret (Martin, Gaffan, & Williams, 1999; Vollmer, Iwata, Duncan, & Lerman, 1993). At times, difficulty in interpretation of results may be due to undifferentiated response patterns. That is, if SIB occurs at similar rates across all functional analysis conditions, it is not clear if the behavior is automatically reinforced, controlled by multiple sources of reinforcement, influenced by carryover effects from one condition to another, controlled by extraneous (uncontrolled) variables, or some combination. To evaluate whether undifferentiated results indicate automatically reinforced behavior, some researchers have suggested conducting numerous consecutive alone or no consequence conditions to see if SIB persists (e.g., Ellingson et al., 2000). The logic is that if behavior is socially reinforced it should extinguish during alone or no consequence because it does not contact the social reinforcement. To evaluate whether behavior is multiply controlled, previous research has systematically evaluated treatments across each function (e.g., Borrero & Vollmer, 2006, Smith, Iwata, Vollmer, & Zarcone, 1993). In addition, if the participant has difficulty discriminating the conditions, it is recommended to use distinct stimuli with each condition (e.g., different therapists, different colored shirts, etc.). Descriptive analyses can be used to identify potentially idiosyncratic variables that are correlated with behavior and can then be incorporated into the functional analysis.

In summary, functional analysis is considered to be a standard in the behavioral assessment of SIB. Furthermore, previous research has shown that typical functional analysis procedures may be adapted to accommodate time constraints and other previously cited limitations. Functional analysis research or individualized functional analyses provide a direct link between assessment and treatment development.

Behavioral Treatment

Treatments designed to reduce SIB typically involve withholding reinforcers following behavior (extinction), delivering reinforcers following the omission of behavior (differential reinforcement of other behavior), delivering reinforcers following appropriate behavior (differential reinforcement of alternative behavior), delivering reinforcers independent of behavior (noncontingent reinforcement), or some combination of these approaches. In addition to those procedures, other treatments for SIB include general skill building via reinforcement and prompting procedures, and punishment. A brief description of each approach and its potential advantages and disadvantages is described below as follows.

Extinction

Procedurally, extinction involves withholding reinforcers that were previously delivered following behavior (Catania, 1998). Extinction results in a gradual decrease in the likelihood of behavior (Skinner, 1938). In addition to the gradual decrease in behavior (main effect of extinction), the procedure is also commonly associated with a number of side effects sometimes collectively referred to as an extinction burst (Lerman & Iwata, 1996). These side effects may include temporary increases in rate, intensity, aggression, and the number of topographical variations of problematic behavior (including both novel and previously reinforced forms). Other patterns associated with extinction include spontaneous recovery (temporary increases in behavior as a result of re-introducing the individual to the extinction context after a time away from the extinction context) and disinhibition (a temporary increase in previously extinguished behavior as a result of the introduction of novel stimuli). An example of spontaneous recovery is SIB that was extinguished during the school week returning on a Monday following the weekend. An example of disinhibition is an increased rate of SIB associated with the introduction of new teachers or therapists, new routines, or general schedule disruptions. Although commonly reported in basic research, to date no SIB treatment studies have reported disinhibition (Lerman & Iwata, 1996).

Extinction may be considered a treatment on its own, but is usually a component within a larger treatment package. The specific form of the extinction procedure may appear different depending on the source of reinforcement being withheld (Iwata, Pace, Cowdery et al., 1994). For example, extinction of behavior maintained by social positive reinforcement in the form of attention would likely involve minimizing attention

toward the individual following instances of SIB (e.g., Lovaas & Simmons, 1969). Conversely, extinction of SIB maintained by social negative reinforcement in the form of escape from demands would involve continued presentation of demands following problem behavior (e.g., Iwata, Pace, Kalsher, Cowdery, & Cataldo, 1990). In either case, extinction necessitates that the reinforcers no longer follow behavior.

When reinforcement for SIB is socially mediated, it is usually possible for the care-provider to at least minimize reinforcement. However, when SIB is automatically reinforced it is more difficult to withhold reinforcement because it is not directly controlled by a care-provider. Nonetheless, the procedure known as "sensory extinction" provides a model for extinction of automatically reinforced behavior (Rincover, 1978). For example, Iwata, Pace, Cowdery & Mittenberger (1994) implemented extinction of one individual's head-banging by placing a helmet on the individual's head. Rates of SIB decreased markedly when the helmet was worn. Presumably, the helmet served to attenuate the sensation caused by head-banging because the individual was still able to engage in the response (and did, initially) while only the products of the response changed. Therefore, the response decreased when its reinforcing consequences were no longer available. Similar effects have been reported with gloves (for hand biting) and other protective equipment.

Extinction has an advantage of being a conceptually simple method for producing response suppression. It is straightforward logic to withhold the reinforcer for SIB. Another advantage of using extinction is that the reinforcer for SIB is no longer present in the situation to occasion behavior as a discriminative stimulus (Thompson, Iwata, Hanley, Dozier, & Samaha, 2003). In some treatment procedures involving reinforcement, there mere presentation of the previously reinforcing stimulus sets the occasion for SIB.

Apart from the possibility of negative side effects (discussed previously), one disadvantage of extinction is that its effectiveness may be reduced depending on the schedule of reinforcement that was previously in place for SIB. For example, if SIB were previously reinforced on an intermittent schedule then extinction can in some circumstances take longer to have an effect (Lerman, Iwata, Shore, & Kahng, 1996). Another disadvantage of extinction is that reinforcers accidentally delivered during treatment may increase behavior either because they serve as discriminative stimuli

(Thompson et al., 2003) or as intermittent reinforcement when presented following behavior. In addition, extinction should not be recommended in isolation if the reinforcers strengthening behavior cannot be adequately withheld in the face of increased rate, intensity, and variability of the response (i.e., the extinction burst). Intermittent reinforcement during (attempted) extinction may also serve to reinforce new and more intense topographies of SIB that occur during an extinction burst. In addition, extinction itself provides no specific means to increase appropriate behavior. However, the risks and effects associated with the extinction burst may be reduced if extinction is used as one feature of a multi-component intervention.

As a final note on extinction, it is worth mentioning that the commonly discussed side effects (e.g., extinction bursts) may not be as common as once believed. Researchers have examined the prevalence of extinction bursts observed during therapeutic evaluations of extinction. Lerman and Iwata (1995) examined 113 sets of data involving extinction. The results showed that 24% of the cases were associated with an increase in responding during any of the first three sessions of extinction relative to the previous baseline. In a subsequent study, Lerman, Iwata, and Wallace (1999) examined of 41 sets of data and found that 39% showed increases in responding during the first three sessions of extinction. However, side-effects of extinction were only observed in 20% of cases when extinction was combined with other procedures.

Differential Reinforcement of Other Behavior

Differential reinforcement of other behavior (DRO) is the delivery of reinforcement following periods of time in which the target behavior (in this case, SIB) has not occurred (Miltenberger, 2008). There are numerous variations of the DRO procedure. With a resetting DRO, occurrences of SIB have the effect of resetting the current interval such that the amount of time between the previous response and the delivery of the reinforcer is always fixed (Vollmer & Iwata, 1992). With nonresetting DRO, individuals either earn or lose the next upcoming reinforcer depending on whether or not SIB has occurred during the current interval (Repp, Deitz, & Deitz, 1976). Two sub-variations of

nonresetting DRO can be considered: In whole interval DRO, reinforcers are delivered contingent on the absence of behavior throughout the entire interval; in momentary DRO (Repp, Barton, & Brulle, 1983) the delivery of reinforcers is made contingent on the absence of behavior at the moment of observation (usually at the end of the interval).

Treatments involving DRO to reduce behavior reinforced by social positive reinforcement (e.g., attention) involve the delivery of attention only following periods of time in which the problem behavior does not occur (e.g., Vollmer & Iwata, 1992). Likewise, treatments to reduce behavior reinforced by social negative reinforcement (e.g., escape from academic demands) involve the temporary removal of academic materials following intervals in which the target response does not occur (Kodak, Miltenberger, & Romaniuk, 2003; Roberts, Mace, & Daggett, 1995). For treatments to reduce behavior reinforced by automatic reinforcement, potent alternative reinforcers (e.g., preferred items identified using a preference assessment) need to be used because the functional reinforcer cannot be adequately manipulated by the therapist to ensure (a) that the individual obtains the reinforcer following every eligible interval and (b) that the individual does not obtain the reinforcer following ineligible intervals (although, in a noteworthy exception Goh et al., 1995 identified the reinforcer for automatically reinforced hand-mouthing and delivered that reinforcer noncontingently to decrease the behavior).

One potential advantage of DRO is that, when combined with extinction, it may attenuate some of the potential side effects of extinction. That is, unlike with pure extinction, the individual still has some access to the reinforcer. However, DRO has been associated with aggression (Lennox, Miltenberger, & Donnelly, 1987) and emotional behavior (Cowdery, Iwata, & Pace, 1990). DRO has other noteworthy disadvantages. One, the procedure may result in low rates of reinforcement if rates of the target response remain high. In such cases DRO is functionally equivalent to extinction and in turn may produce side-effects similar to the extinction burst. Two, DRO does not explicitly promote appropriate alternative behavior. Although appropriate behavior may indeed occur during intervals in which SIB does not occur, the procedure neither ensures that appropriate behavior occurs nor that other inappropriate behavior does not occur during reinforced intervals. Three, whole interval DRO may be difficult to administer because it requires constant observation by the therapist. Constant observation may be unrealistic in situations where therapists may need to attend to other children (e.g., classrooms) or other duties. Four, when arbitrary reinforcers are used (as is often the case with behavior maintained by automatic reinforcement), DRO is relatively ineffective because the success of the intervention depends on the ability of the arbitrary reinforcers to compete with the reinforcers maintaining problem behavior (Carr & Durand, 1985; Cowdery et al., 1990). Five, DRO is highly sensitive to treatment integrity failures. For example, even if the care-provider correctly withholds the reinforcer with 95% integrity, that means SIB would be reinforced following 1 out of every 20 occurrences which is equivalent to a variable ratio (VR) schedule of reinforcement. Variable-ratio schedules are known to produce high rates of behavior (Ferster & Skinner, 1957).

Differential Reinforcement of Alternative Behavior

Differential reinforcement of alternative behavior (DRA) is a treatment to reduce problem behavior by strengthening a specific desired response (or responses) to compete with the target response, in this case SIB (Miltenberger, 2008). In DRA, reinforcers are presented following occurrences of the appropriate alternative behavior and reinforcers are typically withheld following occurrences of SIB (like DRO, DRA is often used in combination with extinction). One variation of DRA is sometimes called *functional communication training* (FCT) when the alternative behavior takes the form of a conventional communication response and can be used to obtain the same reinforcer previously maintaining problem behavior (Carr & Durand, 1985; Durand & Carr, 1991). The form of the appropriate behavior may be determined by considering the abilities of the student (in terms of their existing communicative repertoire) and the readiness of the community to respond appropriately to the communicative response.

As a treatment to reduce problem behavior reinforced by social positive reinforcement (in the form of attention), FCT would consist of providing brief attention following each appropriate request. Likewise, to reduce problem behavior reinforced by social negative reinforcement (in the form of escape from task

demands), FCT would consist of providing a momentary reprieve from the work materials. For example, if the individual were to sign "break" during an instructional sequence, the therapist might quickly remove the task materials and turn away from the individual for 30 s. Marcus and Vollmer (1995) investigated the use of DRA to reduce a girl's disruptive behavior reinforced by social negative reinforcement in the form of escape from demands. In one condition, breaks were provided following appropriate requests. In another condition, breaks were provided following compliance with the academic demands. Both conditions produced decreases in disruptions; however, compliance remained low in the condition in which requests were reinforced by a break and compliance increased in the condition in which breaks were provided following compliance. Thus, it is important to consider DRA procedures that do not necessarily reinforce communication per se, but that target some other specific replacement behavior.

Differential reinforcement of alternative behavior offers certain advantages when extinction cannot be implemented. That is, parameters of reinforcement such as quality, amount, delay, and ratio-requirement for both problem and appropriate behavior can be manipulated to favor appropriate behavior (Hoch, McComas, Johnson, Faranda, & Guenther, 2002; Horner & Day, 1991; Neef & Lutz, 2001; Vollmer, Roane, Ringdahl, & Marcus, 1999; Worsdell, Iwata, Hanley, Thompson, & Kahng, 2000). Baum (1974) described the matching law, a quantitative description of behavior that can account for variations in reinforcement parameters. The matching law predicts that, in situations in which two responses are available (e.g., problem and appropriate behavior), more behavior will be allocated toward the response associated with higher frequencies, higher quality, higher quantity, and lower delays. When applied to problem behavior, if a parent must provide attention following problem behavior (e.g., SIB that would produce immediate tissue damage), the parent could provide brief, lower quality attention following SIB (e.g., minimal physical guidance or blocking) as compared to following appropriate requests. For less serious problem behavior, delays and ratio-requirements could also be manipulated. For example, a parent might only provide attention following a brief delay after every other instance of problem behavior as compared to providing attention immediately after every instance of appropriate behavior.

In addition to the advantages described above, DRA specifically arranges for the strengthening of appropriate behavior while reducing competing inappropriate behavior. Furthermore, DRA may be somewhat easier to implement relative to DRO because therapists need only react to the individual's behavior and not also a timer. Effects of DRA in the form of FCT may also be more likely than effects of other procedures to persist outside of the treatment environment if the communicative response is likely to produce the maintaining reinforcer in other environments (such as with the use of conventional speech). One disadvantage of DRA, at least in the form of FCT, is that, for some individuals, a punishment component may be necessary in order for severe problem behavior to be suppressed (Fisher et al., 1993; Hagopian, Fisher, Sullivan, Acquisto, & LeBlanc, 1998).

Noncontingent Reinforcement

Noncontingent reinforcement (NCR) is the time-based presentation of reinforcers independent of behavior (Rescorla & Skucy, 1969). The procedure has effects similar to DRO in that it decreases the target response by reducing the establishing operation controlling behavior (e.g., if lots of attention is already available, there is less need to engage in SIB to get attention). Noncontingent reinforcement also weakens the contingency between the target response and reinforcer delivery, and (if extinction is used in combination) ensures that there is no programmed relation between the problem behavior and reinforcer delivery (Thompson & Iwata, 2005).

In the treatment of severe SIB reinforced by social positive reinforcement in the form of attention, NCR involves the delivery of attention at times independent of behavior (e.g., a brief statement or conversation every 30 s). Vollmer, Iwata, Zarcone, Smith, and Mazaleski (1993a) investigated the use of noncontingent attention to treat SIB reinforced by access to attention. Functional analyses were conducted and showed that each participant's self-injury was reinforced by access to attention. Next, the effects of NCR and DRO were compared using reversal and multielement designs. In both treatment conditions, attention was provided either according to a clock (NCR) or at the end of every interval in which problem behavior

was not observed (DRO). The results showed that both NCR and DRO were effective at reducing self-injury (although, for one participant, DRO produced more immediate and consistent reductions).

In the treatment of SIB maintained by social negative reinforcement in the form of escape from academic demands, NCR involves the brief escape from tasks at set intervals (e.g., a 30 s break every 2 min). Vollmer et al. (1995) evaluated a treatment to reduce problem behavior reinforced by social negative reinforcement. Results from a functional analysis showed that the SIB of two individuals was reinforced by social negative reinforcement. Treatment consisted of brief escape from learning activities independent of the individual's behavior. The results showed that noncontingent escape was effective at reducing problem behavior and that the schedule of escape could be thinned to manageable time intervals (2.5 min for a preschooler and 10 min for an adolescent).

Noncontingent reinforcement has also been shown to reduce socially reinforced SIB even when arbitrary reinforcers were used ("arbitrary" only in the sense that they were not functionally related to the SIB). Fischer, Iwata, and Mazaleski (1997) conducted functional analyses of two individuals' SIB. Results showed that one individual's SIB was reinforced by access to attention and the other's SIB was reinforced by access to preferred materials. Next, preference assessments were conducted to identify additional items that were likely to serve as potent reinforcers. These reinforcers were then delivered noncontingently, which produced decreases in self-injury for both participants.

Procedures known as "environmental enrichment" (Horner, 1980) are related to NCR and have been shown to decrease problem behavior reinforced by social negative reinforcement (e.g., escape from demands) and automatic reinforcement. In the case of behavior reinforced by escape from demands, the inclusion of highly preferred reinforcers in an environment may reduce the motivation to escape the situation. In reducing automatically reinforced behavior, Roscoe, Iwata, and Goh (1998) evaluated NCR to treat automatically reinforced SIB. First, a functional analysis demonstrated that the individuals' self-injury was maintained by automatic reinforcement. Second, preference assessments were conducted to identify highly preferred materials. During treatment, individuals had free access to the preferred materials throughout the session. The results showed decreased SIB for all participants.

Noncontingent reinforcement procedures have several important advantages. First, the rate of reinforcement is controlled by the therapist and does not adjust with changes in the target response. Second, NCR is relatively easy to implement because reinforcers are delivered according to a clock. Therapists do not need to constantly attend to the individual in order to implement the procedure correctly. Third, NCR is effective across a range of functions and topographies.

Noncontingent reinforcement is associated with two main disadvantages: (a) NCR does not specifically promote adaptive behavior and (b) NCR has been shown on rare occasion to strengthen behavior as a result of accidental pairings between behavior and reinforcer delivery. However, the first problem can be addressed insofar as NCR can be combined with DRA to reinforce adaptive behavior (Marcus & Vollmer, 1996, Goh, Iwata, & DeLeon, 2000). The second problem can be addressed by including a momentary DRO component to ensure that the SIB and reinforcer are not coupled on a consistent basis (Lindberg, Iwata, Kahng, & DeLeon, 1999).

Skill Acquisition of Replacement Behavior

Another approach is to "treat" SIB is by building a host of replacement skills via reinforcement procedures including shaping, chaining, and modeling. The notion is that the more extensive the adaptive repertoire, the less time an individual has to engage in SIB. This approach is contrasted with DRA insofar as no specific skill or set of skills is targeted as a direct functional replacement for SIB. Rather, the approach is based on the premise that the ability to communicate generally, engage in appropriate leisure activity, engage ins work or academic ability in some way supplants the likelihood of engaging in SIB. The approach is consistent with basic research on the matching law, which suggests that individuals should allocate their behavior toward reinforcers that are more frequent and easier to obtain. One form of the matching law, single-alternative matching (de Villiers, 1977), describes the relation between engaging in one response, the reinforcers available for that response, engaging in all other responses, and all other available reinforcers. For individuals who engage in SIB, response allocation may be considered a "choice" between engaging in SIB and engaging in anything else (the term choice is used here in a technical sense and is not intended to imply that the individual wants to engage in SIB). From the perspective of the matching law, a person may be less likely to engage in SIB if reinforcers for other behavior are more readily available. It follows then that SIB (or other forms of severe problem behavior) may be suppressed by teaching individuals new ways of obtaining reinforcement. That is, by increasing the reinforcers available for "doing anything else," the relative payoff for engaging in SIB will be reduced.

Punishment

Punishment is the suppression of behavior as a result of the presentation or removal of stimuli following behavior (Miltenberger, 2008). The presentation of stimuli following behavior that produces a decrease in behavior is positive punishment and has taken numerous forms including aversive odors (e.g., Altman, Haavik, & Cook, 1978), visual screening (e.g., Jordan, Singh, & Repp, 1989), aversive taste (e.g., Friman & Hove, 1987), and even contingent shock. For example, Linscheid, Iwata, Ricketts, Williams, and Griffin (1990) evaluated a device that delivered contingent shock following severe SIB with individuals for whom previous treatments were unsuccessful. Contingent-shock produced nearly immediate suppression of behavior in every case. Despite its effectiveness, such applications remain controversial.

Negative punishment involves the removal of stimuli following behavior that produces a decrease in behavior. Examples of negative punishment include timeout and response cost. Timeout is the removal of the opportunity to earn reinforcers following behavior. Response cost is the removal of previously earned or already held reinforcers (Weiner, 1962). Burchard and Barrera (1972) evaluated the use of response cost and time out to reduce the inappropriate behavior (e.g., swearing, property destruction, negative interactions) of six adolescents with mild developmental disabilities. Response cost consisted of removing previously earned token reinforcers and time out consisted of sitting on a bench in a designated area. Both procedures produced decreases in inappropriate behavior.

One advantage of punishment as a treatment for problem behavior is that it can be implemented without reference to the operant function of behavior (Azrin & Holz, 1966) or when the operant function cannot be identified (Linscheid et al., 1990). Similarly, punishment can be used to reduce automatically reinforced behavior because a therapist can deliver punishment without control over the reinforcers strengthening behavior. A principal disadvantage of punishment procedures is that they may be misused. For example, a therapist's own use of punishment to reduce severe SIB may generalize to less severe behavior like talking-out-of-turn or incorrect academic behavior. Another disadvantage is that certain punishment procedures (especially those that involve painful or noxious stimuli) may evoke or elicit behavior counter-productive to treatment. For example, some punishment procedures have been shown to produce aggression (Azrin, Hutchinson, & Hake, 1966) and emotional behavior (Lerman & Vorndran, 2002). In addition, use of punishment may produce other effects like avoidance of the individuals and context associated with punishment (Azrin, Hake, Holz, & Hutchinson, 1965). Some of the problems associated with punishment have been used to suggest that punishment procedures should not be used (Meyer & Evans, 1989). On the other hand, others have argued that individuals should have a right to an effective treatment (Van Houten et al., 1988) or that the side effects of punishment are not necessarily more severe than those of differential reinforcement procedures (Vollmer, 2002). In other words, at times it may be considered unreasonable to continue to implement an ineffective treatment when other procedures (i.e., punishment procedures) could be effective. Perhaps in the most severe and intractable cases dangerous SIB could be immediately suppressed via punishment while other (more widely accepted) treatments could be incorporated. Of course careful peer review and proper ethics training would be a prerequisite to usage of punishment procedures, or for that matter any procedures designed to reduce dangerous SIB.

Conclusion

Self-injury is a dangerous form of behavior that occurs in some individuals diagnosed with autism. A majority of evidence supports the notion that SIB is at least in part learned behavior. Behavioral assessment methods are designed to identify reinforcers maintaining SIB so that more effective treatments can be developed. Although assessment components have advantages and disadvantages, collectively the idea is to link the assessment information directly to treatment development. The most commonly used treatments involve withholding reinforcers following SIB (extinction) and presentation of reinforcers when SIB does not occur or when some alternative response occurs (differential reinforcement). It is important to consider the overall skill repertoire of the individual and to teach replacement behavior even if it is not directly or functionally related to SIB. In addition, although controversial, there may be some severe cases where punishment should be considered in the best interest of the individual. In any case of dangerous SIB, peer review is recommended so that the decision-making process of the practitioner is suitably aided by input from colleagues.

References

Altman, K., Haavik, S., & Cook, J. W. (1978). Punishment of self-injurious behavior in natural settings using contingent aromatic ammonia. *Behaviour Research and Therapy, 16,* 85–96.

Arndorfer, R. E., Miltenberger, R. G., Woster, S. H., Rortvedt, A. K., & Gaffaney, T. (1994). Home-based descriptive and experimental analysis of problem behaviors in children. *Topics in Early Childhood Special Education, 14,* 64–87.

Azrin, N. H., Hake, D. F., Holz, W. C., & Hutchinson, R. R. (1965). Motivational aspects of escape from punishment. *Journal of the Experimental Analysis of Behavior, 8,* 31–44.

Azrin, N. H., & Holz, W. C. (1966). Punishment. In W. K. Honig (Ed.), *Operant behavior: Areas of research and application* (pp. 380–447). New York: Appleton-Century-Crofts.

Azrin, N. H., Hutchinson, R. R., & Hake, D. F. (1966). Extinction-induced aggression. *Journal of the Experimental Analysis of Behavior, 9,* 191–204.

Baum, W. M. (1974). On two types of deviation from the matching law: Bias and undermatching. *Journal of the Experimental Analysis of Behavior, 22,* 231–242.

Bijou, S. W., Peterson, R. F., & Ault, M. H. (1968). A method to integrate descriptive and experimental field studies at the levels of data and empirical concepts. *Journal of Applied Behavior Analysis, 1,* 175–191.

Bodfish, J. W., Symons, F. J., Parker, D. E., & Lewis, M. H. (2000). Varieties of repetitive behavior in autism: Comparison to mental retardation. *Journal of Autism and Developmental Disorders, 30,* 237–243.

Borrero, C. S. W., & Borrero, J. C. (2008). Descriptive and experimental analyses of potential precursors to problem behavior. *Journal of Applied Behavior Analysis, 41,* 83–96.

Borrero, C. S. W., & Vollmer, T. R. (2006). Experimental analysis and treatment of multiply controlled problem behavior: A systematic replication and extension. *Journal of Applied Behavior Analysis, 39*, 375–379.

Borrero, C. S. W., Vollmer, T. R., & Borrero, J. C. (2004). Combining descriptive and functional analysis logic to evaluate idiosyncratic variables maintaining aggression. *Behavioral Interventions, 19*, 247–262.

Burchard, J. D., & Barrera, F. (1972). An analysis of timeout and response cost in a programmed environment. *Journal of Applied Behavior Analysis, 5*, 271–282.

Carr, E. G., & Durand, V. M. (1985). Reducing behavior problems through functional communications training. *Journal of Applied Behavior Analysis, 18*, 111–126.

Catania, A. C. (1998). *Learning* (4th ed.). Englewood Cliffs, NJ: Prentice Hall.

Cooper, L., Wacker, D., Sasso, G., Reimers, T., & Donn, L. (1990). Using parents as therapists to assess the appropriate behavior of their children: Application to a tertiary diagnostic clinic. *Journal of Applied Behavior Analysis, 23*, 285–296.

Cooper, L. J., Wacker, D. P., Thursby, D., Plagmann, L. A., Harding, J., Millard, T., et al. (1992). Analysis of the effects of task preferences, task demands, and adult attention on child behavior in outpatient and classroom settings. *Journal of Applied Behavior Analysis, 25*, 823–840.

Cowdery, G. E., Iwata, B. A., & Pace, G. M. (1990). Effects and side-effects of DRO as treatment for self-injurious behavior. *Journal of Applied Behavior Analysis, 23*, 497–506.

Crawford, J., Brockel, B., Schauss, S., & Miltenberger, R. G. (1992). A comparison of methods for the functional assessment of stereotypic behavior. *Journal of the Association for Persons with Severe Handicaps, 17*, 77–86.

de Villiers, P. (1977). Choice in concurrent schedules and a quantitative formulation of the law of effect. In W. K. Honig & J. E. R. Staddon (Eds.), *Handbook of operant behavior* (pp. 233–287). Englewood Cliffs, NJ: Prentice-Hall.

Derby, K. M., Wacker, D. P., Sasso, G., Steege, M., Northup, J., Cigrand, K., et al. (1992). Brief functional assessments techniques to evaluate aberrant behavior in an outpatient setting: A summary of 79 cases. *Journal of Applied Behavior Analysis, 25*, 713–721.

Dominick, K., Davis, N. O., Lainhart, J., Tager-Flusberg, H., & Folstein, S. (2007). Atypical behaviors in children with autism and children with a history of language impairment. *Research in Developmental Disabilities, 28*, 145–162.

Durand, V. M., & Carr, E. G. (1991). Functional communication training to reduce challenging behavior: Maintenance and application in new settings. *Journal of Applied Behavior Analysis, 24*, 251–264.

Durand, V. M., & Crimmins, D. B. (1988). Identifying the variables maintaining self-injurious behavior. *Journal of Autism and Developmental Disorders, 18*, 99–117.

Ellingson, S. A., Miltenberger, R. G., Stricker, J. M., Garlinghouse, M. A., Roberts, J., Galensky, T. L., et al. (2000). Analysis and treatment of finger sucking. *Journal of Applied Behavior Analysis, 33*, 41–52.

Ferster, C. B., & Skinner, B. F. (1957). *Schedules of Reinforcement.* New York: Appleton-Century-Crofts.

Fisher, W. W., Adelinis, J. D., Thompson, R. H., Worsdell, A. S., & Zarcone, J. R. (1998). Functional analysis and treatment of destructive behavior maintained by termination of "don't" (and symmetrical "do") requests. *Journal of Applied Behavior Analysis, 31*, 339–356.

Fischer, S. M., Iwata, B. A., & Mazaleski, J. L. (1997). Noncontingent delivery of arbitrary reinforcers as treatment for self-injurious behavior. *Journal of Applied Behavior Analysis, 30*, 239–249.

Fisher, W., Piazza, C., Cataldo, M., Harrell, R., Jefferson, G., & Conner, R. (1993). Functional communication training with and without extinction and punishment. *Journal of Applied Behavior Analysis, 26*, 23–36.

Friman, P. C., & Hove, G. (1987). Apparent covariation between child habit disorders: Effects of successful treatment for thumb sucking on untargeted chronic hair pulling. *Journal of Applied Behavior Analysis, 20*, 421–425.

Goh, H., Iwata, B. A., & DeLeon, I. G. (2000). Competition between noncontingent and contingent reinforcement schedules during response acquisition. *Journal of Applied Behavior Analysis, 33*, 195–205.

Goh, H., Iwata, B. A., Shore, B. A., DeLeon, I. G., Lerman, D. C., Ulrich, S. M., et al. (1995). An analysis of the reinforcing properties of hand mouthing. *Journal of Applied Behavior Analysis, 28*, 269–283.

Hagopian, L. P., Bruzek, J. L., Bowman, L. G., & Jennett, H. K. (2007). Assessment and treatment of problem behavior occasioned by interruption of free-operant behavior. *Journal of Applied Behavior Analysis, 40*, 89–103.

Hagopian, L. P., Fisher, W. W., Sullivan, M. T., Acquisto, J. T., & LeBlanc, L. A. (1998). Effectiveness of functional communication training with and without extinction and punishment: A summary of 21 inpatient cases. *Journal of Applied Behavior Analysis, 31*, 211–235.

Harding, J., Wacker, D. P., Cooper, L. J., Millard, T., & Jensen-Kovalan, P. (1994). Brief hierarchical assessment of potential treatment components with children in an outpatient clinic. *Journal of Applied Behavior Analysis, 27*, 291–300.

Hoch, H., McComas, J. J., Johnson, L. J., Faranda, N. J., & Guenther, S. L. (2002). The effects of magnitude and quality of reinforcement on choice responding during play activities. *Journal of Applied Behavior Analysis, 35*, 171–181.

Horner, D. (1980). The effects of an environmental "enrichment" program on the behavior of institutionalized profoundly retarded children. *Journal of Applied Behavior Analysis, 13*, 473–491.

Horner, R. H., & Day, H. M. (1991). The effects of response efficiency on functionally equivalent competing behaviors. *Journal of Applied Behavior Analysis, 24*, 719–732.

Hutchinson, R. R. (1977). By-products of aversive control. In W. K. Honig & J. E. R. Staddon (Eds.), *Handbook of Operant Behavior* (pp. 415–431). Englewood Cliffs, NJ: Prentice Hall.

Iwata, B. A. (2005). *Functional analysis screening tool.* Gainesville, FL: The Florida Center on Self-Injury.

Iwata, B. A., Dorsey, M. F., Slifer, K. J., Bauman, K. E., & Richman, G. S. (1994). Toward a functional analysis of self-injury. *Journal of Applied Behavior Analysis, 27*, 197–209. Reprinted from Analysis and Intervention in Developmental Disabilities, 2, 3–20, 1982.

Iwata, B. A., Pace, G. M., Cowdery, G. E., & Miltenberger, R. G. (1994). What makes extinction work: An analysis of procedural form and function. *Journal of Applied Behavior Analysis, 27*, 131–144.

Iwata, B. A., Pace, G. M., Dorsey, M. F., Zarcone, J. R., Vollmer, T. R., Smith, R. G., et al. (1994). The functions of self-injurious behavior: An experimental-epidemiological analysis. *Journal of Applied Behavior Analysis, 27*, 215–240.

Iwata, B. A., Pace, G. M., Kalsher, M. J., Cowdery, G. E., & Cataldo, M. L. (1990). Experimental analysis and extinction of self-injurious escape behavior. *Journal of Applied Behavior Analysis, 23*, 11–27.

Jordan, J., Singh, N. N., & Repp, A. C. (1989). An evaluation of gentle teaching and visual screening in the reduction of stereotypy. *Journal of Applied Behavior Analysis, 22*, 9–22.

Kahng, S. W., Iwata, B. A., Fischer, S. M., Page, T. J., Treadwell, K. R. H., Williams, D. E., et al. (1998). Temporal distributions of problem behavior based on scatter plot analysis. *Journal of Applied Behavior Analysis, 31*, 593–604.

Kahng, S., Abt, K. A., & Schonbachler, H. E. (2001). Assessment and treatment of low-rate high-intensity problem behavior. *Journal of Applied Behavior Analysis, 34*, 225–228.

Kodak, T., Miltenberger, R. G., & Romaniuk, C. G. (2003). The effects of differential negative reinforcement of other behavior and noncontingent escape on compliance. *Journal of Applied Behavior Analysis, 36*, 379–382.

Lennox, D. B., Miltenberger, R. G., & Donnelly, D. R. (1987). Response interruption and DRL for the reduction of rapid eating. *Journal of Applied Behavior Analysis, 20*, 279–284.

Lerman, D. C., & Iwata, B. A. (1993). Descriptive and experimental analysis of variables maintaining self-injurious behavior. *Journal of Applied Behavior Analysis, 26*, 293–319.

Lerman, D. C., & Iwata, B. A. (1995). Prevalence of the extinction burst and its attenuation during treatment. *Journal of Applied Behavior Analysis, 28*, 93–94.

Lerman, D. C., & Iwata, B. A. (1996). Developing a technology for the use of operant extinction in clinical settings: An examination of basic and applied research. *Journal of Applied Behavior Analysis, 29*, 345–382.

Lerman, D. C., Iwata, B. A., Shore, B. A., & Kahng, S. (1996). Responding maintained by intermittent reinforcement: Implications for the use of extinction with problem behavior in clinical settings. *Journal of Applied Behavior Analysis, 29*, 153–171.

Lerman, D. C., Iwata, B. A., Smith, R. G., Zarcone, J. R., & Vollmer, T. R. (1994). Transfer of behavioral function as a contributing factor in treatment relapse. *Journal of Applied Behavior Analysis, 27*, 357–370.

Lerman, D. C., Iwata, B. A., & Wallace, M. D. (1999). Side effects of extinction: Prevalence of bursting and aggression during the treatment of self-injurious behavior. *Journal of Applied Behavior Analysis, 32*, 1–8.

Lerman, D. C., & Vorndran, C. M. (2002). On the status of knowledge for using punishment: Implications for treating behavior disorders. *Journal of Applied Behavior Analysis, 35*, 431–464.

Lindberg, J. S., Iwata, B. A., Kahng, S., & DeLeon, I. G. (1999). DRO contingencies: An analysis of variable-momentary schedules. *Journal of Applied Behavior Analysis, 32*, 123–136.

Linscheid, T. R., Iwata, B. A., Ricketts, R. W., Williams, D. E., & Griffin, J. C. (1990). Clinical evaluation of the self-injurious behavior inhibiting system (SIBIS). *Journal of Applied Behavior Analysis, 23*, 53–78.

Lovaas, O. I., & Simmons, J. Q. (1969). Manipulation of self-destruction in three retarded children. *Journal of Applied Behavior Analysis, 2*, 143–157.

Mace, F. C., & Lalli, J. S. (1991). Linking descriptive and experimental analyses in the treatment of bizarre speech. *Journal of Applied Behavior Analysis, 24*, 553–562.

Marcus, B. A., & Vollmer, T. R. (1995). Effects of differential negative reinforcement on disruption and compliance. *Journal of Applied Behavior Analysis, 28*, 229–230.

Marcus, B. A., & Vollmer, T. R. (1996). Combining noncontingent reinforcement and differential reinforcement schedules as treatment for aberrant behavior. *Journal of Applied Behavior Analysis, 29*, 43–51.

Martin, N. T., Gaffan, E. A., & Williams, T. (1999). Experimental functional analyses for challenging behavior: A study of validity and reliability. *Research in Developmental Disabilities, 20*, 125–146.

Matson, J. L., & Vollmer, T. R. (1995). *User's guide: Questions About Behavioral Function (QABF)*. Baton Rouge, LA.: Scientific.

McDermott, S., Zhou, L., & Mann, J. (2008). Injury treatment among children with autism or pervasive developmental disorder. *Journal of Autism and Developmental Disorders, 38*, 626–633.

Meyer, L. H., & Evans, I. M. (1989). *Nonaversive intervention for behavior problems: A manual for home and community.* Baltimore: Brookes.

Miltenberger, R. G. (2008). *Behavior Modification: Principles and Procedures* (4th ed.). Belmont, CA: Thompson Wadsworth.

Moore, J. W., & Fisher, W. W. (2007). The effects of videotape modeling on staff acquisition of functional analysis methodology. *Journal of Applied Behavior Analysis, 40*, 197–202.

Neef, N. A., & Lutz, M. N. (2001). A brief computer-based assessment of reinforcer dimensions affecting choice. *Journal of Applied Behavior Analysis, 34*, 57–60.

Northup, J., Wacker, D., Sasso, G., Steege, M., Cigrand, K., Cook, J., et al. (1991). A brief functional analysis of aggressive and alternative behavior in an outclinic setting. *Journal of Applied Behavior Analysis, 24*, 509–522.

O'Neill, R. E., Horner, R. H., Albin, R. W., Sprague, J. R., Storey, K., & Newton, J. S. (1997). *Functional assessment and program development for problem behavior: A practical handbook* (2nd ed.). Pacific Grove, CA: Brooks.

O'Reilly, M. F. (1997). Functional analysis of episodic self-injury correlated with recurrent otitis media. *Journal of Applied Behavior Analysis, 30*, 165–167.

Paclawskyj, T. R., Matson, J. L., Rush, K. S., & Smalls, Y. (2001). The validity of the questions about behavioral function (QABF). *Journal of Intellectual Disabilities, 45*, 484–494.

Repp, A. C., Barton, L. E., & Brulle, A. R. (1983). A comparison of two approaches for programming the differential reinforcement of other behaviors. *Journal of Applied Behavior Analysis, 16*, 435–445.

Repp, A. C., Deitz, S. M., & Deitz, D. E. (1976). Reducing inappropriate behaviors in classrooms and in individual sessions through DRO schedules of reinforcement. *Mental Retardation, 14*, 11–15.

Rescorla, R. A., & Skucy, J. C. (1969). Effects of response-independent reinforcers during extinction. *Journal of Comparative and Physiological Psychology, 67*, 382–389.

Rincover, A. (1978). Sensory extinction: a procedure form eliminating self-stimulatory behavior in developmentally disabled children. *Journal of Abnormal Child Psychology, 6*, 299–310.

Roberts, M. L., Mace, F. C., & Daggett, J. A. (1995). Preliminary comparison of two negative reinforcement schedules to reduce self-injury. *Journal of Applied Behavior Analysis, 28,* 579–580.

Roscoe, E. M., Iwata, B. A., & Goh, H. L. (1998). A comparison of noncontingent reinforcement and sensory extinction as treatments for self-injurious behavior. *Journal of Applied Behavior Analysis, 31,* 635–646.

St. Peter, C. C., Vollmer, T. R., Bourret, J. C., Borrero, C. S. W., Sloman, K. N., & Rapp, J. T. (2005). On the role of attention in naturally occurring matching relations. *Journal of Applied Behavior Analysis, 38,* 429–443.

Sigafoos, J., & Saggers, E. (1995). A discrete trial approach to the functional analysis of aggressive behavior in two boys with autism. *Australia and New Zealand Journal of Developmental Disabilities, 20,* 287–297.

Skinner, B. F. (1938). *The behavior of organisms: An experimental analysis.* Acton, MA: Copley Publishing Group.

Skinner, B. F. (1953). *Science and Human Behavior.* New York: Macmillian.

Sloman, K. N., Vollmer, T. R., Cotnoir, N. M., Borrero, C. S. W., Borrero, J. C., Samaha, A. L., et al. (2005). Descriptive analyses of caregiver reprimands. *Journal of Applied Behavior Analysis, 38,* 373–383.

Smith, R. G., & Churchill, R. M. (2002). Identification of environmental determinants of behavior disorders through functional analysis of precursor behaviors. *Journal of Applied Behavior Analysis, 35,* 125–136.

Smith, R. G., Iwata, B. A., Vollmer, T. R., & Zarcone, J. R. (1993). Experimental analysis and treatment of multiply controlled self-injury. *Journal of Applied Behavior Analysis, 26,* 183–196.

Sturmey, P. (1994). Assessing the functions of aberrant behaviors: a review of psychometric instruments. *Journal of Autism and Developmental Disorders, 24,* 293–304.

Thompson, R. H., & Iwata, B. A. (2001). A descriptive analysis of social consequences following problem behavior. *Journal of Applied Behavior Analysis, 34,* 169–178.

Thompson, R. H., & Iwata, B. A. (2005). A review of reinforcement control procedures. *Journal of Applied Behavior Analysis, 38,* 257–278.

Thompson, R. H., Iwata, B. A., Hanley, G. P., Dozier, C. L., & Samaha, A. L. (2003). The effects of extinction, noncontingent reinforcement, and differential reinforcement of other behavior as control procedures. *Journal of Applied Behavior Analysis, 36,* 221–238.

Touchette, P. E., MacDonald, R. F., & Langer, S. N. (1985). A scatter plot for identifying stimulus control of problem behavior. *Journal of Applied Behavior Analysis, 18,* 343–351.

Van Houten, R., Axelrod, S., Bailey, J. S., Favell, J. E., Foxx, R. M., Iwata, B. A., et al. (1988). The right to effective behavioral treatment. *Journal of Applied Behavior Analysis, 21,* 381–384.

Vaughan, M. E., & Michael, J. L. (1982). Automatic reinforcement: An important but ignored concept. *Behaviorism, 10,* 217–227.

Vollmer, T.R., Iwata, B. A., Duncan, B. A., & Lerman, D. C. (1993). Extensions of multielement functional analysis using reversal-type designs. *Journal of Developmental and Physical Disabilities, 5,* 311–325.

Vollmer, T.R. Roane, H. S. Ringdahl, J. E. & Marcus, B. A. (1999). Evaluating treatment challenges with differential reinforcement of alternative behavior. *Journal of Applied Behavior Analysis, 32,* 9–23.

Vollmer, T. R. (2002). Punishment happens: Some comments on Lerman and Vorndran's review. *Journal of Applied Behavior Analysis, 35,* 469–473.

Vollmer, T. R., Borrero, J. C., Wright, C. S., Van Camp, C., & Lalli, J. S. (2001). Identifying possible contingencies during descriptive analyses of severe behavior disorders. *Journal of Applied Behavior Analysis, 34,* 269–287.

Vollmer, T. R., & Iwata, B. A. (1992). Differential reinforcement as treatment for severe behavior disorders: Procedural and functional variations. *Research in Developmental Disabilities, 13,* 393–417.

Vollmer, T. R., Iwata, B. A., Zarcone, J. R., Smith, R. G., & Mazaleski, J. L. (1993a). The role of attention in the treatment of attention-maintained self-injurious behavior: Noncontingent reinforcement and differential reinforcement of other behavior. *Journal of Applied Behavior Analysis, 26,* 9–12.

Vollmer, T. R., Iwata, B. A., Zarcone, J. R., Smith, R. G., & Mazaleski, J. L. (1993b). Within session patterns of self-injury as indicators of behavioral function. *Research in Developmental Disabilities, 14,* 479–492.

Vollmer, T. R., Marcus, B. A., & Ringdahl, J. E. (1995). Noncontingent escape as treatment for self-injurious behavior maintained by negative reinforcement. *Journal of Applied Behavior Analysis, 28,* 15–26.

Wallace, M. D., Doney, J. K., Mintz-Resudek, C. M., & Tarbox, R. S. F. (2004). Training educators to implement functional analyses. *Journal of Applied Behavior Analysis, 37,* 89–92.

Weiner, H. (1962). Some effects of response cost upon human operant behavior. *Journal of the Experimental Analysis of Behavior, 5,* 201–208.

Worsdell, A. S., Iwata, B. A., Hanley, G. P., Thompson, R. H., & Kahng, S. H. (2000). Effects of continuous and intermittent reinforcement for problem behavior during functional communication training. *Journal of Applied Behavior Analysis, 33,* 167–179.

Zarcone, J. R., Rodgers, T. A., Iwata, B. A., Rourke, D. A., & Dorsey, M. F. (1991). Reliability analysis of the motivation assessment scale: A failure to replicate. *Research in Developmental Disabilities, 12,* 349–360.

Chapter 10
Aggression and Noncompliance

James K. Luiselli

Aggression and noncompliance are common problem behaviors displayed by some children with ASD. Aggression in the form of hitting, kicking, and biting can cause serious injury to peers and adults, creating an unsafe learning environment. Furthermore, aggressive behavior interferes with instruction and skill acquisition. The social consequences of chronic aggression also are untoward: the child is avoided, perceived unfavorably, and unlikely to establish friendships. Frequently, children who demonstrate serious aggression are enrolled in restrictive educational settings, sometimes exposed to invasive treatment procedures (e.g., punishment) or ineffective pharmacotherapy.

Like aggression, noncompliance has deleterious effects on learning. A child who has ASD and noncompliant behavior receives inconsistent instruction because she/he does not respond uniformly to requests from a teacher or parent. Noncompliance means that a child will not perform many appropriate behaviors that can be shaped and strengthened through positive reinforcement. Note too that caregivers usually have a poor opinion of children who "refuse" to carry out directions.

This chapter addresses assessment and intervention for aggression and noncompliance. First, I discuss the process of measuring these problem behaviors in applied settings, emphasizing the varied topographies of aggression and noncompliance and different methods for acquiring occurrence data. The next section of the chapter covers functional behavioral assessment (FBA) and functional analysis (FA) methodologies that are critical steps in designing an intervention plan. My subsequent review of intervention covers procedures

that are "matched" to FBA and FA outcomes. Here, I focus on both preventive (antecedent) and behavior-contingent (consequence) procedures that are supported empirically and have good social validity. The chapter concludes with recommendations for formulating, implementing, and evaluating successful intervention plans.

Measurement

Knowing how often aggression and noncompliance occur demands accurate measurement through systematic data collection. Measurement before intervention establishes a baseline by which to evaluate the effects of behavior-change procedures. During intervention, measurement documents response trends, enabling practitioners to make decisions about maintaining, revising, or introducing procedures.

Aggression

Aggression usually consists of distinct responses that can be categorized as "inappropriate physical contact" initiated by a child toward another person. Some representative topographies of aggression are hitting with open palm or closed fist, kicking, biting, pinching, and pulling hair. Many times, a child displays aggression as a single response, for example, "grabbing and squeezing the therapist by the wrists or arms, attempts to head butt the therapist, shoving, pulling hair, and grabbing the therapist's neck with one or both hands" (Progar et al., 2001, p. 70). So defined, practitioners can document frequency of aggression on an event-recording form, summing the total number of responses

J.K. Luiselli (✉)
May Institute, 41, Pacella Park Drive, Randolph, MA, 02368, USA
e-mail: jluiselli@mayinstitute.org

during a fixed-time period (e.g., 6-h school day) or calculating rate of responding during variable recording segments (number of responses/time).

There are situations in which a child exhibits aggression repetitively, making it difficult to record separate responses in isolation. In such cases, data collection can target an "aggressive episode," essentially multiple responses exhibited within a defined period of time. For example, an episode would begin when a child displays the first aggressive response and terminates when aggression ceases for 60 consecutive seconds (Luiselli, 1990). The time between initial response and termination criterion would be recorded so that a "duration per episode" measure is calculated. Frequency alone is an inadequate measure because the duration of an aggressive episode can vary. Accordingly, it is useful to compute the average duration per episode. This type of measurement is valuable when the aggression being recorded is low frequency but high intensity (Kahng, Abt, & Schonbachler, 2001).

Latency-to-first-response is another measure that should be considered when assessing and intervening with a serious behavior such as aggression. Picture a teacher who is confronted with aggression from a child with ASD during 15-min instructional activities. Instead of recording frequency of aggression throughout activities, the teacher would activate a timer when they begin and stop the timer immediately following the first aggressive response. The duration on the timer, or latency-to-first response, would be brief during a baseline phase of evaluation and would increase with effective intervention. The practical advantage of this measurement methodology is that a practitioner does not have to endure repetitive aggression that would be required with frequency recording.

Noncompliance

Noncompliance usually is defined as a child failing to initiate desirable behavior when given a direction or request. It is customary to include a latency criterion such as "noncompliance should be recorded if the specified response does not occur 5 s after stating the instruction." Generally, the instruction-to-response initiation latency is brief but can be adjusted depending on the complexity of instruction and expected behavior from the child.

Frequency of noncompliance can be recorded as long as the number of instructions or requests are held constant. That is, it is reasonable to record noncompliant responses by a child during 10 activities each day and report data as frequency of noncompliance. However, frequency is not an appropriate measure when opportunities to respond vary. To illustrate, a child could be noncompliant with 5 out of 10 instructions on one day and 5 of 20 instructions on another day. Frequency on both days, although identical, is a misleading statistic because it does not consider how many compliance opportunities were presented to the child. Therefore, noncompliance under such conditions should be recorded as a percentage measure.

Noncompliance can occur as a "passive response," as when a child does not carry out an instruction but refrains from challenging behavior. It also is common for noncompliance to occur contemperaneously with a behavior such as aggression. Thus, a child might strike her/his teacher when given an instruction. As discussed later in the chapter, the co-occurrence of aggression and noncompliance has implications for intervention planning and implementation.

Functional Behavioral Assessment and Functional Analysis

Understanding the function or "purpose" of problem behaviors such as aggression and noncompliance is an essential step in formulating an intervention plan (Matson & Minshawi, 2007). Behavior analysts focus on three behavior–environment relationships to explain the role of reinforcement in determining function: (1) pleasurable social or tangible consequences (social positive reinforcement), (2) termination of unpleasant situations (social negative reinforcement), and (3) behavior-elicited (nonsocial) stimulation (automatic reinforcement). Functional behavioral assessment (FBA) and functional analysis (FA) are two methodologies for isolating behavior function.

Functional Behavioral Assessment

FBA is the process of correlating environmental events with problem behaviors. One approach toward FBA relies on *indirect* methods based principally on the subjective reports of care-providers. Instruments such as *Motivation Assessment Scale (MAS)* (Durand & Crimmins, 1988), *Functional Analysis Screening Tool (FAST)* (Iwata, 1995), and *Questions About Behavior Function (QABF)* (Matson & Vollmer, 1995) are informant surveys that target social and nonsocial contingencies responsible for problem behaviors. Cut-off scores derived from surveys are used to endorse one or more sources of control (e.g., attention, tangible, escape, automatic).

The *Functional Assessment Interview (FAI)* (O'Neill, Horner, Albin, Sprague, Storey, & Newton, 1997) is another informant-driven protocol. During an interview conducted by a responsible professional, the informant is asked questions about antecedent and consequence events often associated with occurrence and nonoccurrence of problem behaviors. The *FAI* examines a variety of ecological events (e.g., medical status, sleep patterns, mealtime routines) and interpersonal contacts, thereby producing a comprehensive formulation that guides intervention planning.

Descriptive methods are a second type of FBA, characterized by direct observation of a person under naturalistic conditions. Bijou, Peterson, and Ault (1968) pioneered this approach with their presentation of antecedent-behavior-consequence (A-B-C) data collection. For a child who has aggression and noncompliance, an observer would watch her/him participate in a variety of activities, noting particular events that immediately precede (antecedents) and follow (consequences) the behaviors (Luiselli, 2006). The resulting data then are evaluated to determine whether specific situations reliably predict aggression and noncompliance. In doing so, hypotheses about behavior can be inferred.

Antecedent events can set the occasion for aggression and noncompliance through established stimulus control (Luiselli, 2008). Touchette, MacDonald, and Langer (1985) presented a *scatter-plot* analysis as a first step toward confirming stimulus control over problem behaviors. The recording protocol requires a practitioner to indicate if a child's problem behaviors did not occur, occurred one time, or occurred two times or more during successive 30-min intervals within the day. By reviewing data over several days, "Problem behavior may be correlated with a time of day, the presence or absence of certain people, a social setting, a class of activities, a contingency of reinforcement, a physical environment, and combinations of these and other variables" (Touchette et al., p. 345). Accordingly, intervention can proceed by modifying one or more of these behavior–environment relationships.

Both indirect and descriptive FBA have the advantage of being easily administered by practitioners. From a clinical perspective, it is important to gather information from individuals who are knowledgeable about the child with ASD and to document objectively how often aggression and noncompliance occur and under what conditions. Typically, both assessment methods are performed together, for example, obtaining informant produced impressions about behavior function followed by direct observation and data collection. To reiterate, FBA enables one to form a working hypothesis (e.g., "The child's aggression appears to be escape motivated.") but not a confirmatory "cause and effect" relationship.

Functional Analysis

In contrast to FBA, a FA measures aggression and noncompliance during experimentally manipulated conditions. In the seminal publication on this topic, Iwata, Dorsey, Slifer, Bauman, and Richman (1994) constructed conditions to represent social positive reinforcement, social negative reinforcement, and automatic reinforcement functions. Iwata et al. studied nine children who had developmental disabilities and self-injurious behavior (SIB) during daily 15-min sessions with each session featuring a condition linked to one of four functions:

Social Disapproval. A therapist sat in a room and allowed the child access to toys. The therapist sat away from the child, reading a book or magazine. When the child displayed SIB, the therapist disapproved by stating, "Don't do that, you're going to hurt yourself." This condition provided social attention contingent on SIB.

Academic Demand. A therapist sat in a room with the child and presented her/him with instructional tasks that were difficult to complete. When the child displayed SIB, the therapist removed the task, turned away for 30 s, and then resumed instruction. This condition provided escape from demands contingent on SIB.

Unstructured Play. A therapist sat in a room and allowed the child access to toys. There were no consequences for SIB. Instead, the therapist presented the child with social praise and brief physical contact (hand on shoulder) every 30 s without SIB. "This condition served as a control procedure for the presence of an experimenter, the availability of potentially stimulating materials, the absence of demands, the delivery of social approval for appropriate behavior, and the lack of approval for self-injury" (Iwata et al., 1994, p. 203).

Alone. The child was present in the room without the therapist or access to toys or other potentially stimulating materials. This condition tested for automatic (sensory) reinforcement as a source of control over SIB.

Iwata et al. (1994) found that for six of the nine children, higher frequencies of SIB were associated with a specific experimental condition. When the data from a FA are graphed, the response differentiation among conditions isolates controlling variables. Although Iwata et al. concentrated on SIB, FA methodology has been applied to aggression and noncompliance of children who have a developmental disability including ASD (Hanley, Iwata, & McCord, 2003).

The advantages of FA notwithstanding, it requires greater sophistication than a typical FBA. Another concern is the "ecological validity" of a FA, namely the fact that it is conducted under simulated (analog) conditions that are removed from the natural environment. Hanley et al. (2003) concluded that there has been, "Systematic growth in the use of functional analysis methodology as a primary method of behavior assessment and, more generally, as a means of studying environment–behavior relations" (p. 178). Furthermore, many FAs have been performed in applied settings such as schools, and it appears that the time commitment is no greater than that required for a FBA (Iwata et al., 2000). Practitioners, in fact, can be taught the skills to independently conduct a FA (Moore & Fisher, 2007; Moore et al., 2002). In summary, FA methodologies continue to be refined, adapted to clinical exigencies, and represent the experimental standard when targeting problem behaviors.

Evidence-Based and Empirically Supported Intervention

Detrich (2008) proposed that "the terms evidence-based interventions, evidence-based practices, empirically supported treatments, and best practices have become ubiquitous in education and other human services disciplines" (p. 3). There are different definitions and explanations of these terms but essentially, evidence-based means that scientific information informs decisions about intervention. With respect to aggression

and noncompliance, *evidence-based intervention procedures* would be those derived from research that has sound internal (experimental control) and external (replication) validity. Evidence-based knowledge, in turn, must be translated to the "real world" of practitioners. Evaluation under these circumstances yields *empirically supported intervention procedures.*

This section reviews several evidence-based and empirically supported intervention procedures for aggression and noncompliance. My review is not all inclusive because many procedures have been implemented for these problem behaviors during nearly four decades of applied research (Luiselli, Russo, Christian, & Wilczynski, 2008; Matson, Laud, & Matson, 2004). I emphasize procedures that are linked to behavior-function categorized as (1) social positive reinforcement, (2) social negative reinforcement, and (3) automatic reinforcement. Note that although aggression and noncompliance often are exhibited by children who have ASD, surprisingly there is not a robust literature of intervention research with this clinical population. Accordingly, I have included studies with other diagnostic groups (e.g., children with mental retardation and multiple disabilities) to illustrate certain procedures that with confidence, can be extended to the ASD group.

Before describing specific intervention procedures, it is worthwhile to consider that a single problem behavior can have multiple functions. It is possible, for example, for a child's aggression and noncompliance to be attention-maintained when she/he is playing with peers but escape motivated during academic sessions with a teacher. In such situations, separate intervention plans would have to be designed. Behavior function also can change overtime when problem behaviors contact new sources of reinforcement. Revisions to an intervention plan would be required in these cases.

Social Positive Reinforcement

Aggression and noncompliance that are maintained by social positive reinforcement is evident when the behaviors produce pleasurable attention and/or objects. Because practitioners sometimes respond to problem behaviors by reprimanding or verbally chastising a child, such a consequence will function as reinforcement if the child enjoys this social attention. Similarly, noncompliance will be reinforced if a practitioner allows a child access to preferred objects when she/he does not follow instructions.

After confirming that a child's aggression or noncompliance is maintained by attention or tangible objects, a first-choice intervention would be eliminating these sources of reinforcement through *social extinction*. Procedurally, social extinction operates by not reacting to problem behaviors with verbal comments, nonverbal expressions, or other forms of attention. Recent research has shown that social extinction depends on knowing precisely what constitutes "attention," be it a simple glance toward, physical contact with, or speaking to a child (Kodak, Northup, & Kelley, 2007). Additionally, for social extinction to be effective, identified sources of positive reinforcement must be withheld following every occurrence of aggression and noncompliance.

Social extinction works best when combined with differential positive reinforcement. Kern and Kokina (2008) reviewed several differential positive reinforcement procedures that have been successful in reducing problem behaviors of children with ASD. The *differential reinforcement of other behavior (DRO)* makes pleasurable consequences contingent on the absence of problem behaviors during a specified period of time. *With the differential reinforcement of alternative behavior (DRA)*, particular behaviors and not simply the absence of responding are reinforced. The third procedure, *differential reinforcement of low rate behavior (DRL)*, provides positive reinforcement when problem behaviors do not exceed a predetermined criterion.

Concerning intervention for aggression, various differential positive reinforcement procedures have been effective with children who have ASD when implemented as the only procedure and when combined with other methods (Luiselli & Slocumb, 1984) Noncompliance can be addressed with DRA by positively reinforcing instruction-following (Wilder, Saulnier, Beavers, & Zonneveld, 2008). As reported by Russo, Cataldo, and Cushing (1981), increasing child compliance through reinforcement procedures can effectively reduce co-occurring problem behaviors such as aggression. This outcome is possible when aggression and noncompliance share the same response class.

The preceding discussion highlights the importance of conducting preference assessment before implementing positive reinforcement procedures. Potential reinforcing stimuli for a child can be identified through observation, asking the opinions of care-providers, and

administering a preference survey. However a study by Mueller, Wilczynski, Moore, Fusilier, and Trahant (2001) demonstrates that ideally, reinforcers should be selected through formal assessment of preferences (Piazza, Fisher, Hagopian, Bowman, & Toole, 1996). They measured aggression (hitting, kicking, slapping, biting, pinching, and head butting) by an 8-year old boy with autism, first during an FA and subsequently during an intervention evaluation. The FA confirmed that the boy's aggression was maintained by access to preferred objects. As determined by a preference assessment, giving the boy noncontingent access to high-preference objects was associated with less frequent aggression when compared to middle-preference and low-preference stimuli. Absent a preference assessment, the proper choice of objects to make available during intervention would not have been made.

Noncontingent reinforcement (NCR) is the behavior-independent delivery of pleasurable consequences (Carr & LeBlanc, 2006). NCR actually is imprecise terminology because reinforcement by definition cannot be noncontingent (Skinner, 1948). In practice, NCR is implemented by presenting stimuli on a fixed-time (FT) or variable-time (VT) schedule. Hagopian, Fisher, and Legacy (1994) reported NCR as an effective intervention procedure for attention-maintained problem behaviors (aggression, disruption, self-injury) in 5-year old female quadruplets diagnosed with PDD and mental retardation. Following a baseline phase, a therapist presented social attention to the children on an FT 10s schedule ("dense" schedule condition), then on an FT 5 min schedule ("lean" schedule condition). The "dense" schedule of reinforcement was associated with the largest decrease in problem behaviors, suggesting that at the onset of NCR intervention, the FT schedule should be near continuous. Hagopian et al. (1994) eventually were able to fade the delivery of social attention so that by conclusion of the study, a near-zero rate of problem behaviors was maintained by an FT 5 min schedule.

Functional communication training (FCT), reported initially by Carr and Durand (1985), teaches a child with attention-maintained aggression and noncompliance to contact pleasurable stimuli using an acceptable language response. In depiction, a child who has learned to hit her teacher to obtain a favorite object could be taught to say, "Can I have that toy?" Or, when noncompliance is reinforced by parent attention, an FCT alternative could be, "Talk to me," or "Look what I did." Because language acquisition is a dominant learning objective for children with ASD, it is expected that most practitioners would rank FCT as an acceptable procedure. Recent studies also have shown that FCT can be combined efficaciously with other behavior-deceleration methods (O'Reilly, Cannella, Sigafoos, & Lancioni, 2006).

Social Negative Reinforcement

Problem behaviors that are escape motivated are maintained by social negative reinforcement. Noncompliance, in particular, is demonstrated by many children with ASD during "demanding" educational activities. Some features of teacher–child interaction that provoke noncompliant behavior (sometimes accompanied by aggression) include rate of task delivery (Smith, Iwata, Goh, & Shore, 1995), response effort (Iwata, Pace, Kalsher, Cowdery, & Cataldo, 1990), and objects that have acquired idiosyncratic stimulus control (Carr, Yarbrough, & Langdon, 1997). Social negative reinforcement operates when noncompliance and aggression terminate the nonpreferred interactions.

A procedure termed *escape extinction* (Carr, Newsom, & Binkoff, 1980) maintains an ongoing interaction to prevent negatively reinforcing aggression and noncompliance. In responding to aggression, a practitioner would block and redirect a child from hitting, kicking, and similar responses. Escape extinction for noncompliance might consist of re-presenting instructions until a child follows through appropriately. Although this procedure is matched functionally to escape maintained problem behavior, there are disadvantages because it is not easy to implement, may occasion other negative responses, and necessitates physical contact with a child.

Guided compliance is similar to escape extinction in that a practitioner physically stops the behaviors contingent on escape maintained aggression and noncompliance. Additional intervention then is provided by prompting alternative responses, starting with a gentle touch (partial physical prompt) and increasing the guidance as needed to overcome resistance. Guided compliance usually is implemented several seconds after a child does not initiate a requested behavior and

is withdrawn when the behavior is performed. The effective use of guided compliance should be realized by a child avoiding physical contact with a practitioner by complying with instructions. If a child consistently resists guided compliance or struggles forcefully, the procedure should be reconsidered. Wilder et al. (2008), for example, found that two preschool-age children with autism responded better to a positive reinforcement procedure for compliant behavior than guided compliance when they did not follow instructions.

Whereas escape extinction and guided compliance focus on the consequences of aggression and noncompliance, antecedent intervention manipulates behavior-provoking stimuli and conditions (Luiselli, 2008). One antecedent influence on escape maintained problem behaviors is how a practitioner delivers a verbal instruction. For some children with aggression and noncompliance, it is helpful to reduce the number of instructions they receive as a way to improve compliance and then slowly present more instructions (Zarcone et al., 1993). *With behavioral momentum* (Mace et al., 1988), a child is presented first with instructions that always produce compliance (HPR: high-probability requests) followed by instructions that historically have been associated with poor compliance (LPR: low-probability requests). This sequencing of HPR and LPR is thought to promote stimulus control over compliance. One additional instruction-giving manipulation is to shift from *direct to indirect requests*. For example, Adelinis and Hagopian (1999) were able to eliminate aggression by a 27-year old man who had autism by interrupting his disruptive behavior using a "do" request (e.g., "Sit in a chair.") instead of a "don't" request (e.g., "Don't lie on the floor."). Although the participant in this study was an adult, manipulating verbal instructions to reduce problem behaviors likely can be used with children who have a similar presentation.

Butler and Luiselli (2007) evaluated *noncontingent escape (NCE),* a variant of NCR described previously, as an intervention procedure with a 13-year old girl who had autism, aggression, and poor compliance with academic task requests. Following an FA that verified escape maintained problem behaviors, she was permitted a break from academic activities on a FT-20s schedule that was progressively increased to a FT300s schedule over the course of 18 sessions. Intervention also included instructional fading by which academic requests initially were eliminated and later introduced in small increments. NCE combined with instructional fading essentially eliminated aggression and improved compliance. As programed in this study, NCE usually starts with a frequent FT schedule that overtime becomes more practical by progressively delaying acceptable escape.

FCT also is a function-based intervention procedure for escape-maintained problem behaviors. Johnson, McComas, Thompson, and Symons (2004) evaluated FCT with an 11-year old boy who had autism and displayed aggression (hitting, kicking, pinching, biting, pulling hair) toward his mother and infant brother. An FA conducted in the boy's home revealed that aggression was negatively reinforced by his mother picking up the infant brother and leaving the room. Aggression was reduced to a near-zero rate by teaching the boy to request separation from his mother and brother. Interestingly, the positive effect from FCT was more pronounced when the mother frequently prompted the boy to make requests.

Finally, a study by Peyton, Lindauer, and Richman (2005) highlights the importance of properly assessing the source of control over escape maintained problem behavior before formulating an intervention plan. The participant was a 10-year-old girl with autism and vocal behavior involving a refusal to comply with requests (e.g., "I won't do it."). An FA suggested that noncompliance was reinforced by escaping task demands. One intervention evaluation showed that noncompliant vocal behavior persisted whether demands were or were not accompanied by removal of task materials. When the manner of prompting the girl included a nondirective request (e.g., "I wonder where the --- is.") instead of a direct request (e.g., "Show me the ----."), noncompliance quickly extinguished. Therefore for this child, it was how requests were presented and not demands per se that occasioned the problem behavior.

Automatic Reinforcement

Problem behaviors are automatically reinforced when they occur independent of social consequences. Stereotypy and self-injury are the behavior topographies most often controlled by automatic reinforcement, resulting from either pleasurable sensory stimulation or attenuation of physical discomfort (Lerman & Rapp, 2006). No studies have been reported in which child noncompliance was shown to be maintained by automatic reinforcement. Concerning aggression, Thompson, Fisher, Piazza, and Kuhn (1998) found that hitting, kicking, pinching, and scratching by a 7-year-old boy diagnosed with PDD were attention-maintained, while a separate topography of "grinding" his chin against a person's body was automatically reinforced by tactile stimulation. Intervention for the attention-maintained aggression consisted of FCT and social extinction. The procedures implemented to reduce automatically reinforced aggression included response blocking and giving the child access to alternative forms of chin stimulation. This study is instructive because it shows how multiple aggressive responses can have different sources of operant control and require separate function-based intervention plans.

Future studies should explore other clinical situations in which aggression and noncompliance are automatically reinforced. I have seen two cases where behavior-contingent sensory consequences appeared to reinforce aggression. One case was an adolescent boy with autism who slapped his teacher and parents. Observation and FBA results pointed to audible feedback as the source of reinforcement. That is, the boy displayed aggression because he enjoyed the sound that his slapping produced! The second case was a 6-year-old girl with autism who demonstrated aggression towards peers and adults by pulling their hair. This behavior was evident in many contexts, seemingly maintained by the girl visually inspecting strands of hair that she pulled. Similar to these examples, it is possible that noncompliance also could be automatically reinforced, for example, through physical contact that is provided when a practitioner uses "hand over hand" guidance to prompt responding. Although automatic reinforcement is less likely to be the primary source of control for child aggression and noncompliance (Thompson & Iwata, 2001), all potential influences on behavior should be considered so that practitioners have available the greatest selection of potentially effective intervention procedures.

Intervention Recommendations

The evidence-based and empirically supported procedures reviewed in this chapter give practitioners many options for intervention with children who have ASD, aggression, and noncompliance. Whereas the earliest ABA approaches to aggression and noncompliance were not function-based and often relied on punishment (Luiselli, 2004), our perspective on intervention has widened, emphasizing FBA, FA, antecedent control, and positive behavior support. Aggression and noncompliance certainly are two of the most difficult-to-manage problem behaviors confronting practitioners. Notably, research has endorsed several intervention procedures that are well suited to school, home, and community settings. Nonetheless, there are additional intervention recommendations, which I present in this final section.

Establishing Operations

Establishing operations (EOs) are defined as "events, operations, or stimulus conditions that establish the capacity of classes of consequences to serve as reinforcement and increase the frequency of behaviors that have produced members of these classes in the past" (Friman & Hawkins, 2006, p. 33). In function, EOs relate to states of deprivation and satiation, most evident with food as primary reinforcement. Hunger (a state of deprivation) will increase the reinforcing properties of food and the behavior of food-seeking. Conversely, when a person is not hungry (a state of satiation), food is less reinforcing and food-seeking stops.

Detailed reviews of how EOs influence problem behaviors can be found in McGill (1999) and Friman and Hawkins (2006). Imagine a child with ASD who has attention-maintained aggression. Intervention based on the concept of EOs might consist of giving the child social attention noncontingently on an FT schedule throughout the day. Providing attention this way would function as intervention by eliminating the child's motivation to seek social consequences through aggression. Another example would be a child who shows escape motivated noncompliance during educational activities. Teaching the child to request a "break"

from activities through FCT or having breaks scheduled noncontingently would be another alteration of EOs.

Both *distal events* and *biological* conditions also can function as EOs for problem behaviors by temporarily changing the impact of environmental contingencies. Poor sleep the night before school could result in more frequent escape motivated noncompliance compared to evenings without sleep disturbance (O'Reilly, 1995). A child's aggression towards teachers and parents may increase when she/he has allergy-induced distress (Kennedy & Meyer, 1996) or an ear infection (Luiselli, Cochran, & Huber, 2005; O'Reilly, 1997). Such influences must be assessed so that if applicable, proper behavioral intervention or medical treatment can be applied.

Intervention Integrity

The most carefully formulated and function-based intervention plan can only be effective if practitioners implement it accurately. Intervention integrity refers to procedural fidelity: is a plan carried out as written? For aggression and noncompliance, the concern about intervention integrity is particularly salient because most plans combine antecedent and consequence procedures (Ricciardi, 2006). Furthermore, practitioners typically are responsible for data collection as another component of intervention. The requirement of following a multi-procedural plan and recording data can easily compromise implementation.

Intervention integrity should be assessed routinely by observing practitioners implement procedures and documenting their performance. The observer should have a recording form that lists all procedures comprising the intervention plan and a respective scoring section with integrity measures such as, "implemented as written" and "not implemented as written" (Codding, Feinberg, Dunn, & Pace, 2005). Immediately following observation, the performance results are reviewed with the practitioners, pointing out accurate implementation and correcting misapplication. This performance feedback can be delivered with written comments and/or visual inspection of integrity data (Hagermoser Sanetti, Luiselli, & Handler, 2007). Sufficient research exists supporting these methods for improving intervention integrity (Hagermoser Sanetti & Kratochwill, 2008).

Social Validity

How acceptable to practitioners are intervention procedures targeting aggression and noncompliance? Procedures that are judged poorly can be a further impediment to intervention integrity because a practitioner may be reluctant to apply them conscientiously. Social validity labeled as "consumer satisfaction" has been a concern in ABA for sometime (Wolf, 1978). More recently, Kennedy (2002) proposed that limited maintenance outcomes from behavioral intervention sometimes can be attributed to poor acceptance by practitioners. Clearly, positive results from intervention will not persist if practitioners resist implementation because they "don't like" the procedures.

Cautious attention should be paid to the acceptability of intervention procedures in dealing with children who physically challenge practitioners with aggression and do not follow directions when instructed. Facing actual or threatened aggression, as well as chronic noncompliance, creates a burden that is less apparent with children who do not have serious problem behaviors. Some of the considerations in selecting procedures are whether they require physical contact with a child (e.g., guided compliance, response blocking, physical restraint), include unique precautions (e.g., a practitioner wears protective equipment to prevent injury), or are socially stigmatizing. Asking practitioners to judge procedures on these and similar characteristics speaks to the sustainability of intervention within natural settings (Dunlap, Carr, Horner, Zarcone, & Schwartz, 2008).

Restrictive Procedures

As noted, intervention procedures such as escape extinction and guided compliance require physical contact with a child. *Physical restraint* is another restrictive procedure that has been used as intervention with people who have developmental disabilities and serious problem behaviors (Harris, 1996). When applying physical restraint, one or more practitioners immobilizes a person's voluntary movement. Many times, physical restraint is required to manage unanticipated emergency situations where there is a threat of harm to self, others, and the environment. However, planned physical restraint sometimes is justified as an acceptable behavior-reduction procedure within a comprehensive intervention plan (Federal Statutes and Policies Governing the ICF/MR Program, 2003).

There are several studies in which physical restraint, alone and combined with other procedures, has decreased aggression in people with ASD and related developmental disabilities (Luiselli, Suskin, & Slocumb, 1984; Matson & Keyes, 1988; Rolider, Williams, Cummings, & Van Houten, 1991). However, physical restraint is an invasive procedure that can be misapplied, causing injury to the person being restrained and the people responsible for implementation (Hill & Spreat, 1987). Physical restraint also can provoke additional problem behaviors, seen typically when a person resists or struggles against being immobilized. A further complication is that in some cases, physical restraint could maintain problem behaviors because it functions as positive or negative reinforcement (Favell, McGimsey, & Jones, 1978; Magee & Ellis, 1988). And, although some practitioners may be inclined to use physical restraint because it stops problem behaviors, many view the procedure as unacceptable (Cunningham, McDonnell, Easton, & Sturmey, 2003; McDonnell & Sturmey, 2000).

Acknowledging the disadvantages of physical restraint, it is desirable to reduce implementation to those cases where it is clinically justified. One intervention approach, illustrated in a study by Luiselli, Kane, Treml, and Young (2000), is to modify antecedent conditions that provoke the behaviors requiring restraint. The participants were two boys, 14 and 16 years old, who had PDD and attended a residential school. Both boys were aggressive towards peers and staff (hitting, biting, scratching, kicking). During a 1-month baseline phase, staff implemented several procedures, including physical restraint, according to student-specific intervention plans. The plans had staff deliver pleasurable consequences to the students when they demonstrated positive behavior and did not exhibit aggression. Staff applied physical restraint with the boys when they determined that aggression was unmanageable. Next, intervention was changed so that physical restraint was implemented according to behavior-specific criteria and not arbitrarily determined by staff. A second intervention phase subsequently was evaluated in which several antecedent control procedures were introduced, each designed to reduce the escape function of aggression and in consequence, producing fewer incidents of physical restraint. For one of the students, staff were taught to detect behaviors indicating he was becoming upset and often predicted aggression. Upon observing these precursor behaviors, staff directed the boy to take time away from his group until he was composed. Functional communication training also was provided so that he could request a break from instruction. With the second student, the antecedent procedures were giving him more access to novel activities, reducing sedentary tasks in favor of more preferred interactions with staff, and placing him strategically within groups so that he had less proximity to peers.

Luiselli et al. (2000) found that implementing behavior-specific criterion for physical restraint as the first intervention procedure was ineffective. Subsequently, physical restraint decreased and remained at near-zero frequency when the same criteria were maintained in conjunction with the antecedent intervention procedures. These and similar procedures should remain a priority when physical restraint or other restrictive procedures are considered as behavioral intervention for children with ASD (Lerman, 2008).

Skill Building Intervention

Many children with ASD display aggression and noncompliance because they are unable to contact positive reinforcement through alternative behaviors. In particular, poor social skills contribute greatly to attention maintained and escape motivated problem behaviors. A child who does not socialize appropriately with peers and adults may learn to hit them as a way to elicit attention. Or, being unable to enjoy social interactions could result in escape motivated noncompliance. A logical approach in such circumstances is to teach a child the skills needed to initiate and maintain social interactions.

Machalicek et al. (2008) outlined five categories of social skills that have been studied in intervention research with children who have ASD: conversation, cooperation, nonverbal responding, pivotal behaviors, and play. Various procedures have been evaluated with each of these social skills. *Priming,* as one example, is an antecedent procedure that includes modeling, instruction, and demonstration of behaviors to be performed and reinforced in a later social context (Licciardello, Harchik & Luiselli, 2008; Zanolli & Daggett, 1998). *Peer-mediated* intervention involves teaching typically developing peers to initiate social contact with and engage a child with ASD in mutually pleasurable social exchanges such as conversation and games (Gonzalex-Lopez & Kamps, 1997). More recently, computerized video modeling has become a useful procedure for improving social skills (LeBlanc et al., 2003; Simpson, Langone, & Ayres, 2004). The procedure consists of taping a video sequence of a child with ASD, a peer, or adult performing specific social skills and then showing the tape to the child prior to interaction opportunities. These and other procedures provide a rich selection for practitioners in building adaptive social skills.

Summary

ABA has been instrumental in assessment and intervention for aggression and noncompliance in children who have ASD. Proper assessment begins by operationally defining the behaviors to permit reliable measurement before and during intervention. Functional behavioral assessment (FBA) and functional analysis (FA) should precede intervention in order to isolate controling influences on aggression and noncompliance. Social positive reinforcement, social negative reinforcement, and automatic reinforcement are three categories emphasized in FBA and FA. Some of the evidence-based and empirically supported intervention procedures that can be matched to behavior-function include social extinction, differential positive reinforcement, FCT, NCR, NCE, instructional fading, and modifying verbal directions. Other contributions to effective intervention are studying the role of EOs, assessing procedural fidelity, documenting social validity, monitoring implementation of restrictive methods, and teaching social skills.

References

Adelinis, J. D., & Hagopian, L. P. (1999). The use of symmetrical "do" and "don't" requests to interrupt ongoing activities. *Journal of Applied Behavior Analysis, 32*, 519–523.

Bijou, S. W., Peterson, R. F., & Ault, M. H. (1968). A method to integrate descriptive and experimental field studies at the level of data and empirical concepts. *Journal of Applied BehaviorAnalysis, 1*, 175–191.

Butler, L. R., & Luiselli, J. K. (2007). Escape maintained problem behavior in a child with autism: Antecedent functional analysis and intervention evaluation of noncontingent escape (NCE) and instructional fading. *Journal of Positive Behavior Interventions, 9*, 195–202.

Carr, E. G., & Durand, V. M. (1985). Reducing behavior problems through functional communication training. *Journal of Applied Behavior Analysis, 18*, 111–126.

Carr, J. E., & LeBlanc, L. A. (2006). Noncontingent reinforcement as antecedent behavior support. In J. K. Luiselli (Ed.), *Antecedent control: Innovative approaches to behavior support* (pp. 147–164). Baltimore, MD: Paul H. Brookes Publishing Co.

Carr, E. G., Newsom, C. D., & Binkoff, J. A. (1980). Escape as a factor in the aggressive behavior of two retarded children. *Journal of Applied Behavior Analysis, 13*, 101–117.

Carr, E. G., Yarbrough, S. C., & Langdon, N. A. (1997). Effects of idiosyncratic stimulus variables on functional analysis outcomes. *Journal of Applied Behavior Analysis, 30*, 673–686.

Codding, R. S., Feinberg, A. B., Dunn, E. K., & Pace, G. M. (2005). Effects of immediate performance feedback on implementation of behavior support plans. *Journal of Applied Behavior Analysis, 38*, 205–219.

Cunningham, J., McDonnell, A., Easton, S., & Sturmey, P. (2003). Social validation data on three methods of physical restraint: Views of consumers, staff, and students. *Research in Developmental Disabilities, 24*, 307–316.

Detrich, R. (2008). Evidence-based, empirically supported, or best practice? A guide for the scientist practitioner. In J. K. Luiselli, S. Wilczynski, D. C. Russo & W. P. Christian (Eds.), *Effective practices for children with autism: Educational and behavior support interventions that work* (pp. 3–25). New York, NY: Oxford University Press.

Dunlap, G., Carr, E. G., Horner, R. H., Zarcone, J. R., & Schwartz, I. (2008). Positive behavior support and applied behavior analysis: A familial alliance. *Behavior Modification, 32*, 682–698.

Durand, V. M., & Crimmins, D. B. (1988). Identifying the variables maintaining self-injurious behavior. *Journal of Autism and Developmental Disorders, 18*, 99–117.

Favell, J. E., McGimsey, J. F., & Jones, M. L. (1978). The use of physical restraint in the treatment of self-injury and as positive reinforcement. *Journal of Applied Behavior Analysis, 11*, 225–241.

Federal Statutes, Regulations, and Policies Governing the ICF/MR program. (2003). Retrieved from http://cms.hhs.gov/medicaid/icfmr/icfregs.asp

Friman, P. C., & Hawkins, R. O. (2006). Contribution of establishing operations to antecedent intervention. In J. K. Luiselli (Ed.), *Antecedent control: Innovative approaches to behavior support* (pp. 31–52). Baltimore, MD: Paul H. Brookes Publishing Co.

Gonzalex-Lopez, A., & Kamps, D. M. (1997). Social skills training to increase social interactions between children with autism and their typical peers. *Focus on Autism and Other Developmental Disabilities, 12*, 2–15.

Hagermoser Sanetti, L. M., & Kratochwill, T. R. (2008). Treatment integrity in behavioral consultation: Measurement, promotion, and outcomes. *International Journal of Behavioral Consultation and Therapy, 4*, 95–114.

Hagermoser Sanetti, L. M., Luiselli, J. K., & Handler, M. L. (2007). Effects of verbal and graphic performance feedback on behavior support plan implementation in a public elementary school. *Behavior Modification, 31*, 454–465.

Hagopian, L. P., Fisher, W. W., & Legacy, S. M. (1994). Schedule effects of noncontingent reinforcement on attention-maintained destructive behavior in identical quadruplets. *Journal of Applied Behavior Analysis, 27*, 317–325.

Hanley, G. P., Iwata, B. A., & McCord, B. E. (2003). Functional analysis of problem behavior: A review. *Journal of Applied Behavior Analysis, 36*, 147–185.

Harris, J. (1996). Physical restraint procedures for managing challenging behaviors presented by mentally retarded adults and children. *Research in Developmental Disabilities, 17*, 99–134.

Hill, J., & Spreat, S. (1987). Staff injury rates associated with the implementation of contingent restraint. *Mental Retardation, 25*, 141–145.

Iwata, B. A. (1995). *Functional analysis screening tool (FAST)*. Gainesville, FL: University of Florida.

Iwata, B. A., Dorsey, M. F., Slifer, K. J., Bauman, K. E., & Richman, G. S. (1994). Toward a functional analysis of self-injury. *Journal of Applied Behavior Analysis, 27*, 197–209. Reprinted from Analysis and Intervention in Developmental Disabilities, 2, 3–20, 1982.

Iwata, B. A., Pace, G. M., Kalsher, M. J., Cowdery, G. E., & Cataldo, M. F. (1990). Experimental analysis and extinction of self-injurious escape behavior. *Journal of Applied Behavior Analysis, 23*, 11–27.

Iwata, B. A., Wallace, M. D., Kahng, S., Lindeberg, J. S., Roscoe, E. M., Conners, J., et al. (2000). Skill acquisition in the implementation of functional analysis methodology. *Journal of Applied Behavior Analysis, 33*, 181–194.

Johnson, L., McComas, J., Thompson, A., & Symons, F. J. (2004). Obtained versus programmed reinforcement: Practical considerations in the treatment of escape-reinforced aggression. *Journal of Applied Behavior Analysis, 37*, 239–242.

Kahng, S., Abt, K. A., & Schonbachler, H. E. (2001). Assessment and treatment of low-rate high-intensity problem behavior. *Journal of Applied Behavior Analysis, 34*, 225–228.

Kennedy, C. H. (2002). The maintenance of behavior change as an indicator of social validity. *Behavior Modification, 26*, 594–604.

Kennedy, C. H., & Meyer, K. A. (1996). Sleep deprivation, allergy symptoms, and negatively reinforced behavior. *Journal of Applied Behavior Analysis, 29*, 133–135.

Kern, L., & Kokina, A. (2008). Using positive reinforcement to decrease challenging behavior. In J. K. Luiselli, S. Wilczynski, D. C. Russo & W. P. Christian (Eds.), *Effective practices for children with autism: Educational and behavior support interventions that work* (pp. 413–432). New York, NY: Oxford University Press.

Kodak, T., Northup, J., & Kelley, M. E. (2007). An evaluation of the types of attention that maintain problem behavior. *Journal of Applied Behavior Analysis, 40,* 167–171.

LeBlanc, L., Coates, A., Daneshvar, S., Charlop-Christy, M., Morris, C., & Lancaster, B. (2003). Using video modeling and reinforcement to teach perspective-taking skills to children with autism. *Journal of Applied Behavior Analysis, 36,* 253–257.

Lerman, D. C. (2008). Behavior-contingent (restrictive) intervention: A function-based approach. In J. K. Luiselli, S. Wilczynski, D. C. Russo & W. P. Christian (Eds.), *Effective practices for children with autism: Educational and behavior support interventions that work* (pp. 433–454). New York, NY: Oxford University Press.

Lerman, D. C., & Rapp, J. T. (2006). Antecedent assessment and intervention for stereotypy. In J. K. Luiselli (Ed.), *Antecedent control: Innovative approaches to behavior support* (pp. 125–146). Baltimore, MD: Paul H. Brookes Publishing Co.

Licciardello, C. C., Harchik, A. E., & Luiselli, J. K. (2008). Social skills intervention for children with autism during interactive play at a public elementary school. *Education and Treatment of Children, 31,* 27–37.

Luiselli, J. K. (1990). Reinforcement control of assaultive behavior in a sensory impaired child. *Behavioral Residential Treatment, 5,* 45–53.

Luiselli, J. K. (2004). Behavior support and intervention: Current issues and practices in developmental disabilities. In J. L. Matson, R. B. Laud & M. L. Matson (Eds.), *Behavior modification for persons with developmental disabilities: Treatments and supports* (pp. 33–54). Kingston, NY: NADD.

Luiselli, J. K. (2006). *Antecedent assessment and intervention: Supporting children and adults with developmental disabilities in community settings.* Baltimore, MD: Paul H. Brookes.

Luiselli, J. K. (2008). Antecedent (preventive) intervention. In J. K. Luiselli, S. Wilczynski, D. C. Russo & W. P. Christian (Eds.), *Effective practices for children with autism: Educational and behavior support interventions that work* (pp. 393–412). New York, NY: Oxford University Press.

Luiselli, J. K., Cochran, M. L., & Huber, S. A. (2005). Effects of otitis media on a child with autism receiving behavioral intervention for self-injury. *Child & Family Behavior Therapy, 27,* 51–56.

Luiselli, J. K., Kane, A., Treml, T., & Young, N. (2000). Behavioral intervention to reduce physical restraint of adolescents with developmental disabilities. *Behavioral Interventions, 15,* 317–330.

Luiselli, J. K., Russo, D. C., Christian, W. P., & Wilczynski, S. (eds.). (2008). *Effective Practices for Children with Autism: Educational and Behavior Support Interventions that Work.* New York: Oxford University Press.

Luiselli, J. K., & Slocumb, P. R. (1984). Management of multiple aggressive behaviors by differential reinforcement. *Journal of Behavior Therapy and Experimental Psychiatry, 14,* 343–347.

Luiselli, J. K., Suskin, L., & Slocumb, P. R. (1984). Application of immobilization time-out in management programming with developmentally disabled children. *Child & Family Behavior Therapy, 6,* 1–15.

Mace, F. C., Hock, M. L., Lalli, J. S., West, B. J., Belfiore, P., Pinter, E., et al. (1988). Behavioral momentum in the treatment of noncompliance. *Journal of Applied Behavior Analysis, 21,* 123–141.

Machalicek, W., Davis, T., O'Reilly, M., Beretvas, N., Sigafoos, J., Lancioni, G., et al. (2008). Teaching social skills in school settings. In J. K. Luiselli, S. Wilczynski, D. C. Russo & W. P. Christian (Eds.), *Effective practices for children with autism: Educational and behavior support interventions that work* (pp. 269–298). New York, NY: Oxford University Press.

Magee, S. K., & Ellis, J. (1988). The detrimental effects of physical restraint as a consequence for inappropriate classroom behavior. *Journal of Applied Behavior Analysis, 34,* 501–504.

Matson, J. L., & Keyes, J. (1988). Contingent reinforcement and contingent restraint to treat severe aggression and self-injury in mentally retarded and autistic adults. *Journal of the Multihandicapped Person, 1,* 141–153.

Matson, J. L., Laud, R. B., & Matson, M. L. (2004). *Behavior modification for persons with developmental disabilities: Treatments and supports.* Kingston, NY: NADD Press.

Matson, J. L., & Minshawi, N. F. (2007). Functional assessment of challenging behavior: Toward a strategy for applied settings. *Research in Developmental Disabilities, 28,* 353–361.

Matson, J. L., & Vollmer, T. R. (1995). *User's guide: Questions about behavioral function (QABF).* Baton Rouge, LA: Scientific Publishers.

McDonnell, A. A., & Sturmey, P. (2000). The social validation of three physical restraint procedures: A comparison of young people and professional groups. *Research in Developmental Disabilities, 21,* 85–92.

McGill, P. (1999). Establishing operations: Implications for the assessment, treatment, and prevention of problem behavior. *Journal of Applied Behavior Analysis, 32,* 393–418.

Moore, J. W., Edwards, R. P., Sterling-Turner, H. E., Riley, J., DuBard, M., & McGeorge, A. (2002). Teacher acquisition of functional analysis methodology. *Journal of Applied Behavior Analysis, 35,* 73–77.

Moore, J. M., & Fisher, W. W. (2007). The effects of videotape modeling on staff acquisition of functional analysis methodology. *Journal of Applied Behavior Analysis, 40,* 197–202.

Mueller, M. M., Wilczynski, S. M., Moore, J. W., Fusilier, I., & Trahant, D. (2001). Antecedent manipulations in a tangible condition: Effects of stimulus preference on aggression. *Journal of Applied Behavior Analysis, 34,* 237–240.

O'Neill, R. E., Horner, R. H., Albin, R. W., Sprague, J. R., Storey, K., & Newton, J. S. (1997). *Functional assessment and program development for problem behavior: A practical handbook.* Pacific Grove, CA: Brookes/Cole.

O'Reilly, M. F. (1995). Functional analysis and treatment of escape-maintained aggression correlated with sleep deprivation. *Journal of Applied Behavior Analysis, 28,* 225–226.

O'Reilly, M. F. (1997). Functional analysis of episodic self-injury correlated with recurrent otitis media. *Journal of Applied Behavior Analysis, 30,* 165–167.

O'Reilly, M. F., Cannella, H. I., Sigafoos, J., & Lancioni, G. (2006). Communication and social skills interventions. In J. K. Luiselli (Ed.), *Antecedent control: Innovative approaches to behavior support* (pp. 187–206). Baltimore, MD: Paul H. Brookes Publishing Co.

Peyton, R., Lindauer, S. E., & Richman, D. M. (2005). The effects of directive and nondirective prompts on noncompliant vocal behavior exhibited by a child with autism. *Journal of Applied Behavior Analysis, 38,* 251–255.

Piazza, C. C., Fisher, W. W., Hagopian, L. P., Bowman, L. G., & Toole, L. (1996). Using a choice assessment to predict reinforcer effectiveness. *Journal of Applied Behavior Analysis, 29,* 1–9.

Progar, P. R., North, S. T., Bruce, S. S., DiNovi, B. J., Nau, P. A., Eberman, E. M., et al. (2001). Putative behavioral history effects and aggression maintained by escape from therapists. *Journal of Applied Behavior Analysis, 34,* 69–72.

Ricciardi, J. N. (2006). Combining antecedent and consequence procedures in multicomponent behavior support plans: A guide to writing plans with functional efficacy. In J. K. Luiselli (Ed.), *Antecedent control: Innovative approaches to behavior support* (pp. 227–245). Baltimore, MD: Paul H. Brookes Publishing Co.

Rolider, A., Williams, L., Cummings, A., & Van Houten, R. (1991). The use of a brief movement restriction procedure to eliminate severe inappropriate behavior. *Journal of Behavior Therapy and Experimental Psychiatry, 22,* 23–30.

Russo, D. C., Cataldo, M. F., & Cushing, P. J. (1981). Compliance training and behavioral covariation in the treatment of multiple behavior problems. *Journal of Applied Behavior Analysis, 14,* 209–222.

Simpson, A., Langone, J., & Ayres, K. (2004). Embedded video and computer based instruction to improve social skills for students with autism. *Education and Training in Developmental Disabilities, 39,* 240–252.

Skinner, B. F. (1948). "Superstition" in the pigeon. *Journal of Experimental Psychology, 38,* 168–172.

Smith, R. G., Iwata, B. A., Goh, H. L., & Shore, B. A. (1995). Analysis of establishing operations in self-injury maintained by escape. *Journal of Applied Behavior Analysis, 28,* 515–535.

Thompson, R. H., Fisher, W. W., Piazza, C. C., & Kuhn, D. E. (1998). The evaluation and treatment of aggression maintained by attention and automatic reinforcement. *Journal of Applied Behavior Analysis, 31,* 103–116.

Thompson, R. H., & Iwata, B. A. (2001). A descriptive analysis of social consequences following problem behavior. *Journal of Applied Behavior Analysis, 34,* 169–178.

Touchette, P. E., MacDonald, R. F., & Langer, S. N. (1985). A scatter plot for identifying stimulus control of problem behavior. *Journal of Applied Behavior Analysis, 18,* 343–351.

Wilder, D. A., Saulnier, R., Beavers, G., & Zonneveld, K. (2008). Contingent access to preferred items versus a guided compliance procedure to increase compliance among preschoolers. *Education and Treatment of Children, 31,* 297–305.

Wolf, M. M. (1978). Social validity: The case for subjective measurement or how applied behavior analysis is finding its heart. *Journal of Applied Behavior Analysis, 11,* 203–214.

Zanolli, K., & Daggett, J. (1998). The effects of reinforcement rate on the spontaneous social initiations of socially withdrawn preschoolers. *Journal of Applied Behavior Analysis, 31,* 117–125.

Zarcone, J. R., Iwata, B. A., Vollmer, T. A., Jagtiani, S., Smith, R. G., & Mazaleski, J. L. (1993). Extinction of self-injurious escape behavior with and without instructional fading. *Journal of Applied Behavior Analysis, 26,* 353–360.

Chapter 11
Adaptive and Self-Help Skills

Noha F. Minshawi, Iryna Ashby, and Naomi Swiezy

Independence is a major concern for children with ASD, particularly with the large percentage who also have intellectual disability. This chapter will cover common adaptive and self-help problems those children evince, procedures used to train these skills and potential future research needs.

Introduction

An area of increasing importance in the treatment of children and adults with autism spectrum disorders (ASD) is adaptive skills training. Adaptive skills first came into awareness as the definition of intellectual disability (ID) became further specified in the early 1900s (Doll, 1936). The current American Association of Mental Retardation's (AAMR) definition of ID defines adaptive behavior as being "...expressed in conceptual, social, and practical adaptive skills" (American Association on Mental Retardation, 2002). More specifically, the authors of the *Diagnostic and Statistical Manual of Mental Disorders* (DSM-IV-TR; American Psychological Association, 2000) define adaptive skills deficits in the definition of mental retardation (i.e., ID) as limitations in at least two of eight adaptive behavior domains: Communication, self-care, home living, social/interpersonal skills, work, leisure, health, and safety. In addition, Sparrow, Balla, and Cicchetti (1984) further emphasize the functional nature of adaptive skills by defining adaptive functioning as the development and application of abilities required for gaining personal independence and social sufficiency.

Interest in the assessment and treatment of adaptive skills has increased considerably in recent years due to the focus placed on these behaviors by the DSM-IV-TR (American Psychological Association, 2000), as well as several other factors. One such factor is the increasing importance placed on improving the functional ability of individuals with developmental disorders as opposed to reducing the severity of the symptoms they experience (Winters, Collett, & Myers, 2005). In addition, the realization that reduction in symptomatology does not necessarily result in a corresponding increase in functional skills has further propelled the drive towards more thorough assessments and interventions for adaptive skills (Winters et al., 2005).

The importance of adaptive skills cannot be overemphasized in the lives of individuals with ASD and other developmental disabilities. Adaptive skill development in young children begins the process of developing independence from caregivers. In adulthood, an individual's ability to manage the everyday demands of life determines the degree to which he or she can live independently (Liss et al., 2001). Furthermore, deficits in adaptive skills (specifically communication and daily living skills) are believed to underlie the etiology of severe behavior problems (e.g., aggression, self-injury) in individuals with developmental disabilities (Baghdadli, Pascal, Grisi, & Aussilloux, 2003).

The focus of this chapter is to review methods for teaching adaptive and self-help skills to individuals with ASD that are derived from applied behavior analysis (ABA). The chapter will begin with an overview of the types of adaptive skills deficits seen in individuals with ASD and how these deficits compare with

N. Swiezy (✉)
Clinical Psychology in Psychiatry, Clinical Director,
Christian Sarkine Autism Treatment Center,
Riley Hospital for children, 702 Barnhill Drive, Rm. 4300,
Indianapolis, IN, 46202-5000, USA
e-mail: nswiezy@iupui.edu

J.L. Maston (ed.), *Applied Behavior Analysis for Children with Autism Spectrum Disorders*,
DOI 10.1007/978-1-4419-0088-3_11, © Springer Science+Business Media, LLC 2009

those seen in individuals with other types of developmental disabilities. A review of standardized assessment measures will then follow, as accurate assessment of an individual's strengths and weaknesses is the first step toward designing an effective skills training program. Selection of skills to target, as well as specific techniques used to teach adaptive skills, will also be discussed.

Adaptive Skills Deficits in ASD

Among individuals with ASD, adaptive skills deficits are considered to be of key concern. Two types of adaptive skills, communication and social skills, are part of the diagnostic criteria for ASD and are hallmark characteristics of these disorders. Therefore, it is not surprising that children with ASD have lower adaptive skills than neurotypically developing children. Children with ASD have consistently been shown to demonstrate more severe deficits in adaptive functioning than cognitive functioning. Children with autism have greater deficits in adaptive behavior than children matched for age and intelligence (Carpentieri & Morgan, 1996; Volkmar et al., 1987). Furthermore, children with autism can be differentiated from children with Pervasive Developmental Disorder, Not Otherwise Specified (PDD-NOS) and other developmental disabilities on the basis of their scores on the socialization and daily living skills domains of adaptive behavior instruments (Gillham, Carter, Volkmar, & Sparrow, 2000).

The long-term impact of adaptive skills deficits has been demonstrated in individuals with ASD. In fact, deficits in adaptive behavior become more evident as children with ASD get older (Lord & Schopler, 1989). Jacobson and Ackerman (1990) reported that while children with autism between the ages of 5 and 12 years demonstrated higher scores on measures of daily living skills than children with ID, these differences were not found in adulthood. These authors reported that adults with autism demonstrated significantly fewer daily living skills than adults with ID.

Howlin, Mawhood, and Rutter (2000) reported on a British sample of adults with ASD stating that only 5% of individuals were employed and that 72% had little independence in the area of daily living skills. Furthermore, nearly half of the sample lived in residential facilities and 31% lived with their parents. These

trends have been seen in a North American sample as well. Ballaban-Gil, Rapin, Tuchman, and Shinnar (1996) found that only 11% of adults with ASD held a job (primarily entry-level positions), and 16% worked in sheltered vocational workshops. Approximately half of the individuals in this sample lived in residential placements. Strikingly, Ballaban-Gil et al. (1996) found that even among individuals with average intellectual functioning, 23% still lived in supervised settings.

Adaptive skills take on additional importance in individuals with ASD due to the potential limitations in intellectual or cognitive testing in this population. The relationship between adaptive behavior and intellectual functioning has been researched considerably. In general, a moderate correlation has been reported between adaptive behavior and measures of intelligence (Carpentieri & Morgan, 1996; Dacey, Nelson, & Stoeckel, 1999; Sparrow et al., 1984). In addition, Vig and Jedrysek (1995) reported a higher correlation between intelligence and adaptive skills for children with lower intelligence quotients and diagnoses of Autistic Disorder than for higher functioning children with no comorbid diagnoses.

However, recently researchers have called into question the validity of standardized intelligence tests in determining the intellectual functioning of individuals with ASD. Some researchers have indicated that current measures of intelligence do not accurately assess cognitive potential in individuals with ASD, especially young children (Magiati & Howlin, 2001). Evidence for this argument comes primarily from studies that fail to show consistent correlations between intelligence scores and measures of adaptive behavior (e.g., Magiati & Howlin, 2001; Roberts, McCoy, Reidy, & Cruciti, 1993; Szatmari et al., 2002; Tsatsanis et al., 2003). Assessments of intelligence provide estimates of cognitive potential, whereas measures of adaptive behavior provide information about an individual's current observable behavior. Therefore, focus has begun to shift more towards assessment of adaptive skills in individuals with ASD as opposed to cognitive functioning (Kraijer, 2000).

Assessment of Adaptive Skills

The comprehensive assessment of adaptive skills is an important component to the diagnosis and treatment of nearly all individuals with developmental or mental health disorders. The assessment of adaptive skills should include a combination of techniques in order to provide a comprehensive assessment. Typically, assessment begins with the use of a standardized instrument that assesses multiple domains of adaptive skills. A variety of standardized measures are available for the assessment of adaptive behavior in individuals with intellectual and developmental disabilities. A brief review of three of the primary measures is provided below. Completing a standardized adaptive skills instrument provides clinicians with information on the individual's functioning in a number of broad areas. Specific strengths and weaknesses can be indentified and provide direction for further assessment and treatment, as well as a method of measuring improvement over time.

Following an overview of the individual's adaptive strengths and weaknesses, assessment should then be conducted directly by the clinician under more naturalistic circumstances. Naturalistic observation is an important component to any assessment as it can provide additional information on the individual's actual performance of skills in real-world settings. Direct observation is also crucial for determining which methods of training may be most effective for the individual, as well as providing information on aspects of the individual's environment and learning style that will influence treatment.

Standardized Assessments

Vineland Adaptive Behavior Scales

Since its publication in 1984, the *Vineland Adaptive Behavior Scales (VABS;* Sparrow et al., 1984) has gained respect among clinical and research professionals for the assessment of adaptive behavior of individuals (Balboni, Pedrabissi, Molteni, & Villa, 2001; De Bildt, Kraijer, Sytema, & Minderaa, 2005; Freeman, Del'Homme, Guthrie, & Zhang, 1999; Oakland & Houchins, 1985). The two forms of the scale (the Survey Form and the Expanded Form) cover the areas of adaptive behavior in the following four domains: Communication, Daily Living Skills, and Socialization. In addition, the VABS includes an optional Motor Skills domain, which assesses gross and fine motor skills for children under 6 years old and a Maladaptive

Behavior domain for children over 5 years of age. The Survey Form is intended for screening and assessment based on 297 items, whereas the Expanded Form, which covers 577 items, is intended to be used in rehabilitation or residential treatment programs (Oakland & Houchins, 1985). The administration of both forms of the VABS requires a trained interviewer. The parent or caregiver interviewed should be familiar with the child in order to answer questions that target everyday behavior. Scores are calculated for each domain and then converted to a standardized composite score and an Adaptive Behavior Composite (mean = 100, and standard deviation = 15).

The VABS provides a number of benefits to its users. The VABS assesses actual functional skills and provides a good prediction of social adaptation and long-term outcome (Freeman, Ritvo, Yokota, Childs, & Pollard, 1988). Since time constraints are a reality for many professionals, the flexibility of using the shorter Survey Form (20–60 min to administer), versus the longer Expanded Form (60–90 min to administer) may be beneficial. The comprehensive content of the Survey Form meets the needs of various situations, and a semi-structured method of interviewing allows more freedom in forming questions and eliciting responses from the caregiver (Sparrow et al., 1984). The extensive investigation of the psychometric properties of the VABS and its use in research (Burack & Volkmar, 1992; Kraijer, 2000; Paul et al., 2004; Volkmar et al., 1987) have made the VABS the de facto gold-standard for both clinical and research use.

Vineland Adaptive Behavior Scales-II (VABS-II)

The *Vineland Adaptive Behavior Scales – II* (VABS-II) is a revision of the VABS (Sparrow et al., 1984) that was first released in 2005. Compared to the earlier edition, the VABS-II underwent many changes, including the expansion of the age range. The current version covers from birth to 90 years of age. In addition, the quality of items has been enhanced and the number of items in each domain has been increased (Sparrow, Cicchetti, & Balla, 2005). Similar to the VABS, the VABS-II has 4 domains (Communication, Daily Living Skills, Socialization, and Motor Skills) and 11 subdomains. The current version of the measure contains two survey forms (the Survey Interview Form, which is interview-based, and the Parent/Caregiver Rating Form, which is rating scale-based), as well as the Expanded Interview Form. The Expanded Interview Form contains 577 items and allows for a more thorough assessment of adaptive behavior. This form can be used either by itself or as a follow-up measure to establish the basis for an educational or treatment program (Sparrow et al., 2005).

Administration of the VABS-II Survey Interview Form requires that the interviewer be trained in conducting a semi-structured interview and further computation of results. However, parents or caregivers can independently complete the Rating Form without training as long as they are familiar with the everyday behavior of the individual being assessed. Scoring is conducted in the same manner as for VABS, (mean = 100 and standard deviation = 15).

Finally, the *Vineland Adaptive Behavior Scales, Teacher Rating Form* (VABS-TRF; Sparrow et al., 2005) was developed concurrently with the VABS-II survey forms based on the revision of the *Vineland Adaptive Behavior Scales, Classroom Edition.* This comprehensive measure can be used to assess students from 3 through 21 years old to determine their eligibility for intervention in school settings. The VABS-TRF should be completed by teachers or day-care providers who are familiar with the child and can give an account of his or her behavior in the four broad domains: Communication, Daily Living Skills, Socialization, and Motor Skills. The VABS-TRF is an effective and useful instrument to assess adaptive behavior of students in the classroom (Sparrow et al., 2005).

The American Association of Mental Retardation's Adaptive Behavior Scale – Residential and Community, Second Edition

The American Association of Mental Retardation's Adaptive Behavior Scale – Residential and Community, Second edition (ABS-RC:2; Nihira, Leland, & Lambert, 1993) is the revision of the *AAMR Adaptive Behavior Scales* (Nihira, Foster, Shellhaas, & Leland, 1969) that meets the definition of mental retardation suggested by the American Association of Mental

Retardation in 1992. This comprehensive measure was designed to assess many specific adaptive and maladaptive behaviors in older individuals with mental retardation in residential and community settings (Nihira et al., 1993; Walsh & Shenouda, 1999).

The ABS-RC:2 consists of two parts. Part one covers the areas of personal independence and responsibility in daily living based on the following 10 domains: Independent Functioning, Physical Development, Economic Activity, Language Development, Numbers and Time, Domestic Activity, Prevocational Vocational Activity, Self-Direction, Responsibility, and Socialization. Part Two focuses on social behaviors using four subscales: Social Behavior, Self-Abusive Behavior, Social Engagement, and Disturbing Interpersonal Behavior. In addition, five factors are taken into account across the two parts when determining adaptive and maladaptive behaviors, namely Personal Self-Sufficiency, Community Self-Sufficiency, Personal-Social Responsibility, Social Adjustment, and Personal Adjustment.

A trained professional, should he or she possess a direct knowledge of the individual assessed, can complete the ABS-RC:2. Otherwise, the instrument must be completed via interviewing a person who is well-acquainted with the individual being assessed. Scoring is based on the sum of all items scores for Part One and Part Two. Standard scores for the measure are based on mean of 10 and standard deviation of 3. The standardization sample for the ABS-RC:2 was designed to represent the national population of individuals with developmental disabilities. The measure was standardized on individuals with developmental disabilities (ages 18 through 60+ years), as well as individuals with blindness, deafness, emotional disturbance, learning disability, physical impairments, and speech/language impairments (Nihira et al., 1993).

Scales of Independent Behavior-Revised

The *Scales of Independent Behavior-Revised* (SIB-R; Bruininks, Woodcook, Weatherman, & Hill, 1996) evolved from the *Scales of Independent Behavior,* which used to be a part of the *Woodcock-Johnson Psychoeducational Battery* (Woodcock-Johnson). The current version of the measure is used separately from the Woodcock-Johnson in order to assess functional independence and adaptive functioning of individuals from 3 months to 80+ years in a variety of settings.

The SIB-R can be completed using one of the three available forms: Early Development Form, Short Form, and Comprehensive Form. There is also a variation of the Short Form which assesses adaptive and maladaptive behaviors of individuals with visual impairment. The Early Development Form contains 40 items that are included in Comprehensive Form, designed for children from birth until 5 years old or older individuals with severe developmental disabilities (Msall, 2005). The Short Form also contains 40 items included in the Comprehensive Form and can be used as a screening measure for all ages. Finally, the Comprehensive Form includes 259 items distributed between 14 subscales as a part of one of four adaptive behavior clusters: Motor Skills, Social Interaction and Communication Skills, Personal Living Skills, and Community Living Skills. Maladaptive behaviors are assessed using the Problem Behavior Scale.

The administration of any of the scales of the SIB-R can be conducted either using a semi-structured interviewing technique or by filling out a respondent checklist. The latter is suggested if more than one individual a day needs to be assessed (Bruininks, Woodcook, Weatherman, & Hill, 1996). Extensive training is not required to complete the measure; however, training is needed to score the SIB-R and interpret the results. The SIB-R is an easy-to-use tool to assess adaptive and maladaptive behaviors within a wide range of ages and developmental levels, as well as in a broad variety of settings, such as school, home, or community. In particular, the SIB-R serves well in evaluating basic adaptive skills in younger children with significant delays in cognitive development or in children with ASD (Msall, 2005). The SIB-R can also be used for developing individualized educational plans, determining academic placement, and in research involving adaptive skills (Lecavalier, Leone, & Wiltz, 2006).

Naturalistic Observation

In addition to the standardized assessments available for the measurement of adaptive skills, naturalistic observation is another critical component of a comprehensive evaluation. As was previously mentioned, a reason for continued focus on adaptive skills in indi-

viduals with ASD is that these behaviors are often more easily measured than other symptoms of the disorders. Naturalistic observation is concerned with observing behaviors as they occur spontaneously in the natural environment. Naturalistic observation provides the opportunity to see behaviors as they occur, as opposed to assessing potential or typical behaviors with standardized measures (Kraijer, 2000). In fact, one could argue that there is no better way to assess whether or not a behavior occurs than to observe the individual interacting with his or her environment (Belfiore & Mace, 1994).

Naturalistic observations provide the opportunity to obtain a great deal of information about an individual that may not be captured by standardized, informant-based measures. However, consideration must be given to how naturalistic data is collected in order to obtain a representative sample of the individual's behavior. Some factors to consider in collecting naturalistic data include observing the individual in multiple settings, conducting multiple observations, and observing the individual while he or she is engaged in functional activities (Ogletree & Oren, 1998; Ogletree, Pierce, Harn, & Fischer, 2001).

Selection of Skills to Train

Once a thorough assessment of an individual's current adaptive skills has been conducted, the next step is to determine where to begin training. Because there are often many areas that require training, clinicians, parents, and teachers often are forced to construct a hierarchy of importance to guide their training of adaptive skills. The overall goal of any adaptive skills training program should be to increase the individual's independence. However, training of nearly any adaptive skill will serve this purpose to some degree. Brown, Nietupski, and Hamre-Nietupski (1976) recommend that the "criterion of ultimate functioning" be applied to selecting whether or not a specific skill should be taught. The "criterion of ultimate functioning" according to these authors is whether the individual will be able to function as an adult without being able to perform a specific skill.

Many other factors must be considered when selecting treatment targets. Anderson, Jablonski, Thomeer, and Knapp (2007) highlight the importance of including the child's age, developmental level, presence of learning readiness skills, and the child's interests when selecting which skills to train and in what order. For many parents of children with ASD, the age-appropriateness of an adaptive behavior is an easy way to determine whether or not the behavior should be a training target. While age-appropriateness is one factor that goes into selection of targets, this is often misleading. Development in neurotypical children is not a constant progression; there is a natural flow that is characterized by uneven progress across multiple areas (Bloom & Tinker, 2001). In other words, development of skills in one area may increase while development of skills in another area have reached a temporary plateau. Therefore, considering age-appropriateness only may not lead to choosing the most appropriate training targets (Anderson et al., 2007).

In addition to the age-appropriateness of a skill, its developmental appropriateness should also be taken into consideration (Anderson et al., 2007). Developmental appropriateness takes into account the child's progression through known developmental sequences. For example, a child who cannot yet walk would not be expected to begin running. By following a developmental progression for skill development, the clinician can ensure that the child has the prerequisite skills within a developmental domain. Researchers studying communication and play skill development in children with ASD have found evidence to support following a developmental rather than a chronological (i.e., age) sequence. Children with ASD have been shown to be more likely to acquire skills that were chosen based on the child's current developmental level rather than his or her age (Dyer, Santarcangelo, & Luce, 1987; Lifter, Sulzer-Azaroff, Anderson, & Cowdery, 1993).

Another factor that is important in selecting appropriate adaptive skills targets for children with ASD is the presence of learning readiness skills (Anderson et al., 2007). In other words, has the child learned the behaviors that are necessary in order to learn new skills? Learning readiness skills, according to Anderson et al. (2007), include the following: The child can pay attention to an activity for an extended period of time (e.g., 5–10 min); the child responds to his/her name; the child follows simple instructions; the child can imitate the actions of others; and, the child can make choices (i.e., in order to choose rewards if needed). Without these skills, a child may not be able to benefit fully from adaptive skills training.

Another factor to consider is the child's interests in the selection of intervention targets (Anderson et al., 2007). The child's current interests and emerging abilities can often help clinicians determine which skill to train next. For example, if a child very much enjoys cereal and is attempting to make his or her own bowl in the morning, then training this activity may increase the child's motivation to learn because he or she will be reinforced by the end product of the activity (i.e., getting to eat the cereal). However, some kids with ASD may not show clear preferences or interests, or may show inappropriate ones. Therefore, careful consideration should be given to how interests can be included appropriately, as well as the functionality of the skill (Anderson et al., 2007).

Finally, a clinician must take into account the opinions and priorities of the caregivers when selecting treatment targets (Anderson et al., 2007). Because most individual's with ASD interact with a number of different care providers (e.g., parents, teachers, job coaches, employers) within a number of different settings (e.g., home, school, work), it is important to develop a consensus as to which skills should be taught and in what order. Consensus among caregivers, as well as training of all caregivers, will help to ensure that skill development is promoted across individuals and settings. In addition, careful attention should be given to training skills in the setting that the skills will most often be used. By training in naturalistic settings, we increase the probability that the skill will be maintained long-term (Schreibman & Ingersoll, 2005).

In summary, the selection of which adaptive skills to train must take into account a multitude of variables and factors that may influence the ability of the child to learn the skill, as well as the probability that the skill will be maintained and generalized. It is important to constantly reappraise the appropriateness and utility of specific skills and to make changes to treatment targets as necessary.

Methods for Training Adaptive Skills

The ABA literature is replete with well-studied techniques for training a wide range of behaviors to individuals with developmental disabilities. The breadth of the adaptive skills literature cannot possibly be entirely encapsulated into one brief chapter. Therefore, the focus of this section is to highlight the major training techniques that are used for training adaptive skills in individuals with ASD. Prompting procedures, including graduated guidance and least-to-most prompting, are a cornerstone to ABA and have been applied to adaptive skills training in a variety of studies. In addition, when considering individuals with ASD specifically, attention should also be paid to the errorless learning techniques and environmental adaptations that can be used to increase the success of other forms of training.

Environmental Manipulations

Prior to discussing the numerous strategies used to teach adaptive skills, it is important to consider the role of environmental manipulations when teaching new skills to individuals with ASD. Considering ways in which the environment can be adapted to promote success in individuals with ASD is an important initial consideration when designing a training program. Many individuals with ASD may learn or process information in a different manner than typically-developing individuals. Therefore, adaptations should be made to the environment to suit his or her learning style. Researchers have shown that individuals with ASD may not learn as effectively using observation, imitation, and verbal instructions (Tsatsanis, 2004). However, many individuals with ASD may show strengths in rote memorization skills and learn better when information is presented visually (e.g., O'Riordan, Plaisted, Driver, & Baron-Cohen, 2001; Williams, Goldstein, Carpenter, & Minshew, 2005). In addition, memory for nonverbal material may be relatively less impaired than memory for verbal material (Prior & Chen, 1976). Addressing potential differences in learning style may help to promote more rapid skill acquisition. Two types of environmental adaptations, visual and physical supports, are especially applicable to the teaching of adaptive skills in individuals with ASD.

Visual Supports

The presence of visual information in the environment has been theorized to assist individuals with ASD to organize themselves (Janney & Snell, 2004). Visual information may also provide a sense of structure, stability and consistency in the environment, which may be beneficial to individuals with ASD. As a result, visual supports decrease the dependency on prompting and assistance from others in the environment (Schopler, Mesibov, & Hearsey, 1995).

Visual supports include the use of pictorial or word cues in the environment that serve as instructional or environmental prompts (Quill, 1997). Instructional prompts are those visual supports that aide in language expression or comprehension, whereas environmental prompts assists the individual in developing organizational and self-management skills. When applying visual supports to teaching adaptive and self-help skills, the focus is primarily on the use of visual aids as environmental prompts. These cues can help an individual organize his or her time, as well as allow him or her to anticipate upcoming events so as to be less dependent on the prompting of others (MacDuff, Krantz, & McClannahan, 1993). An added benefit of the use of visual cues in teaching adaptive skills is that visual cues can remain in the environment even after other forms of prompting have been faded to further support the generalization and maintenance of the attained behavior. When used effectively, visual supports have been shown to increase independence and motivation in children and adults with ASD (Dettmer, Simpson, Myles, & Ganz, 2000).

When applied to teaching self-help skills, visual supports are often used in combination with a task analysis to visually represent the steps required to complete the activity. Pierce and Schreibman (1994) demonstrated the use of visual supports combined with task analysis for teaching children with autism several self-help skills, including dressing, making lunch, setting the table, doing laundry, making the bed, and getting a drink. In this study, a task analysis was completed for each skill and then each of the steps in the task analyses were represented by a picture and placed in sequential order in photo books. Training consisted of first having the children discriminate between the pictures in a specific task. The child was then prompted to complete the step depicted by the first picture before gaining access to a reinforcer. This process was continued until the child could independently engage in each of the steps of the task analysis. The presence of the trainer was then gradually faded so that the children eventually completed the entire skill independently. The authors then went on to probe whether the skills would be performed by the children in the absence of the photo books and found variable results, which indicated that the children were assisted by the picture stimuli.

Adaptation of Physical Environment

In addition to visual supports, adapting the physical environment is another form of environmental adaptation that can assist in teaching adaptive skills. One of the areas of deficit that may contribute to learning difficulties in individuals with ASD is problems in processing environmental stimuli (Siegel, 1999). Therefore, providing an environment that minimizes distractions and emphasizes important stimuli may help promote learning (Rogers & DiLalla, 1991). Physical supports have been shown to help individuals with ASD perform skills more successfully (Heflin & Alberto, 2001). Physical supports include a wide variety of adaptations to the environment. For example, items in the environment can be arranged in a manner that reduces distraction and provides order and clear physical boundaries for activities. The environment can be organized in a variety of ways including the use of specific furniture arrangements, carpet squares, or tape.

An example of the use of physical supports in the teaching of adaptive skills can be found in task analysis for vacuuming in Table 1. When first teaching a skill such as this, it may be helpful to require the individual to vacuum only a small segment of flooring to avoid overwhelming the individual. In order to do this,

one can place colored tape on the floor to indicate a square of carpet that should be vacuumed. Over time, vacuuming larger areas can be shaped by gradually increasing the size of the taped portion of flooring. This clear division of the physical environment may allow the individual to navigate his or her environment more easily and independently through an enhanced sense of organization and structure.

Prompting Procedures

When an individual is trying to learn a new skill, it is important that he or she has the opportunity to practice that skill and receive feedback on his or her performance. For individuals with ASD, learning a new skill may not be as simple as observing how others perform the skill and then practicing themselves. Most often, additional assistance is required for the individual to learn the new skill. An effective way to teach a new skill to an individual with autism is to provide additional support in the form of prompts. Prompts are a class of antecedent stimuli that elicit the occurrence of the desired behavior (MacDuff, Krantz, & McClannahan, 2001). Prompts are presented before or after the presence of the discriminative stimuli that will eventually cue the behavior (Foxx, 1982).

Prompts can take a number of different forms, including verbal instructions, gestures, modeling, and any other antecedent stimuli that is used to increase the likelihood that the individual will engage in the desired

Table 1 Examples of task analyses

Brushing teeth	Washing hands	Vacuuming
1. Get toothbrush	1. Turn water on	1. Get vacuum
2. Wet toothbrush	2. Wet hands	2. Take vacuum to yellow square
3. Get toothpaste	3. Put soap on	3. Unwrap cord
4. Put toothpaste on the toothbrush	4. Rub hands together	4. Plug in cord
5. Brush top teeth	5. Rinse hands	5. Turn on vacuum
6. Brush bottom teeth	6. Turn water off	6. Step on button
7. Rinse mouth	7. Get paper towel	7. Pull cord out of way
8. Spit	8. Dry hands	8. Push vacuum back and forth in yellow square
9. Wipe face	9. Throw away paper towel	9. Turn off vacuum
10. Hang towel		10. Push handle up
11. Rinse toothbrush		11. Unplug cord
12. Put toothbrush away		12. Wrap cord around vacuum
		13. Put vacuum away

behavior or response (McClannahan & Krantz, 1999). Verbal prompts are a commonly reported prompt in the ABA literature. Verbal prompts can come in the form of explicit instructions, questions, or single words. Some researchers caution against the exclusive or excessive use of verbal prompts because they can often be difficult to fade and inhibit independence (e.g., Anderson et al., 2007).

Another common prompt is modeling. In modeling, the individual with ASD watches as another person performs the desired behavior. The model being used may be another child or even the parent (Jones & Schwartz, 2004). In addition to in vivo modeling, more research is emerging on the effectiveness of video modeling in teaching adaptive and social skills to individuals with ASD. For example, Keen, Brannigan, and Cuskelly (2007) compared the use of operant conditioning only to operant conditioning plus video modeling in teaching daytime urinary control to children with autism. These authors found that children who also watched the animated toileting videos engaged in a higher frequency of in-toilet urination than those who did not watch the video. In general, it is important to note that before a child can benefit from a model, he or she must first be able to imitate (Ghezzi, 2007).

Two other types of prompting are gestural and manual, or physical, prompts. Gestural prompts include pointing or motioning toward a person, activity, or material that indicates to the individual that a specific response should occur (MacDuff et al., 2001). Gestural prompts are especially useful when teaching nonverbal responses, such as adaptive skills (Ghezzi, 2007). Manual prompting typically entails the trainer using some level of physical guidance to help the trainee perform the desired behavior. Physical prompting can involve hand-over-hand prompting (when initially teaching the correct response), partial physical prompting (when tapping/guiding from the wrist to shoulder area), or full physical (fully guiding from both sides of the body to engage in the task). Manual prompting is often considered to be the most intrusive type of prompting because it requires physical contact between the trainer and the trainee.

An example of the use of physical prompting in teaching adaptive skills comes from Reid, Collier, and Cauchon (1991). These authors compared the use of physical and visual prompts to teach leisure skills to individuals with autism. Participants were taught how to bowl using a combination of verbal and physical

prompts in one condition and a combination of verbal and visual prompts in the other condition. Reid et al. (1991) reported that three of the four participants showed greater improvement in bowling skills in the physical prompting condition. However, an important consideration in this study was that the fourth participant did not improve as much in the physical prompting condition due to an apparent dislike of being touched and tactile defensiveness. This point illustrates the need to consider the characteristics of the learner when selecting prompting techniques.

It is also important to note that prompts are rarely used in isolation. In fact, different types of prompts are frequently used in conjunction in order to elicit the desired response with minimal intrusion. The following discussion of graduated guidance and least-to-most prompting provides examples of the ways in which different types of prompting can be used in conjunction to teach specific skills.

Graduated Guidance

Graduated guidance furthers the use of manual or physical prompts. In graduated guidance, a most-to-least prompting hierarchy is applied to the use of physical prompts. Prompting, therefore, begins with full physical or hand-over-hand prompting to ensure that the child completes the entire behavior. Over time, prompting is faded by gradually decreasing the either the intensity with which physical touch is applied or by moving from hand-over-hand prompting to partial physical and then to gestural prompting. Cooper (1987) further delineates the most-to-least hierarchy by stating that the trainer progress from hand-over-hand prompts to prompting the child's wrist, forearm, elbow, and then shoulder. Graduated guidance is beneficial for the teaching of some adaptive skills because this prompting procedure ensures that the child achieves success and completes the task every trial. Graduated guidance also prevents errors from occurring (McClannahan & Krantz, 1999).

Batu, Ergenekon, Erbas, and Akmanoglu (2004) utilized most-to-least prompting to teach the safety skill of crossing the street to five individuals with developmental disabilities. The prompting hierarchy used included: (1) Trainer holds the participant's arm with both hands while providing verbal prompts (full physical prompting); (2) trainer holds partici-pant's arm with only one or two fingers while provid-ing verbal prompts (partial physical prompting); (3) no physical contact between trainer and participants (verbal prompting only). Using most-to-least prompt-ing, these researchers taught participants to cross the street using an above-street walkway, pedestrian cross walks, as well as crossing the street in areas without traffic signals.

Least-to-most Prompting

While graduated guidance follows a most-to-least pro-gression of prompting, least-to-most systems of prompting are also commonly used. In least-to-most prompting, the stimulus that should naturally elicit the behavior or response is presented to the child without any prompting. The child is then given some time (typically 5–10 s) to respond to the stimulus. If the child does not respond, the trainer may present a gestural prompt and then allow the child to respond. This system is continued with a progression from gestural, to verbal, to modeling, and then finally to a physical prompt. Figure 1 presents a graphic repre-sentation of this hierarchy. Assistance in the form of prompting is gradually increased until the child emits the correct response.

Least-to-most prompting was utilized in combina-tion with video modeling by Murzynski and Bourret (2007) to teach several daily living skills (i.e., folding shirts, folding pants, making sandwiches, and making juice) to two children with autism. The children were initially provided a verbal prompt to engage in the activity (e.g., "fold your shirt"). If the child did not respond within 5 s, the instructor provided a gestural prompt. The prompting hierarchy utilized consisted of a verbal prompt, followed by a gesture, physical guid-ance at the forearm, and hand-over-hand physical guidance (Murzynski & Bourret, 2007). Video model-ing was also combined with least-to-most prompting to teach the skills and was found to be more effective than least-to-most prompting alone.

Least-to-most prompting has been shown to be used more frequently than other instructional methods (Westling & Fox, 2004). The popularity of this prompt-ing method has been suggested to be due to its ease of application (West & Billingsley, 2005). An additional strength of least-to-most prompting is that the child has the opportunity to respond to relevant environmen-tal cues on every trial, as opposed to immediately receiving prompting (Cooper, 1987). However, least-to-most prompting has been shown by researchers to require more trials for learning than most-to-least hier-archies (West & Billingsley, 2005), as well as produc-ing more prompt dependence and errors (Karsh, Repp & Lenz, 1990; Repp, Karsh, & Lenz, 1990).

Least amount of adult involvement ⬇ Most amount of adult involvement	I	Independent	After being given the initial direction or expectation, the child can respond to or complete the task with no further prompt or information.
	G	Gesture	The adult points or motions to the child, activity, or visual cue; no physical contact is made.
	V	Verbal	The adult provides verbal information about the task or the correct response.
	M	Model	The adult demonstrates or provides a completed model of what the child is supposed to do.
	PP	Partial Physical	The adult touches the child (possibly on the arm, elbow, or hand) to assist with the task; requires less involvement than hand-over-hand guidance.
	HOH	Hand-over-hand	The adult physically guides the actions of the child by placing their hands over the hands of the child.
	FP	Full physical	The adult provides physical contact in maneuvering the child to complete required task.

Fig. 1 Example of a least-to-most prompting hierarchy. © 2007 Christian Sarkine Autism Treatment Center. All rights reserved. For questions or permission to use, copy, or distribute, please contact Naomi Swiezy, PhD, HSPP, Clinical Director, Christian Sarkine Autism Treatment Center, Program Director, HANDS in Autism Program, at nswiezy@iupui.edu. Last Revised 08/2007

Prompt Fading

Finally, when discussing the use of any prompting procedure, it is important to consider how the individual will learn to engage in the behavior in the absence of the prompt. Continual use of the same type of prompt may result in the individual becoming dependent on the presence of the prompt as opposed to focusing on the relevant stimuli in the environment that should be evoking the behavior (Cameron, Ainsleigh, & Bird, 1992). Individuals with ASD may be more susceptible to prompt dependence because they may be more likely to respond to irrelevant cues in the environment and not attend to the task itself (Cameron et al., 1992). Therefore, attention must be paid to how a prompt will be faded.

Prompt fading has been defined as the gradual removal of prompts (Kazdin, 2001). A systematic approach to prompt fading allows for an individual to progress towards responding with the highest level of independence and accuracy as possible for him or her (Ghezzi, 2007). Each of the individual types of prompts previously discussed can be faded by gradually reducing the amount of assistance provided. For example, a gestural prompt can be faded by providing less exaggerated movements (Ghezzi, 2007). Graduated guidance provides a general framework for fading physical prompting by changing the intensity and location of physical guidance. It is important to keep in mind that the goal of all training, and adaptive skills training in particular, is to have the individual perform the skill with the maximum degree of independence possible for him or her. Therefore, attention must be paid to selecting the appropriate prompts and also to systematically fading those prompts in order to increase independence.

Task Analysis

The reality of training adaptive skills to individuals with developmental disabilities is that the majority of these skills require the individual to complete a number of discrete behaviors. Task analyses are used to address this difficult issue in training new skills. A task analysis is a method for dividing a larger goal or skill into the concrete, discrete behaviors that comprise the skill (Kazdin, 2001). The goal of a task analysis is to specify the individual steps required to complete an activity, as well as the sequence of steps.

The process of creating a task analysis remains the same regardless of the skill be taught, although the complexity of the task analysis will vary depending on the difficulty of the task being taught. The first step to creating a task analysis is to identify the desired behavior that you wish to teach (e.g., brushing teeth, tying shoes). The next step is to evaluate what the behavior looks like when it is done appropriately. This can be fulfilled by observing other people engaging in the behavior or doing so yourself. All of the steps required should then be written down. It is important at this point to consider the baseline level of skill in the behavior demonstrated by the individual being taught. This will inform the level of specificity required in the task analysis. After the task analysis is tested and revised as needed, the next step is to train the individual on the components of the behavior using prompting and other supports (e.g., errorless learning, visual schedules, reinforcement schedules). Data collection during training usually consists of recording the highest level of prompting required to complete each step in the task analysis in order to assess independence.

An additional component to training a task analysis is the inclusion of visual supports. Visual supports, as previously discussed, can assist with teaching the skill and developing independence. Typically, each step in the task analysis is presented to the individual visually through the use of a written checklist or series of photographs or picture icons. As the individual completes each step of the skill, he or she can be prompted to remove the corresponding picture or check off the step on the checklist. As the prompting of the trainer is faded, the visual supports can remain as a permanent product in the environment to support the maintenance of the skill over time.

Task analysis is a common feature of adaptive skills training programs for individuals with autism and other developmental disabilities. For example, Stokes, Cameron, Dorsey, and Fleming (2004) utilized a task analysis for training personal hygiene to adult males with autism and ID. The goal of the treatment program was to teach the individuals to properly clean themselves after bowel movements. The task analysis included 10 steps: Reach for toilet paper roll, grasp edge, pull at least five sections, tear paper, fold three times, reach around to back side, wipe front to back four times (repeat 3–7 times if required), throw used paper in bowl, flush toilet, close lid. In addition to using the task analysis and prompting the individuals to complete each step, the authors also included correspondence training into the wiping step in order to help the individual decide whether further wipes were necessary. The correspondence training included having the individual say what he was going to do, complete the behavior, and then report as to whether the behavior was completed. All of the individuals in the study learned to perform the task analysis and achieved an acceptable level of hygiene in 22–36 training sessions. Table 1 presents examples of task analyses that have been used to teach three adaptive skills: Brushing teeth, vacuuming, and washing hands.

Shaping

When training new skills in individuals with developmental disabilities, clinicians, parents, and teachers often come across situations where the desired behavior is not a part of the individual's current repertoire or may be only partially present. In these cases, shaping is often utilized to reinforce gradual approximations or partial responses in order to develop the goal behavior (Kazdin, 2001). The process of shaping a behavior begins by providing reinforcement for behaviors in the individual's repertoire that are similar to the goal behavior. Once this initial behavior is occurring consistently, the criterion for earning reinforcement is slightly changed so that reinforcement is now being provided only for a response that is somewhat closer to the goal behavior. Reinforcement for the previous response is terminated and that response is eventually extinguished (Kazdin, 2001).

Bigelow, Huynen, and Lutzker (1993) provided an example of the use of shaping in teaching adaptive skills. Bigelow et al. (1993) taught a 9-year-old female with autism how to appropriately and quickly exit her home in the case of a fire. The goal of the training program was to teach this child to respond to a fire alarm by exiting her house and walking to a meeting place outside. Training began by having a trainer prompt the child from behind to walk 11 feet from the living room out the front door. The child received reinforcement in the form of edibles, praise, and affection from a caregiver waiting outside of the door on each trial. Once the child was able to walk the 11 feet to the door, the

researchers began trials one foot further from the door. Over the course of 12 weeks of training, the researchers were able to shape the child's behavior so that she was walking 22 feet each time she heard the fire alarm. At 6 month follow-up, caregivers reported that the child could walk 40 feet starting from a position where she could not see the door or the waiting caregiver.

Chaining

An issue that further complicates the teaching of adaptive skills to individuals with ASD, is that frequently these skills consist of a sequence of responses (i.e., a chain) that must occur in a specific order for the skill to be completed successfully. For example, in order for an individual to brush his or her teeth, a number of discrete behaviors must occur in a specific order (see Table 1 for a task analysis of brushing teeth). In chaining, the individual would receive hand-over-hand prompting to learn the behavior sequence. Each successive step of the sequence would be taught by providing the lowest level of prompt necessary to complete the initial step with hand-over-hand prompting (or caregiver completion) of the rest of the sequence. Once the initial step was mastered, the next step in the sequence as well as the initial one would be prompted with the lowest level of prompting necessary and the balance of the steps completed with hand-over-hand (or caregiver completion), and so on. Reinforcement is provided when the entire sequence of behaviors has occurred and the end behavior has been successfully completed (e.g., teeth have been brushed).

Chaining is further divided into forward and backward chaining. In forward chaining, behaviors are developed in the order in which they are supposed to occur in the skill sequence. For example, in the task analysis for brushing teeth shown in Table 1, using forward chaining the first behavior to be taught is "get toothbrush." The child would initially be taught hand-over-hand for the whole sequence and then highest level of prompting for the initial followed by hand-over-hand of the rest of the task. Training would then continue to "get toothpaste," "put toothpaste on toothbrush," etc. in the order they appear on the task analysis. Backward chaining consists of starting at the end of the sequence and having the child complete only the last behavior in the sequence. For example, in the task analysis for brushing teeth in Table 1, backward chaining would consist of having the child first complete "rinse toothbrush." The child then receives reinforcement for completing this step of the sequence. Backward chaining gradually moves from the end of the sequence to the beginning so that in time the child is able to complete the entire sequence.

In a recent study, Jerome, Frantino, and Sturmey (2007) used backwards chaining to teach leisure computer skills to adults with autism and ID. A task analysis was conducted to assess the steps necessary to access a specific website starting with turning on the computer and ending with clicking on the website of choice from a search engine webpage. Teaching of the skill began with the use of a most-to-least prompting procedure for the final item on the task analysis (i.e., single click on a website of choice from a search engine website). Training then moved on to the next step in the task analysis once the individual independently completed the final step two consecutive times. The process continued until the individual could complete all 13 steps in the task analysis without prompting. These authors demonstrated how backward chaining combined with prompting can be used to teach a relatively complex skill to individuals with developmental disabilities.

Errorless Learning

Another teaching strategy that should be considered when working with individuals with ASD is errorless learning. Errorless learning is a combination of teaching techniques intended to reduce the likelihood of incorrect responding. These techniques can be used to teach a variety of skills (Mueller, Palkovic, & Maynard, 2007). The six techniques that are included in errorless learning are stimulus fading, stimulus shaping, delayed prompting, response prevention, superimposition with fading, and superimposition with shaping (Mueller et al., 2007).

In errorless learning, fading and shaping are conducted using aspects of the physical stimulus as opposed to the fading of prompts and shaping of a response previously discussed. Stimulus fading is designed to teach the appropriate response by initially presenting only the stimulus associated with the presence of reinforcement (S+), thereby making an error impossible. Once accurate responding to the S+ stimulus is obtained, an

incorrect choice that is not associated with reinforcement (S−) is gradually introduced. Fading of the S− is conducted in a variety of ways, such as gradually changing the intensity, duration, color, or size of the stimulus over time. Eventually, the S+ and S− are presented simultaneously with equal intensity, size, shape, etc. so that the individual must make the proper discrimination in order to earn reinforcement.

Stimulus shaping in errorless learning involves the gradual changing of the physical properties of the stimuli (both the S+ and S−) so that they are eventually physically different from the way in which they first appeared (Mueller et al., 2007). In other words, the initial presentation of the S+ and S− may be items that the child can correctly discriminate between, but over time those items may be changed to completely new items. However, the child maintains the ability to make accurate discriminations. For example, if the child is able to discriminate between the letter "A" and the letter "C," the letter "A" may be gradually be changed into the letter "N" and the "C" may be changed into an "O." Stimulus shaping can also be conducted by gradually increasing the similarity between the target stimuli and a distracter in order to make the discrimination more difficult (McGee, Krantz, & McClannahan, 1986).

The next component of errorless learning is delayed prompting. Delayed prompting is the systematic increase in the amount of time between the presentation of a stimuli and a prompt (Touchette, 1971). Initially, when a stimulus is presented, a prompt is immediately provided to ensure that the child makes the correct response without error. A delay is then introduced between the presentation of the stimulus and the prompt in order to allow the individual with the opportunity to independently make a correct response (Handen & Zane, 1987). Delayed prompting may have a number of advantages, including reducing the likelihood that the child will respond to irrelevant stimuli and ease of implementation (Touchette, 1971).

The other hallmarks of errorless learning are the prevention of incorrect responding, and superimposition with fading and shaping. Response prevention entails the trainer helping the child to avoid making incorrect responses. This can most easily be applied to situations in which the child needs to touch or point to a specific stimulus, such as when teaching a child to discriminate between different coins when teaching currency. If the child is presented with a quarter and a penny and told to touch the penny, the trainer would wait for the child to begin responding. If the child begins to respond incorrectly, such as starting to move towards the quarter, the trainer would physically block the quarter by placing his or her hand over the quarter. Over additional trials, the trainer should have to block the incorrect response less frequently until responding is allocated only to the correct response (Mueller et al., 2007).

Superimposition of fading and shaping are less frequently used components of errorless learning. These procedures do not involve any changes to the stimuli used in training, but instead involve the addition of known stimuli (such as pictures) to help the individual discriminate between unknown stimuli. The known stimuli are then gradually changed until they are completely removed and the individual is left with only the previously unknown stimuli which can now be successfully discriminated. Etzel, LeBlanc, Schilmoeller, and Stella (1981) provided an example of superimposition with stimulus shaping to teach children to read sight words. In this study, the children were presented with sight words that they could not read. However, a picture representing the word was included on the cards to aid the child in reading. Over time, the pictures were gradually shaped so that they were incorporated into one of the letters in the word and then further faded until the picture was no longer present.

Maintenance and Generalization

While the training of new skills is the first requirement to improving adaptive functioning in individuals with ASD, it is also necessary to ensure that skills are generalized and maintained over time. Baer, Wolf, and Risley (1968) discussed the three main steps of a successful treatment program as being first the acquisition of a behavior change; second, the generalization of the behavior change to different settings outside of the initial treatment setting; and third, the maintenance of the behavior change over time. An understanding of the importance of generalization and maintenance in the design of an adaptive skills program is paramount to its ultimate success.

Generalization has been defined as the transfer of a response to a situation or situations other than the one in which the response was initially trained (Kazdin,

2001). Generalization is the stability of behavior change across different settings, stimulus conditions, and environments. Stokes and Baer (1977) classified generalization programming as incorporating three general principles: Exploiting current functional contingencies, training diversely, and incorporating functional mediators.

When Stokes and Baer (1977) wrote about exploiting current functional contingencies, they highlighted the importance of using natural reinforcement and consequences when training new behaviors. One method of accessing natural reinforcement in training adaptive skills is to select skills that the individual is interested in, when appropriate. This ensures that the natural result of completing the skill is reinforcing in and of itself to the individual. In addition, shifting from reliance on edibles to more natural reinforcers, such as social praise, may also increase the likelihood of generalization. Another procedure to consider when discussing contingencies is the reinforcement of instances of generalization. In this case, generalization is considered to be an independent response class and each instance of generalization should be reinforced (Goetz & Baer, 1973).

The second general principle proposed by Stokes and Baer (1977) was that training should be diverse. In other words, training should be conducted with as much flexibility as possible and the rigid, highly-structured, and controlled environments that are frequently characteristic of ABA should be avoided if generalization is a primary goal. Stokes and Osnes (1989) point out that "… focused training frequently has focused effects" (p. 344). Therefore, attention should be paid to diversifying different components of training. The ongoing shift towards more naturalistic training strategies highlights the importance of this generalization principle. Naturalistic procedures include more loosely structured training sessions, varying the stimuli across trials, using a variety of prompts, and incorporating natural reinforcers (Cowan & Allen, 2007). Additional examples of ways to train diversely include using multiple trainers, multiple settings, and making antecedent and consequences less easily discriminated by the individual (Stokes & Osnes, 1989). Applied to the training of adaptive and self-help skills, training diversely can include teaching toileting skills at home and school consistently and simultaneously, utilizing parents, teachers, and other caregivers as trainers, and ensuring access to natural reinforcers by selecting skills that correspond to the individual's interests when appropriate.

The final principle of generalization recommended by Stokes and Baer (1977) is the incorporation of functional mediators. A functional mediator in this case has been defined as a stimulus that facilitates generalization by its presence in the training and generalization environments (Stokes & Osnes, 1989). Social stimuli, such as the presence of the trainer in the generalization environment, can also serve as a functional mediator that can promote generalization of an acquired skill. Furthermore, antecedent strategies such as the use of visual cues can be incorporated into different settings in order to enhance the generalization of skills across settings.

Finally, generalization of skills must be differentiated from the maintenance of those skills. Maintenance is defined as the stability of behavior change over time (Kazdin, 2001). Maintenance and generalization are obviously intertwined and neither can occur in isolation. Therefore, the principles discussed in regards to generalization of skills also apply to their maintenance. An additional factor to consider in promoting maintenance is the manipulation of reinforcement. Intermittent reinforcement schedules result in behaviors that are less susceptible to extinction (Foxx, 1982). The gradual thinning of reinforcement schedules during training may therefore promote maintenance. Delaying access to reinforcers may also aide in the maintenance of skills because many naturally occurring reinforcers, such as money and praise, often do not occur immediately following the occurrence of the behavior or use of the skill (Foxx, 1982).

Conclusion

The purpose of this chapter was to provide an overview of the adaptive skills deficits in individuals with ASD and to outline methods for training these skills successfully. Adaptive skills influence all areas of an individual's functioning and should be a top priority in academic and behavioral interventions. Without appropriate adaptive skills, the ability of an individual to function with maximum independence is greatly reduced. Therefore, the focus of adaptive skills training should be on teaching skills that are functional for the individual and will be utilized in their daily routine

to increase independence. ABA provides a framework and a set of strategies for addressing this skills training and for promoting their maintenance and generalization. ABA methods also allows for the consideration of learning styles and individualization of supports for the most efficient and effective skill acquisition.

References

American Association on Mental Retardation. (2002). *The AAMR definition of mental retardation*. Retrieved April 4, 2006, from http://www.aamr.org/Policies/faq_mental_retardation.shtml.

American Psychological Association. (2000). *Diagnostic and statistical manual of mental disorders-text revision* (4th ed.). Washington, DC: Author.

Anderson, S. R., Jablonski, A. L., Thomeer, M. L., & Knapp, V. M. (2007). *Self-help skills for people with autism: A systematic teaching approach*. Bethesda: Woodbine House, Inc.

Baer, D. M., Wolf, M. M., & Risley, T. (1968). Some current dimensions of applied behavior analysis. *Journal of Applied Behavior Analysis, 1*, 91–97.

Baghdadli, A., Pascal, C., Grisi, S., & Aussilloux, C. (2003). Risk factors for self-injurious behaviors among 222 young children with autistic disorders. *Journal of Intellectual Disability Research, 47*(8), 622–627.

Balboni, G., Pedrabissi, L., Molteni, M., & Villa, S. (2001). Discriminant validity of the Vineland Scales: Score Profiles of individuals with mental retardation and a specific disorder. *American Journal on Mental Retardation, 106*(2), 167–172.

Ballaban-Gil, K., Rapin, I., Tuchman, R., & Shinnar, S. (1996). Longitudinal examination of the behavioral, language, and social changes in a population of adolescents and young adults with autistic disorder. *Pediatric Neurology, 15*, 217–223.

Batu, S., Ergenekon, Y., Erbas, D., & Akmanoglu, N. (2004). Teaching pedestrian skills to individuals with developmental disabilities. *Journal of Behavioral Education, 13*(3), 147–164.

Belfiore, P. J., & Mace, F. C. (1994). Self-help and community skills. In J. L. Matson (Ed.), *Autism in children and adults: Etiology, assessment, and intervention* (pp. 193–211). Belmont, CA: Brooks/Cole.

Bigelow, K. M., Huynen, K. B., & Lutzker, J. R. (1993). Using a changing criterion design to teach fire escape to a child with developmental disabilities. *Journal of Developmental and Physical Disabilities, 5*(2), 121–128.

Bloom, L., & Tinker, E. (2001). The intentionality model and language acquisition: Engagement, effort, and the essential tension in development. *Monographs of the Society for Research in Child Development, 66*(4), 1–91.

Brown, L., Nietupski, J., & Hamre-Nietupski, S. (1976). The criterion of ultimate functioning. In M. A. Thomas (Ed.), *Hey don't forget about me: New directions for serving the handicapped* (pp. 2–15). Reston: Council for Exceptional Children.

Bruininks, R. H., Woodcook, R. W., Weatherman, R. F., & Hill, B. (1996). *Scales of independent behavior-revised*. Itasca, IL: Riverside.

Burack, J., & Volkmar, F. (1992). Development of low and high functioning autistic children. *Journal of Child Psychology and Psychiatry, 33*, 607–616.

Cameron, M. J., Ainsleigh, S. A., & Bird, F. L. (1992). The acquisition of stimulus control of compliance and participation during an AD routine. *Behavioral Residential Treatment, 7*, 327–340.

Carpentieri, S., & Morgan, S. B. (1996). Adaptive and intellectual functioning in autistic and nonautistic retarded children. *Journal of Autism and Developmental Disorders, 26*(6), 611–620.

Cooper, J. O. (1987). Stimulus control. In J. O. Cooper, T. E. Heron & W. L. Heward (Eds.), *Applied behavior analysis* (pp. 299–326). Columbus: Merrill.

Cowan, R. J., & Allen, K. D. (2007). Using naturalistic procedures to enhance learning in individuals with autism: A focus on generalized teaching within the school setting. *Psychology in the Schools, 44*(7), 701–715.

Dacey, C. M., Nelson, W. M., & Stoeckel, J. (1999). Reliability, criterion-related validity and qualitative comments of the Fourth Edition of the Stanford-Binet Intelligence Scale with a young adult population with intellectual disability. *Journal of Intellectual Disability Research, 43*(3), 179–184.

De Bildt, A., Kraijer, D., Sytema, S., & Minderaa, R. (2005). The psychometric properties of the Vineland Adaptive Behavior Scales in children and adolescents with mental retardation. *Journal of Autism and Developmental Disorders, 35*(1), 53–62.

Dettmer, S., Simpson, R. L., Myles, B. S., & Ganz, J. B. (2000). The use of visual supports to facilitate transitions of students with autism. *Focus on Autism and Other Developmental Disabilities, 15*(3), 163–169.

Doll, E. (1936). Current thoughts on mental retardation. *Journal of Pscyho-Anesthenics, 41*, 33–49.

Dyer, K., Santarcangelo, S., & Luce, S. C. (1987). Developmental influences in teaching language forms to individuals with developmental disabilities. *Journal of Speech and Hearing Disorders, 52*, 335–347.

Etzel, B. C., LeBlanc, J. M., Schilmoeller, K. J., & Stella, M. E. (1981). Stimulus control procedures in the education of young children. In S. W. Bijou & R. Ruiz (Eds.), *Behavior modification: Contribution to education* (pp. 3–37). Hillsdale, NJ: Erlbaum.

Foxx, R. M. (1982). *Increasing behaviors of severely retarded and autistic persons*. Champaign, IL: Research Press.

Freeman, B. J., Ritvo, E. R., Yokota, A., Childs, J., & Pollard, J. (1988). WISC-R and Vineland Adaptive Behavior Scale scores in autistic children. *Journal of the American Academy of Child and Adolescent Psychiatry, 27*(4), 428–429.

Freeman, B. J., Del'Homme, M., Guthrie, D., & Zhang, F. (1999). Vineland Adaptive Behavior Scale scores as a function of age and initial IQ in 210 autistic children. *Journal of Autism and Developmental Disorders, 29*(5), 379–384.

Ghezzi, P. M. (2007). Discrete trials teaching. *Psychology in the Schools, 44*(7), 667–679.

Gillham, J., Carter, A., Volkmar, F., & Sparrow, S. (2000). Toward a developmental operational definition of autism. *Journal of Autism and Developmental Disorders, 30*(4), 269–278.

Goetz, E. M., & Baer, D. M. (1973). Social control of form diversity and the emergence of new forms in children's block building. *Journal of Applied Behavior Analysis, 6*, 105–113.

Handen, B. L., & Zane, T. (1987). Delayed prompting: A review of procedural variations and results. *Research in Developmental Disabilities, 8*, 307–330.

Heflin, L. J., & Alberto, P. A. (2001). Establishing a behavioral context for learning for students with autism. *Focus on Autism and Other Developmental Disabilities, 16*(2), 93–101.

Howlin, P., Mawhood, L., & Rutter, M. (2000). Autism and developmental receptive language disorder – a follow-up comparison in early adult life. II: Social, behavioral, and psychiatric outcomes. *Journal of Child Psychology and Psychiatry, 41*(5), 561–578.

Jacobson, J. W., & Ackerman, L. J. (1990). Differences in adaptive functioning among people with autism and mental retardation: Comparison over nine years. *Mental Retardation, 29*, 315–321.

Janney, R. E., & Snell, M. E. (2004). *Teachers' guides to inclusive practices: Modifying schoolwork* (2nd ed.). Baltimore: Brookes.

Jerome, J., Frantino, E. C., & Sturmey, P. (2007). The effects of errorless learning and backward chaining on the acquisition of internet skills in adults with developmental disabilities. *Journal of Applied Behavior Analysis, 40*, 185–189.

Jones, C. D., & Schwartz, I. S. (2004). Siblings, peers, and adults: Differential effects of models for children with autism. *Topics in Early Childhood Special Education, 24*(4), 187–198.

Karsh, K. G., Repp, A. C., & Lenz, M. W. (1990). A comparison of the task demonstration model and the standard prompting hierarchy in teaching word identification to persons with moderate retardation. *Research in Developmental Disabilities, 11*, 395–410.

Kazdin, A. E. (2001). *Behavior modification in applied settings* (6th ed.). Belmont, CA: Wadsworth/Thomson Learning.

Keen, D., Brannigan, K. L., & Cuskelly, M. (2007). Toilet training for children with autism: The effects of video modeling. *Journal of Developmental and Physical Disabilities, 19*(4), 291–303.

Kraijer, D. (2000). Review of adaptive behavior studies in mentally retarded persons with autism/pervasive developmental disorder. *Journal of Autism and Developmental Disorders, 30*(1), 39–47.

Lecavalier, L., Leone, S., & Wiltz, J. (2006). The impact of behaviour problems on caregiver stress in young people with autism spectrum disorders. *Journal of Intellectual Disability Research, 50*(3), 172–183.

Lifter, K., Sulzer-Azaroff, B., Anderson, S. R., & Cowdery, G. (1993). Teaching play activities to preschool children with disabilities: The importance of developmental considerations. *Journal of Early Intervention, 17*, 139–159.

Liss, M., Harel, B., Fein, D., Allen, D., Dunn, M., Feinstein, C., et al. (2001). Predictors and correlates of adaptive functioning in children with developmental disorders. *Journal of Autism and Developmental Disorders, 31*(2), 219–230.

Lord, C., & Schopler, E. (1989). The role of age at assessment, developmental level, and test in the stability of intelligence scores in young autistic children. *Journal of Autism and Developmental Disorders, 19*(4), 483–499.

MacDuff, G., Krantz, P., & McClannahan, L. (1993). Teaching children with autism to use pictographic activity schedules: Maintenance and generalization of complex response chains. *Journal of Applied Behavior Analysis, 26*, 89–97.

MacDuff, G. S., Krantz, P. J., & McClannahan, L. E. (2001). Prompts and prompt-fading strategies for people with autism. In C. Maurice, G. Green & R. Foxx (Eds.), *Making a difference: Behavioral intervention for autism* (pp. 37–50). Austin, TX: PRO-ED.

Magiati, I., & Howlin, P. (2001). Monitoring the progress of pre-school children with autism enrolled in early intervention programmes. *Autism, 5*(4), 399–406.

McClannahan, L. E., & Krantz, P. J. (1999). *Activity schedules for children with autism: Teaching independent behavior.* Bethesda: Woodbine House.

McGee, G., Krantz, P., & McClannahan, L. (1986). An extension of incidental teaching procedures to reading instruction for autistic children. *Journal of Applied Behavior Analysis, 19*, 147–157.

Msall, M. E. (2005). Measuring functional skills in preschool children at risk for neurodevelopment disabilities. *Mental Retardation and Developmental Disabilities Research Reviews, 11*, 263–273.

Mueller, M. M., Palkovic, C. M., & Maynard, C. S. (2007). Errorless learning: Review and practical application for teaching children with pervasive developmental disorders. *Psychology in the Schools, 44*(7), 691–700.

Murzynski, N. T., & Bourret, J. C. (2007). Combining video modeling and least-to-most prompting for establishing response chains. *Behavioral Interventions, 22*, 147–152.

Nihira, K., Foster, R., Shellhaas, M., & Leland, H. (1969). *AAMD Adaptive Behavior Scale.* Washington, DC: American Association on Mental Deficiency.

Nihira, K., Leland, H., & Lambert, N. (1993). *The American Association of Mental Retardation's Adaptive Behavior Scale – Residential and Community* (2nd ed.). Austin, TX: PRO-ED.

O'Riordan, M. A., Plaisted, K. C., Driver, J., & Baron-Cohen, S. (2001). Superior visual search in autism. *Journal of Experimental Psychology: Human Perception and Performance, 27*(3), 719–730.

Oakland, T., & Houchins, S. (1985). A review of the Vincland Adaptive Behavior Scales, Survey Form. *Journal of Counseling and Development, 63*, 585–586.

Ogletree, B. T., & Oren, T. (1998). Structured yet functional: An alternative conceptualization of treatment for communication impairment in autism. *Focus on Autism and Other Developmental Disabilities, 13*(4), 228–233.

Ogletree, B. T., Pierce, K., Harn, W. E., & Fischer, M. A. (2001). Assessment of communication and language in classical autism: Issues and practices. *Assessment for Effective Intervention, 27*, 61–71.

Paul, R., Miles, S., Cicchetti, D., Sparrow, S. S., Klin, A., Volkmar, F. R., et al. (2004). Adaptive behavior in autism and pervasive developmental disorder-not otherwise specified: Microanalysis of scores on the Vineland Adaptive Behavior Scales. *Journal of Autism and Developmental Disorders, 34*(2), 223–228.

Pierce, K. L., & Schreibman, L. (1994). Teaching daily living skills to children with autism in unsupervised settings through pictorial self-management. *Journal of Applied Behavior Analysis, 27*(3), 471–481.

Prior, M., & Chen, C. (1976). Short-term and serial memory in autistic, retarded, and normal children. *Journal of Autism and Childhood Schizophrenia, 6*(2), 121–131.

Quill, K. A. (1997). Instructional considerations for young children with autism: The rationale for visually cued instruction. *Journal of Autism and Developmental Disorders, 27*(6), 697–714.

Reid, G., Collier, D., & Cauchon, M. (1991). Skill acquisition by children with autism: Influence of prompts. *Adapted Physical Activity Quarterly, 8*(4), 357–366.

Repp, A. C., Karsh, K. G., & Lenz, M. W. (1990). Discrimination training for persons with developmental disabilities: A comparison of the task demonstration model and the standard prompting hierarchy. *Journal of Applied Behavior Analysis, 23*(1), 43–52.

Roberts, C., McCoy, M., Reidy, D., & Cruciti, F. (1993). A comparison of methods of assessing adaptive behaviour in preschool children with developmental disabilities. *Australia and New Zealand Journal of Developmental Disabilities, 18*(4), 261–272.

Rogers, S. J., & DiLalla, D. L. (1991). A comparative study of the effects of a developmentally based instructional model on young children with autism and young children with other disorders of behavior and development. *Topics in Early Childhood Special Education, 11*(2), 29–47.

Schopler, E., Mesibov, G. B., & Hearsey, K. (1995). Structured teaching in the TEACCH system. In E. Schopler & G. Mesibov (Eds.), *Learning and cognition in autism* (pp. 243–267). New York: Plenum Press.

Schreibman, L., & Ingersoll, B. (2005). Behavioral interventions to promote learning in individuals with autism. In F. R. Volkmar, R. Paul, A. Klin & D. Cohen (Eds.), *Handbook of Autism and Pervasive Developmental Disorders* (Assessment, Interventions, and Policy 3rd ed., Vol. II, pp. 882–896). Hoboken, NJ: John Wiley & Sons, Inc.

Siegel, B. (1999). Autistic learning disabilities and individualized treatment for autistic spectrum disorders. *Infants and Young Children, 12*(2), 27–36.

Sparrow, S. S., Balla, D. A., & Cicchetti, D. V. (1984). *Vineland Adaptive Behavior Scales, Interview Edition, survey form manual.* Circle Pines, MN: American Guidance Service.

Sparrow, S. S., Cicchetti, D. V., & Balla, D. A. (2005). *Vineland Adaptive Behavior scales: Second edition (Vineland II), Survey interview form/caregiver rating form.* Circle Pines: AGS Publishing.

Stokes, T. F., & Baer, D. M. (1977). An implicit technology of generalization. *Journal of Applied Behavior Analysis, 10*(2), 349–367.

Stokes, T. F., & Osnes, P. G. (1989). An operant pursuit of generalization. *Behavior Therapy, 20*, 337–355.

Stokes, J. V., Cameron, M. J., Dorsey, M. F., & Fleming, E. (2004). Task analysis, correspondence training, and general case instruction for teaching personal hygiene skills. *Behavioral Interventions, 19*(2), 121–135.

Szatmari, P., Merette, C., Bryson, S. E., Thivierge, J., Roy, M. A., Cayer, M., et al. (2002). Quantifying dimensions in autism: A factor-analytic study. *Journal of the American Academy of Child and Adolescent Psychiatry, 41*(4), 467–474.

Touchette, P. E. (1971). Transfer of stimulus control: Measuring the moment of transfer. *Journal of the Experimental Analysis of Behavior, 15*(3), 347–354.

Tsatsanis, K. D. (2004). Heterogeneity in learning style in Asperger syndrome and high-functioning autism. *Topics in Language Disorders, 24*(4), 260–270.

Tsatsanis, K. D., Dartnall, N., Cicchetti, D., Sparrow, S. S., Klin, A., & Volkmar, F. R. (2003). Concurrent validity and classification accuracy of the Leiter and Leiter-R in low-functioning children with autism. *Journal of Autism and Developmental Disorders, 33*(1), 23–30.

Vig, S., & Jedrysek, E. (1995). Adaptive behavior of young urban children with developmental disabilities. *Mental Retardation, 33*(2), 90–98.

Volkmar, F. R., Sparrow, S. S., Goudreau, G., Cicchetti, D. V., Paul, R., & Cohen, D. J. (1987). Social deficits in autism: An operational approach using the Vineland Adaptive Behavior Scales. *Journal of the American Academy of Child & Adolescent Psychiatry, 26*(2), 156–161.

Walsh, K. K., & Shenouda, N. (1999). Correlations among the Reiss Screen, the Adaptive Behavior Scale Part II, and the Aberrant Behavior Checklist. *American Journal of Mental Retardation, 104*(3), 236–248.

West, E. A., & Billingsley, F. (2005). Improving the system of least prompts: A comparison of procedural variations. *Education and Training in Developmental Disabilities, 40*(2), 131–144.

Westling, D. L., & Fox, L. (2004). *Teaching students with severe disabilities* (3rd ed.). Columbus: Merrill.

Williams, D. L., Goldstein, G., Carpenter, P. A., & Minshew, N. J. (2005). Verbal and spatial working memory in autism. *Journal of Autism and Other Developmental Disorders, 35*(6), 747–756.

Winters, N., Collett, B. R., & Myers, K. M. (2005). Ten-year review of rating scales VII: Scales assessing functional impairment. *Journal of the American Academy of Child & Adolescent Psychiatry, 44*(4), 309–338.

Chapter 12
Generalization and Maintenance

Angela M. Arnold-Saritepe, Katrina J. Phillips, Oliver C. Mudford, Kelly Ann De Rozario, and Sarah Ann Taylor

It is often reported that children with ASD do not readily generalize and maintain skills. As such it is of particular importance that practitioners specifically address these issues when developing interventions. This chapter will review and discuss generalization and maintenance within the current ABA research.

Introduction

The past 20 years has seen a marked increase in the quantity of research literature investigating the effectiveness of interventions for people with autism spectrum disorders (ASD). Much of this research has been conducted in applied behavior analysis (ABA), however, many reported interventions do not include information or data on generalization and maintenance of behavior change. The importance of this is self-evident, as an intervention that increases or decreases a behavior is of little use if the behavior change is not observed in a variety of settings and fails to continue after the intervention period has ended.

This chapter seeks to outline why generalization across settings, stimuli, people, and time can be particularly difficult for children with ASD and to review strategies for promoting generalization and maintenance. We did not conduct a comprehensive review of generalization and maintenance in published ASD intervention research. Instead, the available literature was sampled to provide examples of the various strategies that are used to promote generalization and maintenance. Recommendations are provided for practitioners on how to plan for generalization and maintenance.

What is Generalization and Maintenance?

As ABA developed, generalization of behavior change was included as one of the field's defining characteristics (Baer, Wolf, & Risley, 1968). Behavior change was said to have generalized if it lasted over time, occurred in many environments, or spread to related behaviors. These three aspects of generalized behavior change (i.e., across time, settings, and behaviors) were later stressed by Stokes and Baer (1977) when they defined generalization as "… the occurrence of relevant behavior under different nontraining conditions (i.e., across subjects, settings, people, behaviors, and/or time) without the scheduling of the same events in those conditions as has been scheduled in the training conditions. Thus, generalization may be claimed when no extra training manipulations are needed for extra training changes; or may be claimed when some extra manipulations are necessary, but their cost or extent is clearly less than that of the direct intervention." (p. 350).

Generalization is an integral part in the development of any behavioral plan as it allows for the behavior that is being taught to occur (or not occur) under different, nontraining conditions. It is clearly an advantage to take what we are taught and apply it appropriately in a novel situation. For example, if we were unable to generalize then every time we bought a new pair of shoes we would have to relearn how to tie our shoelaces.

A. Arnold-Saritepe (✉)
Applied Behavior Analysis Program, Department of Psychology (Tamaki Campus), University of Auckland, Private Bag 92019, Auckland, New Zealand
e-mail: a.arnold-saritepe@auckland.ac.nz

J.L. Maston (ed.), *Applied Behavior Analysis for Children with Autism Spectrum Disorders*, DOI 10.1007/978-1-4419-0088-3_12, © Springer Science+Business Media, LLC 2009

Discrimination or Generalization?

When teaching a child to point to a picture of a cat upon hearing the word "cat", we are teaching discrimination. When the child hears the word "cat," the child touches the picture of the cat in the book that is being read, and we praise or otherwise reinforce the child for touching the correct picture. The act of the child touching the picture of the cat is called a discriminated operant. The child has made a discrimination and the behavior of touching the picture of the cat, the discriminated operant, occurs more frequently under the antecedent condition of the adult saying "cat," than it does at any other time. Because the discriminated operant, touching the cat, occurs at a higher frequency when we say "cat," the response is said to be under stimulus control. The relationship of the stimulus to the discriminated operant comes from the three-term contingency – antecedent, behavior, and consequence. In the example above, the antecedent is the adult saying the word "cat," the behavior is the child touching the picture of the cat, and the consequence is the delivery of a reinforcer. If the child were to touch something else on the page, the consequence would not be reinforcement, but error correction or extinction to decrease the likelihood of that behavior occurring again.

The adult has taught the relationship to the child "when you see *this* cat in *this* picture book and I say "cat," your touching the cat will result in reinforcement". Touching the picture of the cat is more likely to occur in the presence of the discriminative stimulus, the spoken word "cat." This is a discrimination, however, it is limited to the adult saying "cat" in the presence of that picture of that cat in that book. Other people may say "cat" to the child in the presence of the same book in the same or other settings. Others may also say "cat" in the presence of other pictures or photos of cats, or actual cats in multiple settings. Cats come in many forms, big, small, fat, and furry and the adult may also say "cat" tomorrow or next week.

A successful program for socially significant behavior change requires more than that the individual performs exactly the same topography of behavior, in the identical stimulus context as in a tightly controlled training setting, and with the intervention program remaining in place. Real success will include that the intervention has produced generalization of change across a range of functional response forms in a wide variety of settings

and maintenance (i.e., generalization beyond the termination of the original training program).

Generalization

The occurrence of generalization without additional training manipulations is consistent with the historical understanding that generalization was a passive phenomenon. Generalization was not something that was trained. It was something that just happened. If generalization did not occur, it was assumed that the teaching processes had managed to maintain particularly good control of the stimuli and the responses involved, thus producing little variability in behavior.

Stokes and Baer (1977) questioned the view that generalization was a passive phenomenon by which behavior change in the training setting (e.g., one-to-one therapist–child teaching in a distraction-free room) with specified antecedent stimuli (e.g., particular materials and therapist's script) "naturally" transferred to other settings and stimulus contexts. Put another way, is generalization a desirable outcome that often naturally comes with no extra effort on the part of the therapist or ABA programmer? From their review of ABA research to that time, Stokes and Baer (1977) concluded that behavior analysts should assume that socially important generalization never comes "for free." Baer et al. (1968) had made similar arguments several years earlier. They recommended that plans for generalization be incorporated in interventions rather than assuming that generalization would occur and mourning if it did not. Thus, programming actively for generalization has long been encouraged.

The passive view of generalization is implicit in the following statements: "Children with autism learn OK, but do not generalize what they have learned" {oft-said by anonymous therapists (year dot to present)}; and, "It is sometimes assumed that application [of a behavioral intervention] has failed when generalization does not take place in any widespread form." (Baer et al., 1968, p. 96). In the first example, children are, and/or autism is, the implied source of failed generalization. In the second example, the blame is on the intervention. Sometimes, these sources of failure are conflated, e.g., "... and inability (of children with autism) to use trained skills outside school are some of the shortcomings critics attribute to ABA" (Wallis, 2006).

A contrasting approach, consistent with proactive recommendations of Baer et al. (1968) and Stokes and Baer (1977), would attribute successful generalization to well-planned, well-designed, and well-implemented procedures to promote generalization. A failure of generalization would be blamed not on the child, or autism, or the intervention per se, but on the inadequacies in generalization planning, design, and implementation.

Before further discussing how to promote generalized behavior change, it is necessary to understand the different terms used to describe generalization.

The following paragraphs define and provide examples of the three basic forms of generalized behavior change: Stimulus generalization, response generalization, and response maintenance, in addition to other types of generalized outcome.

Stimulus generalization is said to have occurred when the likelihood of the behavior increases in the presence of a stimulus or setting as a result of being reinforced in the presence of a different stimulus or setting (Martin & Pear, 2003). In our example above, if the child were to touch the picture of the same cat in a different book upon hearing the word "cat," this would be stimulus generalization. Further examples would be touching the same cat on flash cards, or on computer screens. Touching similar cats (cats with physical similarity – similar colors, size) is also an example of stimulus generalization. As with animals, we (humans) have evolved such that when two stimuli have a large degree of physical similarity the more likely it is that stimulus generalization will occur between them. However, is the child likely to touch a lion, or a hairless cat? Perhaps not, as the child may not have learned the complete stimulus class "cat." A further example of stimulus generalization occurs when we teach a child to wash their hands. Stimulus generalization is very useful in this case as we want our learner to wash their hands in a new situation that is different in some way to the teaching setting (different bathrooms) and stimuli (different taps, soap dispensers, towels).

Response generalization is shown when the learner emits a new, untrained behavior that is functionally equivalent to the behavior that was trained (Cooper, Heron, & Heward, 2007). For example, our child who learnt receptive identification of the cat by pointing to the picture of the cat now responds to the adult saying "cat" by handing over the correct picture. Pointing to and handing over a picture are functionally equivalent as they demonstrate receptive identification of the cat

and will both result in reinforcement. In the example of our hand washer, if they were to dry their hands by wiping them on their pants this would be response generalization. Drying ones hands on ones pants is not necessarily desirable. However, drying hands on ones pants does have the same function as using a towel, as it results in getting one's hands dry.

Response maintenance occurs when the learner continues to perform the trained behavior after the intervention responsible for the behavior has ceased. How long a newly learned behavior maintains in a person's life depends on how useful it is to them and whether natural contingencies in the environment continue to reinforce it. Our learner should be able to point to a picture of a cat in response to the word "cat" years after it has been taught, and the presence of dirty hands should result in the response of hand washing for the rest of the person's life.

In addition to stimulus and response generalization and response maintenance, other generalized outcomes (e.g., generalization across subjects and stimulus equivalence) have been reported in the ABA literature. Having taught one child to wash their hands, if another child in the same house, who was not directly taught, started washing their hands too, this would be an example of generalization across children.

Stimulus equivalence occurs when correct responding to untrained stimulus–stimulus relations occurs. Sidman (1971) provided the first example of an equivalence class among arbitrary stimuli in a boy with mental retardation. Prior to the study, the boy could match pictures to their spoken names and name pictures. After being taught to match written names to spoken names the boy could, without additional training, match written names to pictures, match pictures to written names, and say the written words. The result of learning one stimulus–stimulus relation was the emergence of three other relations without direct training. Sidman and Tailby (1982) described this in the logical formulation: If A = B and B = C, then A = C. Potentially, this would be advantageous in programming and curriculum design for children with ASD. In theory, if A is the spoken word "cat," B is the picture of a cat, and C the written word cat, we could train the stimulus relations spoken word "cat" to picture and picture to written word CAT, then spoken word "cat" to written word CAT would emerge without further training. Eikeseth and Smith (1992) found naming of visual stimuli (Greek letters) to enhance the development of three-member (name and two visual stimuli; Greek letters and their written name) equivalence classes for one preschool child and to have mixed benefits with three other children.

Desirability of Generalized Behavior Change

Is generalized behavior change always desirable? Not necessarily, as sometimes we are seeking discrimination rather than generalization. For example, following the establishment of the discrimination "cat," if our cat learner were to point to a dog in the presence of someone saying "cat" we would say they have overgeneralized. Cats and dogs after all do have some physical similarities. If our learner was to touch every black and white object they saw, in response to the spoken word "cat," faulty stimulus control would have occurred. The target behavior has come under the control of an irrelevant feature of the antecedent stimulus. It just so happens that our learner was taught cat in the presence of picture of a black and white cat.

As practitioners, we should always assume that there is no such thing as free generalization. This applies even more when working children with ASD who are often described as having difficulty in generalizing behavior change.

Generalization and ASD

In teaching a child with ASD to identify a cat upon hearing the word "cat", practitioners anecdotally report that when different adults present the same discriminative stimulus ("cat") or when a different pictorial example of a cat is shown, errors occur. This difficulty with generalization has been attributed to insistence to sameness (Horner, Dunlap, & Koegel, 1988; Lovaas, Koegel, & Schreibman, 1979; Rincover & Koegel, 1975), stimulus overselectivity (Lovaas, Schreibman, Koegel, & Rehm, 1971), and/or lack of motivation (Horner et al., 1988).

One of the behaviors identified as being symptomatic of autism is "restricted, repetitive, and stereotypic patterns of behavior, interests, and activities" (American

Psychiatric Association, 2000, pp. 70–75). Insistence on sameness may hinder the child's success in generalizing the target behavior across settings, time, and people (Horner et al., 1988; Lovaas et al., 1979; Rincover & Koegel 1975). When aspects of the generalization setting are different in any form from the setting that the child was trained in, the change in stimuli can inhibit the transfer of skills. Thus, different pictures of cats or cats in different forms (e.g., photos on a television screen) would result in errors. The likelihood that the child will only ever see one representation of a cat is extremely low. Furthermore, even a slight change in the stimulus, such as the pictured cat being at a different angle, could also hinder generalization, as this seemingly trivial change can be significant to a child with ASD.

Stimulus overselectivity has also been identified as playing a role in the difficulty children with autism have in generalizing behavior. Stimulus overselectivity is best defined as when a learner selects particular aspects of the stimulus to make the discrimination that may, or may not, be relevant (Lovaas et al., 1971). For example, a child, who only recognized cats when they had a white left front paw (the trained cat had a white left front paw), would be said to be overselective in making the discrimination "cat or not-cat". Children with autism have been found to be more likely to respond to selected aspects of a complex stimulus compared with typically developing children, who respond to multiple aspects (Lovaas et al., 1971). Schreibman and Lovaas (1973) found that children with autism were able to discriminate between male and female dolls. However, when the clothes and other characteristics of the dolls were changed the majority of the children with autism were no longer able to make the discrimination. This was not the case for typically developing children. Further testing revealed that the reason for lack of generalization was due to the children with autism selecting irrelevant item(s), such as the doll's shoes, as the discriminative stimulus to determine gender. Stimulus overselectivity has been shown to affect a child's ability to generalize their target behavior(s). If the target behavior is only under the control of limited aspects of the antecedent stimuli during training, it is possible that these aspects will not be present in another setting (Lovaas et al., 1979).

Lack of motivation may also be a factor for children with autism failing to generalize (Horner et al., 1988; Koegel & Egel, 1979; Koegel & Mentis, 1985).

It has been said that children with autism have low levels of responding when in contact with intermittent reinforcers (Horner et al., 1988; Koegel & Mentis, 1985). When in an environment that does not produce reinforcers for every instance of correct behavior, children with autism may become "unmotivated" to emit the behavior, thus resulting in a decrease and extinction of the target behavior. Furthermore, learned helplessness has also been reported as a factor for children being unmotivated to respond (Horner et al., 1988; Koegel & Egel, 1979; Koegel & Mentis, 1985). A decreased level of responding is observed because of constant failure at new tasks. Children quickly learn that reinforcement is only available when a correct response is delivered, and not for every response. So, when presented with a new task the learner with autism may become unmotivated as they are reinforced only for correct responses that are less likely to occur.

Although the research outlined above suggests that children with autism have some specific limitations with regard to generalization, it does not mean that the behavior changes that occur within the increasing or decreasing programs cannot be generalized. As stated in the earlier section, the failure to see generalization is not a failure of an intervention or a child and their diagnosis, but rather the failure of the person planning the intervention to program for generalization.

Current Practices

It is the purpose of this section to report on the current practice of generalization strategies with specific reference to research with children with autism. Intervention articles published in the *Journal of Applied Behavior Analysis* from 2003 to present {Vol. 36 – Vol. 41(2)} with children with ASD as the participants were reviewed. Forty-three articles were identified. Generalization and maintenance were not measured in 42% of the reviewed articles. This is a dismal finding given that the importance of generalization and maintenance has been emphasized for 40 years. Generalization was programmed for in 26% of articles, with the techniques of programming common stimuli and multiple exemplar training (these terms are defined below) being the most popular. A further 32% of articles measured generalization and/or maintenance. The measurement of

generalization without programming for it has been described as "train and hope" (Stokes & Baer, 1977). Training and hoping is characterized by the measurement of generalization across responses, experimenters, settings, and time after a behavior change has been effected because of intervention. Generalization is not actively sought; it is just welcomed should it occur.

It is clear that the majority of researchers do not report planning for generalization. Even though researchers do not always attend to generalization, it can never be ignored by responsible practitioners.

Strategies to Promote Generalization

As previously discussed, if we are to increase the likelihood of generalized behavior change, it is necessary to plan systematically for the desired outcome. This requires selecting target behaviors that are functional and will come under naturally occurring reinforcement contingencies in the environment, specifying all environments where the target behavior (stimulus generalization) should occur, and in all forms that it should occur (response generalization). Returning to our example of cat identification, the desired outcome is for our learner to recognize all cats in all forms (e.g., pictures, photos, live, textual) in all settings (e.g., home, grandparents' house, school, outside) – stimulus generalization – and to be able to receptively identify cats, expressively identify cats, and sort cats into categories – response generalization. Identifying all the behaviors that need to be changed and all the settings and situations, in which the behavior should occur, requires a fair amount of planning. However, without a *systematic* plan the practitioner will be relying on the train-and-hope approach and generalization that does occur may not be desired. Furthermore, if we are going to all the bother of changing behavior, we should ensure that it will maintain in the natural environment and that it will occur in all forms and relevant environments.

Strategies for promoting generalized behavior change were categorized under nine general headings by Stokes and Baer (1977).

1. Train and Hope
2. Sequential Modification
3. Introduce to Natural Maintaining Contingencies
4. Train Sufficient Exemplars

5. Train Loosely
6. Use Indiscriminable Contingencies
7. Program Common Stimuli
8. Mediate Generalization
9. Train "To Generalize"

Other authors have extended and re-categorized the nine proposed approaches to generalization (e.g., Cooper et al., 2007; Stokes & Osnes, 1989). However, we will use Stokes and Baer's original terminology because of its clarity and inclusiveness.

The following sections explain and provide examples of each generalization strategy with reference to children with autism. Despite train-and-hope being the common practice, it will not be discussed further as it is not a strategy to promote generalization.

Sequential Modification

As with train-and-hope, sequential modification addresses generalization only after behavior change has occurred (Stokes & Baer, 1977). That is, an intervention is conducted, behavior change occurs, generalization is probed for and then, if generalization has not occurred to the desired, settings, stimuli, and/or behaviors it is trained. This would be akin to teaching a child to receptively identify a cat by pointing to one flashcard of a cat in one setting. After the desired response is being emitted, pointing to the cat in response to the instructor saying "cat," generalization probes would be conducted with different cats in flashcard and other forms in the same and different settings.

Kamps, Potucek, Lopez, Kravits, and Kemmerer (1997) used a multiple probe design across activities to measure the effects of introducing peer networks and reinforcement of social interaction for three young boys with autism. The intervention was introduced in a sequential fashion across four activities for each student while baseline conditions remained in effect for two activities. For two of the participants, generalization of social interactions was observed in at least one untrained activity. The authors do not report whether the intervention was introduced to the activities or for participants for which generalization did not occur. Generalization was more likely to occur in similar social settings, when the generalization activity was scheduled soon after the trained activity, and when the materials between activities were similar.

Introduce to Natural Maintaining Contingencies

In order for behavior to continue to occur outside the training environment, it must continue to make contact with its maintaining contingencies. Therefore, when planning for generalization a practitioner must work to *maximize* the contact the behavior will have with natural contingencies. The practitioner, therefore, should consider the target behavior, possible natural contingences, and alternative strategies if the natural contingencies are not strong enough (Baer, 1999).

One way of achieving this is to ensure that there are natural contingencies in the generalization setting that the behavior will contact. When selecting a target behavior a practitioner should consider what the learner would achieve for emitting the behavior in the natural setting. If the behavior is not going to result in reinforcement at a high enough rate, or is going to require too much effort to emit, then it is unlikely that the behavior will occur in the natural setting (Baer, 1999).

In conjunction with ensuring that the target behavior has a natural consequence, the practitioner must also ensure that the behavior occurs in a manner that allows it to make contact with reinforcement. This requires the practitioner to consider the most appropriate topographical form of the behavior. Harchik, Harchik, Luce, and Sherman (1990) found that although the phrase "check it out," to gain attention, was appropriate and received praise in the home setting, it did not receive praise in the school setting and, instead, often lead to a reprimand. In addition to considering the topography of the behavior, a practitioner must also ensure that the behavior is trained until it is accurate and occurring often enough, long enough, fast enough, and with enough magnitude to obtain reinforcement (e.g., Tiger, Bouxsein, & Fisher, 2007). For example, it is unlikely that a peer's greeting behavior will be maintained if following their "good morning" greeting the second child takes 30 s to respond. The peer, who made the initial greeting, will have probably left by this time, thus removing the opportunity for either child to receive reinforcement. For those behaviors that do have a natural consequence but do not occur often enough, long enough, fast enough and with enough magnitude to obtain reinforcement, it may be beneficial to start training with a contrived reinforcer (e.g., Jones, Feeley, & Takacs, 2007).

Baer and Wolf (1970) used the term "behavior trap" to describe how natural contingences can result in significant and efficient behavior change that maintains over time without intervention. Despite there being little research on behavior traps, it is worthwhile to describe the concept. A behavior trap has four essential features. First, it is necessary that the consequence for initially entering the behavior trap is something reinforcing. The second is that the individual has, in his/her repertoire, the response required to enter the behavior trap, and the response does not require much effort to emit. The third feature is that once in the trap there are a number of contingencies that interact with each other to ensure that the individual acquires, extends, and maintains the targeted skills. Finally, a behavior trap will continue to reinforce behavior change without an intervention because the individual will show minimal satiation effects (Alber & Heward, 1996).

Some behavior traps occur naturally. For example, if parents teach their child to say please and thank you at mealtimes those behaviors may be trapped by social reinforcement from their grandparents for using old-fashioned manners. Alber and Heward (1996) outlined several steps for developing effective behavior traps. First, the practitioner must identify an appropriate target behavior. This means a behavior that is important, has natural consequences, is able to be practiced frequently, and is easily emitted. Second, the practitioner must identify the reinforcer for entering the behavior trap (e.g., look at the individual's interests). Third, the practitioner must now create or set the behavior trap. This requires making sure the child will emit the behavior and therefore come into contact with the initial reinforcer. Fourth, the practitioner should continually be assessing the behavior change to ensure that the trap is effective.

Alber and Heward (1996) provide a number of examples of how to create behavior traps within a classroom. For example, the teacher identifies that her student is having difficulty interacting socially with her peers. Increased and generalized peer interaction is sought. The student is very good on computers and enjoys playing games on them. The teacher asks the student to teach one of the other children how to play a game based on a topic that is mutually liked by both children. Once both are competent in the game, the teacher asks the two students to work together to find out other information on the game. During this time, the teacher assesses the children's amount and type of interaction during prescribed learning time and outside of this time.

An alternative, when the natural reinforcement is low, is to "wake up" any potential natural reinforcement in the environment (Baer, 1999). This is especially important if the schedule cannot be thinned to a point that the natural contingencies will take effect (e.g., Tarbox, Wallace, & Tarbox, 2002). One way to increase the natural reinforcement that is available in the generalization setting is for the practitioner to recruit others to help generalize and maintain the behavior. The techniques vary from merely drawing people's attention to the intervention and/or behavior to more explicit instructions and training. Tarbox et al. (2002) used parent training to ensure continued treatment gains obtained with an intervention that was designed to decrease object mouthing by a child with autism. The treatment involved the provision of prompted toy play in conjunction with response blocking. Initial attempts by therapists to thin the schedule of response blocking in the natural setting were somewhat successful. However, this success was not maintained when the schedule was thinned further. In response to this outcome, the mother was trained to implement the initial procedure at home. The training consisted of explanations of the rationale, descriptions, modeling of the procedure, and feedback based upon actual implementation. This training resulted in near-zero levels of the behavior. As well as parents, research has also been conducted where peers (e.g., Kamps et al. 1997) and staff (e.g., Arco & Millet, 1996) have been recruited to maintain the behavior in the natural environment.

Where possible, it is often more advantageous to teach the child to recruit reinforcement. For example, Durand and Carr (1992) found that teaching children to gain attention in an appropriate manner (e.g., "Am I doing good work?") was equally as effective as time out in decreasing behavioral excesses maintained by access to attention. However, the results of a generalization test to a naive trainer showed that the communicative response groups' behavior remained low, while the time out groups' behavior increased. Although it would be possible to train the naive trainer to implement the timeout procedure, it is much more cost effective to train the children and have them assisted in generalizing the behavior. Harchik et al. (1990) taught four boys with autism to ask questions and make requests in order to increase the amount of praise they received from adults. All the children learnt to ask the questions and make requests and used these skills over a number of different settings and activities.

A review of the maintenance data showed that the original levels were maintained for at least 3 weeks, at which time data collection stopped. One limitation that was noted with this research was that there was no corresponding decrease in attention-seeking behaviors. This may have been because the children's requests for praise did not always result in praise. This limitation draws attention for the need to consult all interested parties when considering target behaviors to maximize the chances of the behavior contacting the natural contingencies and generalizing.

There appears to be consensus (e.g., Baer, 1999; Cooper et al., 2007; Stokes & Baer, 1977; Stokes & Osnes, 1989) on the need for practitioners to program to capture natural contingencies when designing interventions to change both behavioral excesses and deficits. Indeed, it is possible that a number of interventions that have shown generalization and/or maintenance without any programming will have done so because the behavior has inadvertently come into contact with natural contingences (e.g., Carr & Darcy, 1990).

Train Sufficient Exemplars

Training sufficient exemplars was described by Stokes and Baer (1977) as the most prominent generalization strategy in the literature. In teaching a generalizable lesson, often only one exemplar is taught to mastery with no generalization beyond what has been specifically taught. Training sufficient exemplars involves teaching another, another, and another exemplar of the same generalizable lesson until generalization occurs on its own sufficiently to teach the lesson. For example, when teaching the receptive identification of cats, we may teach with a picture of one cat. After this has been mastered, and there is no evidence of generalization to other cat pictures, another cat exemplar would be taught, then another, and then another until the learner can identify cats of all different forms e.g., photos of cats, live cats, different colored cats, cats standing in different positions, and different species of cats. Laushey and Heflin (2000) conducted a study to increase the social skills in two kindergarten children with autism. Each child attended a mainstream kindergarten class where a buddy system was developed in which each student with autism was paired with a typical peer to engage in play and conversation. As part of

the generalization training, multiple stimulus examples were provided by rotating the pairing so that the participants were with a different peer each day. The pairing of the participant with multiple peers provided them with opportunity to respond correctly to different peers. Results showed that the participants increased their social skills significantly with many of their peers. A generalization probe conducted at follow-up showed that the social skills had generalized across settings also, as one participant maintained a high level of interaction with peers in his first grade class.

Fiorile and Greer (2007) programmed for generalization among four children with autism after it was found that tact training (experimenter presentation of item, and vocal tact) did not result in a naming repertoire. Fiorile and Greer provided multiple examples of the stimuli (pictures of and actual objects), alternating between match, point, and tact for a set of objects during instruction. Once mastery was met, generalization probes showed that the children had acquired naming of stimuli in trained sets as well as the capability to name from tact instruction alone.

When promoting generalization by training with multiple stimulus and response examples, it is necessary to conduct a generalization probe in an untrained setting or with untrained people following initial training. If the child is successfully able to emit the target behavior in untrained examples, then generalization has occurred. However, if the child does not, training should then be conducted in the probe setting or with more examples. Generalization probes should again follow with further untrained examples until the child is able to emit the target behavior proficiently with untrained examples (Stokes & Baer, 1977).

Train Loosely

In training loosely, the behavior analyst plans to randomly alter irrelevant aspects of the training setting that may inadvertently acquire stimulus control over the child's newly learned behavior (Campbell & Campbell, 1982). When training the receptive identification of a cat, the practitioner will randomize the position of the correct picture; teaching will occur with many different teachers, in many different rooms, and at a desk, as well as when sitting on the floor. Stokes and Baer (1977) recommended that practitioners use loose teaching by varying random stimuli in the training setting such as temperature, tone of voice, trainers, and noise level in addition to further examples. One of the aims of teaching loosely is that the participant's target behavior is not controlled by unwanted stimuli. Rincover and Koegel (1975) found that their participants' behavior did not generalize to an untrained setting because of the children responding to unintended stimuli (hand movements) instead of the planned discriminative stimuli (verbal commands). Teaching loosely is also useful for avoiding any "surprises" that the child may encounter in the generalization setting (Cooper et al., 2007; Horner et al., 1988). By varying the different stimuli in the training setting, there is a high possibility that the child may experience some, if not all, of these stimuli in other untrained settings. When training loosely, it is important during planning to take note of the different irrelevant antecedent stimuli and vary them at different times of the day and as unpredictably as possible (Baer, 1999).

Use Indiscriminable Contingencies

It has been identified that practitioners should strive to select behaviors that have naturally occurring contingencies although these contingencies are sometimes weak (i.e., lean schedules of reinforcement or delayed reinforcement). In situations such as this, the chances of generalization occurring is enhanced if the contingencies that mark the presence or absence of the availability of reinforcement for the behavior are unclear, i.e., indiscriminable. Practitioners should program indiscriminable contingencies once the behavior has been mastered and before the intervention is removed from all settings. When an indiscriminable contingency is in place, the child should not receive immediate reinforcement for every response but only for some responses. This is called intermittent reinforcement and is obtained through a process known as schedule thinning. Research shows that behavior that is reinforced on an intermittent schedule is more resistant to extinction, and as such should be more likely to generalize (Stokes & Baer, 1977).

Koegel and Rincover (1977) were among the first to investigate the effects of manipulating the contingencies within the intervention and natural setting to make them less discriminable. The participants were children with autism between 7 and 13 years of age. The intervention consisted of teaching the children nonverbal imitation and following verbal instruction. In the initial study, Koegel and Rincover found that two of the children showed generalization but failed to maintain their behavior and one failed to generalize at all. In the second experiment, they found that children given continuous reinforcement for their behavior during treatment did initially generalize to the alternative setting. However, the behavior quickly extinguished. They found that the thinner the schedule during treatment (the more correct responses that were not reinforced) the more resistant the behavior was to extinction in the generalization setting. In addition, they found that if a schedule was thinned and paired with noncontingent reinforcement in the natural setting, generalization over time was further enhanced.

Program Common Stimuli

Generalization can also be promoted by making the training setting similar to the generalization setting. Programming common stimuli requires the training environment to contain stimuli comparable to those in the generalization setting (Stokes & Baer, 1977). For example, in teaching the receptive identification of cats, our goal may be for the child to point to pictures of cats in a book during circle time in their preschool class. If we were promoting generalization through the programming of common stimuli, we would create a similar environment for training purposes. This may involve using the teacher as the instructor, simulating circle time by having peers present during training, turn-taking responses, and using the same materials as those in the classroom. If the common stimuli are well chosen, functional, and salient during training, the likelihood of generalization will be enhanced (Stokes & Baer, 1977).

Petursdottir, McComas, McMaster, and Horner (2007) used programming common stimuli to increase social interactions for a 5-year-old preschool child with autism with his peer tutoring partners following a tutoring session. Their intervention involved scripted peer tutoring in a reading activity with and without programming common stimuli. Three classmates were selected as peer tutors for the reading activity and observations were carried out to determine the frequency of social interactions between the participant and his tutoring partners during free play. Common stimuli were programmed by incorporating the same play activities into the peer tutoring reading activity sessions as were used in free play sessions. The social interactions in the reading activity generalized to the free play when common stimuli were programmed compared to when they were not.

Before programming common stimuli, it is important to determine the significant stimuli. When teaching children with multiple handicaps to order food at a fast food restaurant, van den Pol et al. (1981) determined that the significant stimuli could include one or multiple stimuli such as the menu board, price of items, and the person at the counter. The practitioner would program common stimuli by placing models of the menu board and price of items in the training setting to increase the probability of facilitating generalization of fast food ordering from one setting to another (Cooper et al., 2007; Horner et al., 1988; van den Pol et al., 1981).

Mediate Generalization

Generalization may be facilitated by arranging a mediating stimulus (e.g., a person or object) to ensure generalization of behavior change from the instructional setting to the generalization setting. This may be done by contriving a mediating stimulus that prompts or aids the child's performance of the target behavior (Stokes & Baer, 1977). A mediating stimulus may be added to the instructional setting or may be naturally present in the generalization setting. The stimulus must reliably prompt the target behavior during instruction and must be transportable to all important generalization settings (Baer, 1999). Examples of mediating stimuli used with children with autism include people (e.g., Goldstein & Wickstrom, 1986), cue cards (e.g., O'Neill & Sweetland-Baker, 2001), photographic activity schedules (e.g., MacDuff, Krantz, & McClannahan, 1993), and the Picture Exchange Communication System (PECS; Bondy & Frost, 1994).

People are highly successful as mediating stimuli as they move from setting to setting and often provide reinforcement for many behaviors (Cooper et al., 2007). Goldstein and Wickstrom (1986) used a peer-mediated intervention to increase interactions among three preschoolers who displayed autistic-like behav-

iors. Two typical preschoolers were taught strategies to facilitate interactions with the target participants (e.g., gaining eye contact and prompting requests). The peers were then also present as mediating stimuli in non-training sessions. During maintenance sessions, all teacher prompts were removed, and results showed interactions to remain at levels higher than baseline.

O'Neill and Sweetland-Baker (2001) used functional communication training (FCT) to reduce escape-maintained disruptive behavior with two students with autism. During instruction (e.g., writing), students were prompted to touch a small "BREAK" card for a 30-s break from task demand. In generalization settings (other tasks such as cleaning and putting items away) the card was present but no prompting occurred. Generalization was demonstrated across most untrained tasks, with reductions in disruptive behavior and increases in unprompted break requests.

A further method to mediate generalization is to teach the child self-management skills. Self-management involves the child themselves applying behavior change tactics to produce a desirable change in the target behavior (Cooper et al., 2007). Self-management can involve the child observing and recording their own behavior (self-monitoring or self-recording), comparing their performance to a pre-determined criterion (self-evaluation), and administering reinforcement (self-reinforcement).

Self-management has been used with children with autism to decrease off-task behavior (e.g., Coyle & Cole, 2004), improve social responses (e.g., Koegel, Koegel, Hurley, & Frea, 1992), teach daily living skills (e.g., Pierce & Shreibman, 1994), and increase appropriate play in unsupervised settings (e.g., Stahmer & Shreibman, 1992). Some mediating stimuli, such as photographic activity schedules (e.g., MacDuff et al., 1993), may also include self-management techniques.

Coyle and Cole (2004) evaluated the effect of video self-modeling and self-monitoring on off-task behavior in three boys with autism. During the intervention, children were first required to watch a video that showed them engaging in on-task behavior. Children were then trained in self-monitoring and were required to record behavior in the classroom as "working" or "not working" at the end of 30-s intervals. The teacher provided reinforcement (including colored stickers and popcorn) for appropriate behavior. Results showed a large decrease in off-task behavior during the intervention that was maintained during follow-up sessions.

As well as a mediating stimulus, a photographic activity schedule also allows for self-management, as it allows children to administer their reinforcement after completing a series of tasks. A photographic activity schedule depicts activities that a child must complete, in order, before having access to a reinforcer. The schedule serves as a prompt to complete the tasks and is easily transportable as it is typically kept in a small binder. MacDuff et al. (1993) used photographic activity schedules with four boys aged 9–14 years with autism to increase on-task and on-schedule behavior. The children were required to complete three activities (including Lego™, games, and handwriting worksheets) before having access to reinforcers (snack, puzzle, and TV). Generalization was assessed by replacing two of the original tasks with similar tasks in the boy's schedules. Results showed sustained on-task and on-schedule behavior across lengthy response chains that generalized to novel tasks. Photographic activity schedules have also been used to teach daily living skills e.g., getting dressed, making lunch, and doing laundry (Pierce & Shreibman, 1994).

Train to Generalize

Possibly, the most simple way to attempt to obtain generalization is to ask the child to generalize. Stokes and Baer (1977) suggested that practitioners could obtain cost-effective generalization by using systematic instructions to inform the learner on what is required in other situations. In order to generalize in this manner, an individual would require prerequisite skills, such as listening skills and the ability to follow rules. However, despite many children with ASD having these skills, there does not appear to be any literature as to the effectiveness of the intervention with this population.

Another way of training to generalize may be reinforcing response variability (Stokes & Baer, 1977). The idea is that that if practitioners can increase variability in responding, they would obtain response generalization. In addition, the increase in variations should then create more contact with natural reinforcement, and thus the response class will be more likely to be maintained in the natural environment. The basic and applied literature has a number of articles that show that response variability can be increased using either extinction and/or direct reinforcement (Lee, Sturmey, & Fields, 2007). Despite this, the research with children with autism, especially in applied situations, is not as extensive. Two studies (Lee, McComas, & Jawor, 2002; Lee & Sturmey, 2006) have investigated the effects of lag schedules on variability in children with autism.

Lag schedules involve reinforcing a response if it is different from the preceding responses. For example, a Lag 1 response schedule would require that the current response be different from the previous response, but not necessarily different from the response that had occurred two responses ago. In comparison, a Lag 2 response schedule would require that the current response be different from the two previous responses, but not different from the third previous response. Lee et al. (2002) investigated the effects of a Lag 1 schedule on responding to social questions. They found that two 7-year-old boys with autism had an increase in the percentage of trials with varied and appropriate responding when posed the questions "what do you like to do?" These results generalized across people and settings, even though reinforcement was not contingent upon variations in responding in these sessions. However, generalization was not maintained when the Lag 1 schedule was not in place in the alternative setting. The authors suggested that the teaching situation might have been serving as a cue for varied behavior. A third participant, a 27-year-old male with autism, failed to show similar results in response to the question "how are you?" The researchers suggested that this was due to the question failing to occasion varied responding or the ineffectiveness of reinforcement. Interestingly, of the two boys who achieved varied responding, one of the boys used 19 novel responses while the other only used four novel responses. Despite this difference, the second boy was able to obtain similar levels of reinforcement to the first boy, because he merely alternated between responses.

Lee and Sturmey (2006) replicated these results with three teenagers who had a diagnosis of autism. They found that two of the three participants showed increased variations when a lag-1 schedule was in place irrespective of the presence of preferred items in the environment (a suspected confound from the previous research). In addition, they also found that while one participant showed a variety or responses, the other alternated between responses. The research by Lee and colleagues has demonstrated that variability can be increased in individuals with autism; however, they acknowledge that more research is needed on the clinical utility of these procedures.

Extinction occurs when reinforcement is no longer provided for a behavior that previously resulted in reinforcement. One of the known side effects of extinction is increased variability in behavior. There appears to be little research on this topic with children with autism. Grow, Kelley, Roane, and Shillingsburg (2008) placed problem behaviors on extinction to induce response variability in FCT responses in three children with autism. Typically, when problem behaviors are put on extinction, the functional alternative that is reinforced is either an existing response or an instructor-selected alternative. The results showed that placing problem behavior on extinction was effective in producing alternative behaviors during FCT.

Stokes and Baer (1977) state that although training an individual to generalize may be an effective tool to ensure generalization, ideally we would want the learner to generalize not only their behavior but also the ability to generalize. They labeled individuals who had been taught this skill as "generalized generalizers." Both the techniques outlined above have received very little research, especially with children with autism, and there does not appear to be any research on "generalized generalizers."

Planning for Generalized Outcomes

In this section, we make recommendations to practitioners regarding *planning* for generalization. The planning is undertaken as part of the development of any plan for behavior change at the outset, not as an afterthought. An intervention plan for a referred behavior should include consideration of desired generalization across behaviors, stimuli, settings, and time, with the last being maintenance of behavior change in the future beyond the intervention. In our experience of planning for generalization in clinical and/or educational applications of ABA or teaching others how to plan, we have previously relied on the "generalization map" designed by Drabman, Hammer, and Rosenbaum (1979). The map presented a conceptual model for categorizing domains of generalization addressed in the ABA research literature. Studies were categorized by

the presence or absence of generalization across participants, behaviors, settings, and time and all the combinations thereof; 16 categories in all. The generalization map may be most helpful for designing research studies concerning generalization, which was its developers' purpose. We have found it helpful as a conceptual model, but less so as a practical tool in planning generalization in individual applied (or clinical) applications. Hence, we have designed a "generalization planner" for applied use (see Fig. 1).

The top panel in Fig. 1 explains recommended domains of generalization to be considered when planning interventions at a relatively conceptual level. The middle panel shows a generalized schema for planning. The bottom panel shows a hypothetical example of the use of the planner for teaching receptive identification of the noun "cat". From left to right, the planner first prompts the behavior analyst to write in a name for the class of behaviors to be changed. Second, to plan for generalization across the variety of response forms that are functionally equivalent, a list is made of all the topographies (forms) of referred behavior that are to be changed. If the intervention aims to teach new desirable forms of behavior that are related, these will be listed as exemplified in the bottom panel. If the intervention also aims to reduce problem behaviors, they will be listed. Third, in planning for generalization across stimuli, the range of materials required to perform the desired generalized behavior are listed. The naturally occurring antecedent stimuli for appropriate performance of the desired behavioral responses need to be considered here. What can be predicted to be naturally maintaining reinforcers (consequent stimuli) following withdrawal of arbitrary or contrived instructional reinforcers are included conceptually in considering generalization across stimuli. Fourth, the range of settings, in which behavior change is to occur, is listed. For children with ASD, obvious examples are home, school, and community settings. However, in planning for generalization for an individual child's behavior change program, these settings need to be specified. For example, in which particular classroom and at which particular school does raising hand to obtain attention need to occur to replace screaming? Another example might be: What is the name of the health center where the child needs to sit still while her ears are examined for otitis media? Fifth, under the heading of "social

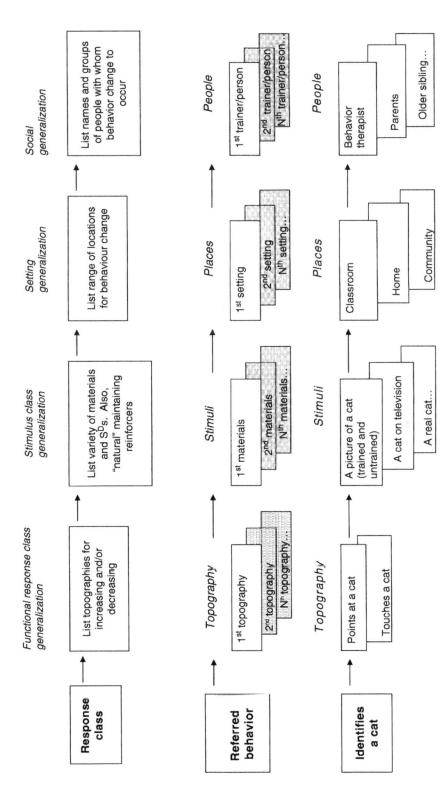

Fig. 1 Generalization planner showing domains of generalization (*top panel*), generalization planning schema (*middle panel*) and hypothetical use of the planner in teaching identification of the stimulus class "cat" (*bottom panel*)

generalization," we recommend that the program designer list the names of people in whose presence the changed behavior is to occur, e.g., which family members, teaching staff, and/or health care providers.

From where are the lists of response class members, stimuli, settings, and people typically obtained? They are from post-referral (but pre-intervention) interviews with the child with ASD where possible, all those who care about and for the child, and from direct observations by the behavior analyst in the child's natural environments. Interviews may be guided by the "generalization planner" (Fig. 1). Observations of the child's behaviors is likely to add information about the forms of response to be targeted, e.g., what form of verbal behavior the child uses (verbal, vocal, signs, gestures, PEC, etc.). Observations in the child's natural current and likely future environments, including peers, will enhance information about instructional and naturally occurring stimuli surrounding the desired behaviors.

At this point in planning, the analyst has exhaustive lists to place in the boxes as in Fig. 1. Before intervention commences, however, prioritization among response class members, stimulus materials, settings, and people needs to be undertaken. Prioritization is best negotiated, with guidance from the behavior analyst, with those informants who contributed to the lists during the interviews. The inclusion of the child, if possible, and parents in decision-making procedures of this type may be required by law in some jurisdictions. With regard to generalization planning for a particular intervention, a starting point has to be decided, e.g., what is the best setting in which to determine if the proposed intervention is effective and perhaps fine-tune it before generalizing to a new setting? In addition, at what point does the intervention end? Though we have planned for and measured behavior change in new settings, what would we expect to happen when an unidentified setting occurs a year after the intervention? Intervention should end when the reinforcing contingencies that naturally occur in the environment take over, thus the behavior should transfer to the new setting a year later without any need for reintroduction of the intervention. To provide further guidance in the use of the planner, a case example from clinical practice is provided below.

Case Example

Client Information

James is an 18-year-old male who attends a school for children with special needs. He has previously been diagnosed with autism and moderate mental retardation. He resides in a group home and spends every other weekend in his family home. James has presented with a number of challenging behaviors over the years including; swearing, hitting others, enuresis, tearing own clothing, and throwing objects.

Referral Question

James was referred to a behavior analyst because of an increase in disruptive behavior in the classroom. Classroom staff reported that the group home was also having difficulty managing James's behavior.

Behavior Assessment

Through the process of interviews with all caregivers and observation of James in all three key settings, the behavior analyst was able to identify the following target behaviors; spitting, throwing objects (particularly food at meal times), hitting staff and others, poking staff and others, swearing, and putting objects in own ear. A functional assessment revealed that all target behaviors occurred to provide James with attention in the form of reprimands, joking comments, cajoling to not misbehave, and other negative comments from staff.

Intervention

As high rates of target behaviors were observed, a schedule of noncontingent reinforcement (positive statements) on a fixed time, 1-min, signaled by a timer, was the recommended intervention. Staff was also provided with information on the rate of praise and other positive statements made to James. Staff and family were consulted about the feasibility of this intervention, and as all the disruptive behaviors had the same function, it was agreed to work on them all at once. Measures of James's engagement in school tasks and other activities were at low levels.

Planning for Generalization

As a part of intervention development, a generalization planner (Fig. 2) was completed. Topographically different behaviors of the same function were grouped for intervention. The maintaining stimuli were identified and the locations of the targeted behavior were listed in the order of intervention. It was decided that generalization strategy of sequential modification would be most effective in this case because of the differences between settings in which the behavior was observed. The classroom was targeted first as rates of behavior were high and fewer staff were involved. The family home was to be the second-to-last place of intervention as disruptive behavior showed low rates at baseline, possibility because of the high level of attention and greater choice of activities provided in that environment.

Results

At the time of writing, a marked decrease in disruptive behavior in the classroom had occurred. Furthermore, James became more engaged in school tasks and activities. During a follow-up observation the timer, which prompted staff to reinforce was not in use, however, disruptive behaviors remained low and staff attention to positive behaviors high. The timer and the fading of the strict timing is an example of indiscriminable contingencies. Intervention was not required in the playground as a generalization probe showed a decrease in disruptive behavior in this environment. This was most probably due to the classroom staff, who had been trained in the intervention, always being present, thus mediating generalization. Other school staff had observed the intervention and engaged in it without training. It was necessary to introduce the intervention to residential staff and the noncontingent reinforcement had resulted in a decrease in disruptive behavior

in that environment as well. A probe conducted in the taxi showed disruptive behavior still occurred. This intervention area will be the next topic to be reviewed. It is hypothesized that when a generalization probe is conducted during community outings low levels of disruptive behaviors will occur there as James is always with caregivers (mediators).

Concluding Summary and Recommendations

Several hypotheses have emerged as to why children with autism appear to have difficulty generalizing skills learnt between settings, people, behavior, and/or time. Insistence on sameness, stimulus overselectivity, and lack of motivation in teaching environments are more reflective of inadequate teaching practices rather than inherent flaws of children with autism. There is a considerable volume of research available within the applied behavior analytic domain that provides us with strategies to address generalization and maintenance of behavior. The application of this technology has been sorely lacking. Our limited review of the current literature found 42% of intervention research articles not measuring generalization and maintenance, in fact many of these did not even mention it. The cause for considered and well-planned generalization is not enhanced by ABA textbooks leaving discussion of this important topic to the final chapters when students' ability to absorb information is reduced (e.g., Cooper et al., 2007). It is our belief that if a behavior is worthy of modification then surely it is worthy of a little extra effort to ensure that it maintains in the learner's repertoire for years to come and that they are able to generalize the skill across settings, people, and behaviors as necessary. After all, very few of us remain in the same residence surrounded by the same people and same experiences all of our lives. Indeed, with regards to consideration of pivotal skills, one might consider being a generalized generalizer an imperative skill. Given how long it takes for children to learn some skills, taking the effort to ensure appropriate and ongoing generalization is necessary to create cost effective and socially valid results.

The section "Strategies to Promote Generalization" discussed eight strategies to promote generalization.

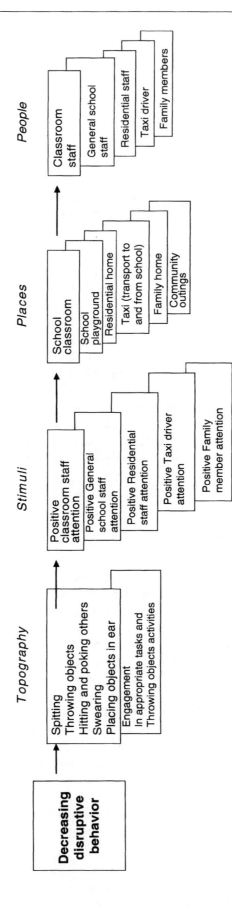

Fig. 2 Generalization planner for James' disruptive behavior

From this group of strategies, it is helpful to consider which will be most effective in generalizing behavior change for the client. Furthermore, it is imperative that the natural maintaining contingencies be determined. Why should a child continue to brush his teeth after the backward chaining procedure, with most to least prompts, and a contrived reinforcer, once the skill is learnt and the interventionists go away? We might continue to clean our teeth into adulthood because the result of not doing so is bad breath and unhealthy, grimy teeth, which are hygienically and socially unacceptable. A child with autism may not be motivated by these factors, so perhaps placing tooth brushing into a chain of morning behaviors that culminates in cartons on TV before school or work may be sufficient. In an environment devoid of positive naturally maintaining contingencies, it is the role of the behavior analyst to promote their establishment before withdrawing from the environment. As behavior analysts, it is not sufficient for us to sit by and wait for generalization to occur; it is our goal to make meaningful and socially significant changes in the lives of children with autism.

References

Alber, S. R., & Heward, W. L. (1996). "GOTCHA!" Twenty five behavior traps guaranteed to extend your students' academic and social skills. *Intervention in School and Clinic, 31*, 285–289.

American Psychiatric Association. (2000). *Diagnostic and statistical manual of mental disorders* (4th ed. Text Revision.). Washington DC: Author

Arco, L., & Millet, R. (1996). Maintaining instructional behavior after on-the-job training with process-based performance feedback. *Behavior Modification, 20*, 300–320.

Baer, D. M. (1999). *How to plan for generalization* (2nd ed.). Austin, TX: Pro-Ed.

Baer, D. M., & Wolf, M. M. (1970). The entry into natural communities of reinforcement. In R. Ulrich, T. Stachnik & J. Mabry (Eds.), *Control of human behavior* (Vol. 2, pp. 319–324). Glenview, IL: Scott, Foresman.

Baer, D. M., Wolf, M. M., & Risley, T. R. (1968). Some current dimensions of applied behavior analysis. *Journal of Applied Behavior Analysis, 1*, 91–97.

Bondy, A., & Frost, L. (1994). The picture exchange communication system. *Focus on Autistic Behavior, 9*, 1–19.

Campbell, C. R., & Campbell, K. S. (1982). Programming "loose training" as a strategy to facilitate language generalization. *Journal of Applied Behavior Analysis, 15*, 295–301.

Carr, E. G., & Darcy, M. (1990). Setting generality of peer modeling in children with autism. *Journal of Autism and Developmental Disorders, 20*, 45–59.

Cooper, J. O., Heron, T. E., & Heward, W. L. (2007). *Applied behavior analysis* (2nd ed.). Upper Saddle River, NJ: Pearson Education.

Coyle, C., & Cole, P. (2004). A videotaped self-modelling and self-monitoring treatment program to decrease off-task behaviour in children with autism. *Journal of Intellectual and Developmental Disability, 29*, 3–15.

Drabman, R. S., Hammer, D., & Rosenbaum, M. S. (1979). Assessing generalization in behavior modification with children: The generalization map. *Behavioral Assessment, 1*, 203–219.

Durand, V. M., & Carr, E. G. (1992). An analysis of maintenance following functional communication training. *Journal of Applied Behavior Analysis, 25*, 777–794.

Eikeseth, S., & Smith, T. (1992). The development of functional and equivalence classes in high-functioning autistic children: The role of naming. *Journal of the Experimental Analysis of Behavior, 58*, 123–133.

Fiorile, C. A., & Greer, R. D. (2007). The induction of naming in children with no prior tact responses as a function of multiple exemplar histories of instruction. *Analysis of Verbal Behavior, 23*, 71–87.

Goldstein, H., & Wickstrom, S. (1986). Peer intervention effects on communicative interaction among handicapped and non-handicapped preschoolers. *Journal of Applied Behavior Analysis, 19*, 209–214.

Grow, L. L., Kelley, M. E., Roane, H. S., & Shillingsburg, M. A. (2008). Utility of extinction-induced response variability for the selection of mands. *Journal of Applied Behavior Analysis, 41*, 15–24.

Harchik, A. E., Harchik, A. J., Luce, S. C., & Sherman, J. A. (1990). Teaching autistic and severely handicapped children to recruit praise: Acquisition and generalization. *Research in Developmental Disabilities, 11*, 77–95.

Horner, R. H., Dunlap, G., & Koegel, R. L. (1988). *Generalization and maintenance: Life-style changes in applied settings.* Baltimore, MD: Paul H. Brookes Publishing.

Jones, E. A., Feeley, K. M., & Takacs, J. (2007). Teaching spontaneous responses to young children with autism. *Journal of Applied Behavior Analysis, 40*, 565–570.

Kamps, D. M., Potucek, J., Lopez, A. G., Kravits, T., & Kemmerer, K. (1997). The use of peer networks across multiple settings to improve social interaction for students with autism. *Journal of Behavioral Education, 7*, 335–357.

Koegel, R. L., & Egel, A. L. (1979). Motivating autistic children. *Journal of Abnormal Psychology, 88*, 418–426.

Koegel, L. K., Koegel, R. L., Hurley, C., & Frea, W. D. (1992). Improving social skills and disruptive behavior in children with autism through self-management. *Journal of Applied Behavior Analysis, 25*, 341–353.

Koegel, R. L., & Mentis, M. (1985). Motivation in childhood autism: Can they or won't they? *Journal of Child Psychology and Psychiatry, 26*, 185–191.

Koegel, R. L., & Rincover, A. (1977). Research on the difference between generalization and maintenance in extra-therapy responding. *Journal of Applied Behavior Analysis, 10*, 1–12.

Laushey, K. M., & Heflin, L. J. (2000). Enhancing social skills of kindergarten children with autism through the training of multiple peers as tutors. *Journal of Autism and Developmental Disorders, 30*, 183–193.

Lee, R., McComas, J. J., & Jawor, J. (2002). The effects of differential and lag reinforcement schedules on varied verbal responding by individuals with autism. *Journal of Applied Behavior Analysis, 35,* 391–402.

Lee, R., & Sturmey, P. (2006). The effects of lag schedules and preferred materials on variable responding in students with autism. *Journal of Autism and Developmental Disorders, 36,* 421–428.

Lee, R., Sturmey, P., & Fields, L. (2007). Schedule-induced and operant mechanisms that influence response variability: A review and implications for future investigations. *Psychological Record, 57,* 429–455.

Lovaas, O. I., Koegel, R. L., & Schreibman, L. (1979). Stimulus overselectivity in Autism: A review of research. *Psychological Bulletin, 86,* 1236–1254.

Lovaas, O. I., Schreibman, L., Koegel, R. L., & Rehm, R. (1971). Selective responding by autistic children to multiple sensory input. *Journal of Abnormal Psychology, 77,* 211–222.

MacDuff, G. S., Krantz, P. J., & McClannahan, L. E. (1993). Teaching children with autism to use photographic activity schedules: Maintenance and generalization of complex response chains. *Journal of Applied Behavior Analysis, 26,* 89–97.

Martin, G., & Pear, J. (2003). *Behavior modification: What it is and how to do it* (7th ed.). Upper Saddle River, NJ: Prentice Hall.

O'Neill, R. E., & Sweetland-Baker, M. (2001). Brief report: An assessment of stimulus generalization and contingency effects in functional communication training with two students with autism. *Journal of Autism and Developmental Disorders, 31,* 235–240.

Petursdottir, A., McComas, J., McMaster, K., & Horner, K. (2007). The effects of scripted peer tutoring and programming common stimuli on social interactions of a student with autism spectrum disorder. *Journal of Applied Behavior Analysis, 40,* 353–357.

Pierce, K. L., & Shreibman, L. (1994). Teaching daily living skills to children with autism in unsupervised settings through pictorial self-management. *Journal of Applied Behavior Analysis, 27,* 471–481.

Rincover, A., & Koegel, R. L. (1975). Setting generality and stimulus control in autistic children. *Journal of Applied Behavior Analysis, 8,* 235–246.

Schreibman, L., & Lovaas, O. I. (1973). Overselective response to social stimuli by autistic children. *Journal of Abnormal Child Psychology, 1,* 152–168.

Sidman, M. (1971). Reading and auditory-visual equivalences. *Journal of Speech and Hearing Research, 14,* 5–13.

Sidman, M., & Tailby, W. (1982). Conditional discrimination vs. matching to sample: An expansion of the testing paradigm. *Journal of the Experimental Analysis of Behavior, 37,* 5–22.

Stahmer, A. C., & Shreibman, L. (1992). Teaching children with autism appropriate play in unsupervised environments using a self-management treatment package. *Journal of Applied Behavior Analysis, 25,* 447–459.

Stokes, T. F., & Baer, D. M. (1977). An implicit technology of generalization. *Journal of Applied Behavior Analysis, 10,* 349–367.

Stokes, T. F., & Osnes, P. G. (1989). An operant pursuit of generalization. *Behavior Therapy, 20,* 337–355.

Tarbox, J., Wallace, M. D., & Tarbox, R. S. F. (2002). Successful generalized parent training and failed schedule thinning of response blocking for automatically maintained object mouthing. *Behavioral Interventions, 17,* 169–178.

Tiger, J. H., Bouxsein, K. J., & Fisher, W. W. (2007). Treating excessively slow responding of a young man with Asperger syndrome using differential reinforcement of short response latencies. *Journal of Applied Behavior Analysis, 40,* 559–563.

Wallis, C. (2006, May 7). A tale of two schools. Time Magazine. Retrieved September 1, 2008, from http://www.time.com/time/magazine/article/0.9171.1191852.00.html

van den Pol, R. A., Iwata, B. A., Ivancic, M. T., Page, T. J., Neef, N. A., & Whitley, F. P. (1981). Teaching the handicapped to eat in public places: Acquisition, generalization and maintenance of restaurant skills. *Journal of Applied Behavior Analysis, 14,* 61–69.

Chapter 13
Training Issues Unique to Autism Spectrum Disorders

Linda A. LeBlanc, Nicole Gravina, and James E. Carr

Intensive early intervention training, discrete trials, transitions to new settings, environments and people, tactile defensiveness, difficulty initiating interactions and other factors specific to ASD will be covered. An emphasis on being aware of these specialized problems and how ABA methods have been developed to address them will be reviewed.

Training Issues Unique to Autism Spectrum Disorders

Behavioral researchers have created a substantial literature on staff training in human-service settings for individuals with developmental disabilities (Parsons, Reid, & Green, 1996; Reid & Green, 1990; Reid, Parsons, Lattimore, Towery, & Reade, 2005; Reid et al., 2003; Schepis & Reid, 1994). This literature illustrates the importance of providing effective initial training, either live or by video (Macurik, O'Kane, Malanga, & Reid, 2008) and clear and potentially public feedback (Parsons & Reid, 1995; Reid & Parsons, 1996; Wilson, Reid, & Korabek-Pinkowski, 1991). In addition, curriculum manuals are available for training both direct support staff and supervisory staff to provide effective positive behavior supports (Reid & Parsons, 2007). Providing behavioral interventions to individuals with autism spectrum disorders (ASDs) presents many of the same training and management challenges encountered in all human-

service environments (e.g., high turnover, low pay, small training budgets), so the resources mentioned above are pertinent and useful; however, the characteristics of ASDs and associated behavioral interventions pose several unique challenges.

Behavioral characteristics common to the diagnostic profiles of ASDs can create challenges in service provision and staff training. For example, unusual sensitivity to change in environments and behavioral rigidity (Tidmarsh & Volkmar, 2003) necessitate an unusually high degree of consistency across treatment implementers and environments. Most individuals with an ASD will have multiple providers across multiple settings, potentially including their family, school staff, home staff, and eventually work-support staff. Ensuring that behavioral procedures are implemented consistently across settings is logistically difficult but critically important as even small changes in implementation could result in the loss of treatment gains for an individual with an ASD. The greatest difficulties can arise with transitions from one environment and support system to the next (e.g., elementary to middle school, high school to supported employment) unless training is coordinated across environments (Stoner, Angell, House, & Brock, 2007).

In addition to the difficulties created by characteristic features of ASDs, certain aspects of behavioral interventions and the direct support staff who implement them can also complicate training. One unique aspect of behavioral intervention for individuals with an ASD is the exceptional level of precision required to effectively implement highly structured early and intensive behavioral intervention (EIBI). Many EIBI models use extensive strategies and infrastructures to promote treatment fidelity (e.g., Davis, Smith, & Donahoe, 2002; Smith, Donahoe, & Davis, 2001). However, many therapists and parents still have

L.A. LeBlanc (✉)
Department of Psychology, Auburn University, 226 Thach Hall, Auburn, AL, USA 36849
e-mail: leblanc@auburn.edu

difficulty achieving and maintaining optimal levels of procedural fidelity (Johnson & Hastings, 2002; Symes, Remington, Brown, & Hastings, 2006). In addition, the shortage and costs of experienced MA and PhD-level professionals with specific expertise in EIBI and ASDs often result in management of programs by under-qualified individuals (Love, Carr, Almason, & Petursdottir, 2009). It is relatively unique to EIBI that many parents choose to serve as the primary coordinators and supervisors of their child's programming by economic and logistical necessity rather than because of a strong background in behavior analysis and personnel management.

Ideally, we recommend that program coordinators of services for individuals with ASDs should have strong backgrounds in the disorders, behavioral treatment, staff training, and performance management. These recommendations are admittedly difficult to achieve. Thus, the purpose of the present chapter is to guide the program supervisor through several of the most common and challenging training issues unique to providing services to individuals with ASDs and to offer some potential solutions and resources for creating organizational performance improvement. The remainder of this chapter is structured according to three categories of common training issues. For each issue, the most likely problems are described along with basic recommendations for solutions and additional resources that practitioners and program coordinators might pursue.

Issue One: Workforce and Organizational Challenges

As is the case with the workforce in many disability-related human services, this group is often underpaid for the relative difficulty and social importance of their jobs. Direct-service providers are responsible for everyday personal care and physical activities and are also the primary implementers of instructional programs, behavior management programs, and data collection systems. Despite the importance of these tasks to the well-being of those with disabilities, direct-service staff in disability services are paid an average wage of only $7.97 in the United States (Wage Rates:...And Could We Care Less?, n.d.), though the demand for EIBI staff has driven wages higher for this subset of providers. In general, low wages often result in a workforce

with a lower overall level of education and higher rates of adverse conditions leading to absenteeism and high turnover (Hirschfield, Schmitt, & Bedeian, 2002; Lakin & Larson, 1992).

The rate of turnover in the workforce for EIBI programs is often high for several other reasons besides wages, including: (a) job difficulty associated with the technical precision requirements for instruction with this population, (b) the high risk of injury due to aggression or other problem behavior, and (c) the strong appeal of higher education for many of the very best direct-service staff. In programs serving individuals with ASDs there are typically extensive training requirements prior to initiating contact with the consumer. These training requirements make every instance of turnover costly to the employer in terms of both time and financial resources (Larson & Hewitt, 2005). In-home programs may have particularly limited resources for adjusting to employee absenteeism resulting in loss of therapeutic services when staff members are unavailable for their scheduled shifts.

There are several potential solutions to the difficulties associated with workforce issues and the solutions begin with effective personnel selection (Larson & Hewitt, 2005). Agencies should determine the most difficult-to-train skills they deem essential to providing effective services and hire new employees based on the presence of those skills. For example, communicating effectively and empathetically with parents may be a more difficult skill to train compared to conducting a preference assessment, so staff might be screened for those social skills. Highly engaging incidental or naturalistic teaching may be more difficult to train than structured discrete-trial instructional procedures, so staff might be screened for play skills and the ease with which they notice and use natural learning opportunities. Having interviewees demonstrate these targeted skills in practice scenarios during the interview process is considered superior to other selection procedures in predicting future performance (Campion, 1972).

Designing Effective Training

When hiring is complete, training systems that create an efficient transfer of knowledge and development of skills for new staff are critical (Larson & Hewitt, 2005). Prior to the first day of work, staff should be provided with background information on the organization and services. Testing their knowledge over those materials may provide incentives for new employees to review the information thoroughly. It may also be more efficient to determine the skills the new staff have already mastered so time is not wasted on skills that do not require extensive training.

In addition, to making materials available for review, active-response training procedures such as Behavioral Skills Training (BST) are quite effective for teaching staff new skills (e.g., Fleming, Oliver, & Bolton, 1996). Rather than passively listening to lectures or watching videos, training should involve interactive components such as modeling and role-playing with performance feedback until a preset performance criterion is met (e.g., 80% accurate; 100% accurate on a critical component). When face-to-face instruction is not feasible, interactive computer training that requires the viewer to answer questions and make evaluations has been demonstrated to be more effective than lecture (Williams & Zahad, 1996) and reading (Eckerman et al., 2002). Additionally, video presentation has proven as effective as and more efficient than live training for behavioral intervention plan implementation, though live training was rated more highly by staff (Macurik et al., 2008). See Reid and Green (1990) for excellent additional recommendations for designing your initial training procedures.

Another effective training tool is viewing and scoring videos of performance of the targeted procedures. Video can provide an effective and immediate strategy for training new procedures without lengthy delays for arranging group-training opportunities. Self-evaluation of videotaped performance can enhance awareness of error patterns and evaluating someone else's performance has been demonstrated to improve the same performance of the evaluator (Alvero & Austin, 2004). Videos are particularly useful for direct service staff who work in environments with little supervision as they allow for direct objective feedback to the performer and supervisor feedback and performance consequences that might not otherwise be available. When using video as a training tool, carefully select the skills for which demonstration of subtle features is critical.

Maintaining Staff Performance

After the necessary skills have been acquired, the environment must support their use without creating substantial additional costs or effort for the employer or supervisor. Low-cost incentives such as supervisor feedback and praise are highly effective at improving and maintaining performance (Alvero, Bucklin, & Austin, 2001) and have no additional monetary cost. Praise is most effective when it directly follows monitoring of performance and when it is directly contingent upon and descriptive of aspects of the performance (Komaki, Desselles, & Bowman, 1989). Performance-contingent feedback and praise are closely linked with job satisfaction (Podsakoff & Schriescheim, 1985) and job satisfaction is often associated with employee retention (Eskildsen & Dahlgaard, 2000). Therefore, praise of effective performance can be a high-impact organizational tool because it directly relates to improving and maintaining performance, improving job satisfaction, and minimizing turnover without extensive additional cost to the employer.

Other low cost incentives that can be utilized to reinforce maintenance of skills include access to ongoing training, schedule flexibility, small tangible rewards, and small bonus payments. Research on monetary incentives has indicated that even very small financial incentives produce increases in performance equivalent to those produced by comparatively larger financial incentives (Dickinson & Gillette, 1993). Therefore, small bonus payments or entering staff into a raffle for an opportunity to win a desirable prize are reasonable alternatives when funding for incentives is negligible. If performance-based pay is a possibility for an organization, see Abernathy (1996) for a guide to creating pay-for-performance systems.

Managing Performance Problems

When staff members have difficulty performing their job efficiently and effectively (e.g., poor data collection, poor procedural implementation), a common misconception is that more training is required to correct the performance problem. However, training is only likely to produce improvements if performance problems are the result of lack of knowledge or understanding. Several other factors may come into play and affect performance such as fluctuating motivational levels and equipment problems.

Mager (1997) suggests that a supervisor consider whether, with a strong enough incentive, the employee could perform the task perfectly. If the answer is no, it is likely a training issue. If the answer is yes, it is likely a motivation issue. Additional training is unlikely to impact problems that are motivational in nature. For example, an EIBI instructor may know how to implement a procedure correctly but over time may elect to use a shortcut because it is faster or easier. There may be no immediately evident consequences to using the shortcut, although its use may adversely impact treatment outcome in the long term. For example, failure to follow correct prompt fading procedures may result in immediate skill performance, but could later result in prompt dependence and slower skill acquisition. The staff member may not recognize that the deviation from the protocol is related to the latter problem, which suggests a different type of training is needed. The instructor may need to learn more about the potential long-term impact of his or her performance rather than only about accurate implementation of the procedure. In addition, direct consequences for accurate implementation may be needed to supplement the relatively delayed natural consequences that often cannot be linked to one specific employee (i.e., the child has several instructors, the same instructor works with children who do not develop prompt dependence in spite of similarly faulty prompting procedures).

Factors other than motivation or deficit training can also affect performance. Austin (2000) developed the Performance Diagnostic Checklist for determining potential causes of performance issues. One portion of the checklist identifies training factors due to knowledge and skills. The remaining items on the checklist identify challenges in three areas – antecedents and information, equipment and processes, and consequences. Examples of the way antecedents may negatively impact performance would be misplaced data sheets leading to no data and stalled progress because a program does not specify mastery or prompt fading criteria. Examples of deficiencies in equipment and processes that may impact performance include running out of reinforcers during instruction, nonportable communication or data collection systems, or data collection systems that are not well-suited to the task and therefore are not used. One of the most common and frustrating problems with poor implementation of the Picture Exchange Communication System (PECS) intervention is that the communication book remains out of reach on a shelf or does not get regularly transported from home to school or work.

Lastly, just as consequences are extremely important in teaching and maintaining client behavior, they are equally important for developing and maintaining staff behavior. Staff might deviate slightly from a teaching procedure and not notice the change in their own behavior. If the consumer does not provide immediate feedback (e.g., confusion, problem behavior), the slight deviation may continue because there are no immediate consequences to deter the change. This phenomenon is referred to as procedural drift. Many staff work under minimal supervision in home-based programs, residential facilities, and schools, which means that supervisors may not provide sufficient feedback on performance to maintain adherence to specific procedures. For example, a staff member may know that antecedent-behavior-consequence data should be recorded after each occurrence of problem behavior, but he may wait to record until the end of the day because the data sheet is not readily accessible. This data collection strategy may not produce many errors if the problem behavior is infrequent but the quality of the data may decrease with this strategy as the frequency of problem behavior increases and they become more difficult to remember.

We acknowledge the fact that many clinical supervisors and coordinators (including parents) do not receive formal education in organizational behavior management. Nonetheless, careful attention to staff training, maintenance, and performance management is critical for the long-term success of any ASD intervention effort. See Daniels and Daniels (2004) and Reid (1998) for additional information on performance management.

Issue Two: Detection and Management of Subtle Behavioral Patterns

After hiring, training, and retaining a sufficient number of well-qualified staff, the next task for the program coordinator will be teaching those individuals a wide range of difficult and subtle repertoires in order to ensure delivery of effective services. Effective teaching of individuals with ASD requires one to use precise sequences of discriminative stimuli, prompts, and consequences while constantly tracking the type of instructions given, the degree of prompting required, and the response of the learner (Green, 1996; Smith, 2001).

Effective management of prosocial and problem behavior requires one to detect the emergence of subtle behavioral patterns and employ preventative strategies such as prompting alternative behaviors before problems arise. Many program supervisors teach the implementation of specific skills (e.g., least-to-most prompt hierarchies, PECS, functional communication training) according to available manuals. However, most supervisors do not directly target generalized repertoires such as detecting, preventing, and reporting problems, which can drastically improve the overall quality of services.

The ability of direct service staff to quickly detect developing patterns of problem behavior allows them to maximize the usefulness and efficiency of the clinical supervision they receive (Komaki et al., 1989). However, effective detection, reporting, and prevention of important environmental events require discrimination of subtle factors in the midst of many irrelevant background events. Problem behaviors are often so salient that they overshadow the important environmental conditions with which they are correlated, resulting sometimes in a seemingly random pattern. Teaching staff constantly surveying aspects of the physical environment (e.g., minimal attention, loud noises) and their own behavior (e.g., prompt types, allowing response-contingent escape) as potential determinants of problem behavior can result in quicker and more accurate detection of important patterns, potentially facilitating prevention.

Development of problem behavior is common for individuals with developmental disabilities and even young typically developing children. The most common functions of problem behavior are (a) escape from ongoing unpleasant stimuli (e.g., difficult task demand), (b) attention from others, (c) access to preferred tangibles, and (d) sensory or automatic reinforcement (Iwata et al., 1994). In addition to these more common functions of problem behavior, two unique functions are likely for individuals with an ASD due to the characteristics of the disorders (Tidmarsh & Volkmar, 2003). Repetitive behavior and restricted patterns of interests and preferences can lead to problem behavior maintained by disruption of rituals or by daily transitions (Reese, Richman, Belmont, & Morse, 2005; Reese, Richman, Zarcone, & Zarcone, 2003).

A strong preference for a certain chain of behavior, placement of objects, or complex interaction pattern (e.g., verbal rituals) can lead to aggression or tantrums when the pattern is disrupted until the ritual is eventually accommodated (Murphy, Macdonald, Hall, & Oliver, 2000). Rituals evolve from repetitions of patterns, so the beginning of a ritual may not be particularly noticeable unless one is vigilant for its development. Subtle contingencies (e.g., escape from a client's mild distress) can gradually shape a care provider's behavior to conform to unstated rituals to avoid more intense problem behavior associated with ritual disruption (LeBlanc & Fisher, 1997). The provider may be unaware that he has begun to carefully avoid disruption of rituals, but that avoidance can actually strengthen rituals and contribute to more intense problem behavior over time as ritual disruption becomes increasingly aversive to the individual with an ASD.

Rituals and resulting problem behavior are typically noticed when rituals and avoidance of ritual disruptions are strongly engrained even more carefully. It is more effective to detect the rituals and avoidance behavior quickly, before rituals become highly ingrained. Systematic exposure to mild and signaled disruptions of the patterns could then be employed to *prevent* the development of intense and complex rituals and the problem behaviors that typically accompany them. Frequent and signaled exposure to unexpected events or changes in patterns can be incorporated into activity schedules using a salient visual stimulus to represent the occurrence of an unknown event. The unknown or unexpected event should initially be highly preferred (e.g., go to a new place to do a favorite activity) and brief. Tolerance of the unexpected events could then be differentially reinforced, with problem behavior never resulting in access to the ritual (or proto-ritual). Over time, the duration of exposure to the unexpected events can be increased and their preference can be shifted from highly preferred to neutral to nonpreferred. This progression should continue until the client can tolerate ritual disruption.

Similarly, transitions from activity to activity can precipitate problem behavior for individuals with ASDs, potentially limiting their community-based opportunities (McCord, Thomson, & Iwata, 2001; Schreibman, Whalen, & Stahmer, 2000; Sterling-Turner & Jordan, 2007). Flannery and Horner (1994) suggest that individuals with ASDs have a uniquely high need for predictability. If naturally occurring cues for upcoming transitions are not salient to the individual with an ASD, then transitions may be experienced as highly unpredictable environmental changes. If teaching staff attend to a change in activities as a potentially important environmental event, it can lead to more rapid identification of this unique function of problem behavior and effective treatment or prevention (Flannery, O'Neill, & Horner, 1995). Sterling-Turner and Jordan reviewed the literature on several viable behavioral interventions for transition-related problem behavior and determined that verbal and auditory cues (e.g., "we will switch activities in 2 min") and salient visual cues (e.g., photos, activity schedules, video priming) may be prove useful if predictability (or lack thereof) was the primary contributing factor for problem behavior.

Regardless of the predictability of an upcoming transition, the behavioral practitioner should be aware of the likelihood that the value of the activities themselves may lead to subtle operant contingencies that support problem behavior (Sterling-Turner & Jordan, 2007). If the transition is from a highly preferred activity to a less preferred activity or from a neutral activity to an aversive activity, problem behavior may still arise despite a clearly signaled transition. The problem behavior is likely to be maintained by the resumption of the prior preferred activity or by avoidance of the upcoming aversive activity and cuing is unlikely to be effective unless extinction is also in effect (i.e., no problem-behavior contingent failure to transition). To detect this type of contingency, staff will need to attend to the occurrence of the transition as an event and also to the probable value of the events for the client. Supplemental strategies to use in these instances include (a) altering the schedule of activities to minimize the contrast in value between contiguous activities, (b) changing aspects of the aversive activities to make them more enjoyable (i.e., curricular revision, inserting pleasant stimuli into unpleasant self-care routines), and (c) differential reinforcement of smooth transitions.

Several training strategies and organizational systems can prove useful in creating a treatment environment that is focused on prevention and is quickly responsive to the development of problems. It is important to explicitly train staff on accurate detection of subtle behavior and environmental events that should trigger increased vigilance on their part. Positive behavior supports curricula such as the one developed by Reid and Parsons (2007) provide instructional resources for the most common environmental anteced-

ents that can contribute to problem behavior – presentation of difficult tasks, low attention or overall stimulation, and unavailability of preferred items. The occurrence of any of those environmental events should be established as a cue to notice any associated problem behavior. Of course, staff should already be trained to not deliver the potentially reinforcing consequences associated with these antecedents (e.g., problem behavior-contingent escape, attention, and tangible items). An unusual pattern of behavior or repetition of a pattern of behavior and transition between events can also be established as a cue for vigilant observation (Flannery et al., 1995).

Training videos can be used to establish the aforementioned events as reliable triggers for data collection and reporting. Videos should include extensive footage of a variety of clients with ASDs in a variety of situations. It is important that many of the situations should *not* depict problem behavior because you want to establish the environmental events rather than problem behavior as the trigger for detection. Set up training sessions in which staff practice recording problem behaviors and appropriate behaviors that occur during or within 2 min of one of the triggers and provide performance feedback (i.e., differential reinforcement of accuracy, corrective feedback for errors). The most likely errors to occur early on are errors of omission where instances of important situations are not detected.

In addition to training for detection of important environment-behavior relations, there should be a system that is easy, intuitive, and automatic when possible for reporting incidents. Reporting is often done informally during team meetings or supervision with emphasis on recently developed or ongoing problem behaviors. There are multiple limitations of reporting that is focused on episodes of problem behavior. First, staff may become reluctant to report for fear of negative evaluation of their performance. Second, and perhaps most importantly, the reporting is not triggered until it is already too late to prevent problem behavior from developing. Setting up a system for low-effort and frequent reporting of important environmental variables can facilitate a quick start on developing solutions to emerging problems.

One strategy a supervisor might use is daily completion of a structured reporting form that prompts identification of the subtle variables mentioned above. By including nomination responses for important environmental events and places to note concerning behaviors, there is a daily reminder to pay attention to those environmental variables and their impact on the individual with an ASD. Note, however, that completion of the form should take less than 3–5 min or low levels of compliance or insufficiently detailed reporting may occur. Once an effective and efficient reporting form is created, make completion and submission of that form as automatic as possible. The form should be completed as part of a regular chain of end-of-shift activities as a standard employee responsibility. Finally, consider using some of the strategies for performance management described earlier (see *Issue One: Workforce and Organizational Challenges*) to facilitate consistent and detailed reporting (e.g., monetary incentives, behavior-specific praise).

Issue Three: Promoting Consistency Across Providers and Environments

Individuals with ASDs, like everyone else, need to function in multiple environments (e.g., school, home, work) and they often require supports to do so effectively. Consistency across caregivers and service providers (e.g., family, in-home staff, school, or work support staff) at any given time is critical to ensure the integrity of behavioral treatment and to minimize problem behavior. Furthermore, transitions from one setting to another are critical junctures for success but individuals with ASDs are particularly susceptible to problems in the transition process (Forest, Horner, Lewis-Palmer, Todd, & McGee, 2004). Consistency during times of transition from one provider to another often requires even more planning and management of additional organizational challenges. Each of these two issues of consistency is addressed below.

Consistency Across Caregivers and Environments

At any point in the life of an individual with ASD, there will be at least two major environments that can strongly impact his quality of life, rate of learning, and level of problem behavior. During childhood and adolescence, the critical environments are likely to be home, school, and daycare or after-school care. During adulthood the critical environments are likely to be an employment setting, home, and the community. In addition, college is more frequently becoming an option for those individuals who respond well to behavioral intervention and/or flourish in their secondary educational setting (Van Bergeijk, Klin, & Volkmar, 2008). Within each major environment, several key players (e.g., home: parents, siblings, grandparents, tutors; school: teachers, aides, principal) should be targeted for consistency of implementation of behavioral supports.

The effects of inconsistency across care providers can be potentially detrimental. Poor consistency in response to problem behavior can establish intermittent schedules of reinforcement, which can be resistant to extinction (Mackintosh, 1974). If teaching and prompting procedures vary too greatly across staff and environments, the likely effects are prompt dependency, confusion and impaired rates of acquisition, and increased problem behavior making procedural integrity an important concern (Belfiore, Fritts, & Herman, 2008; Johnson & Hastings, 2002; Smith et al., 2001). Even mastered self-care tasks such as independent toileting skills can regress if one environment requires independent skill use while another environment does not. It is often difficult to identify inconsistency as the source of problems because individuals in one environment may have limited access to information about intervention and performance in others.

The practitioner can use several strategies to facilitate consistency across implementers of behavioral and instructional supports. Actively monitor procedural integrity using structured checklists for either live or videotaped performance (Smith et al., 2001). Observe performance on a regular basis so that monitoring is viewed as a constant and accepted part of the job rather than as a punitive measure for suspected poor performance (Leblanc, Riccardi, & Luiselli, 2005). Video-based self-monitoring has proved effective for individuals implementing discrete-trial early intervention (Belfiore et al., 2008), which can be particularly useful if the staff has limited direct contact with coworkers or supervisors. Self-monitoring and monitoring by coworkers (Alvero & Austin, 2004) may be combined with supervisor monitoring to reduce the effort of assessing procedural integrity.

Planning for regular and effective communication across sites or across direct service staff within a site is a critical part of promoting consistent services. Design the communication system to include daily, weekly, monthly, and quarterly components as needed for different parts of the system. For example, staff on different shifts with the same consumer should have a method for communicating daily and school-to-home communication should occur on a daily basis for behavioral targets relevant to both environments (e.g., toileting, problem behavior, prompt levels for requests). Other information might be best summarized on a weekly or monthly basis (e.g., overall progress on acquisition goals, changes in behavioral intervention plans) in supervision meetings or by written communication summaries.

Design supervision or team meetings to ensure optimal efficiency and accuracy of information. First, always use a structured agenda to guide the content of the meeting and to specify who is responsible for providing important information. Second, provide a rubric for reporting progress in programs in relation to a well-specified criterion for progress (e.g., 30% change in percent accuracy over 1 week) and mastery (e.g., 90% accuracy over 3 days with two different staff). Have staff list the programs that are progressing well and then focus the majority of supervision time on problem-solving for ones that are not progressing well. Staff should be trained to either provide specific data or a brief targeted report on critical variables that are likely to impact performance on a program (e.g., duration of time delay, exact prompting strategy, error pattern analysis). Third, train staff to report to their supervisor and to each other on three categories of information potentially related to problem behavior: (a) data on the ongoing occurrence of problem behavior for which there is a plan, (b) data on the occurrence of potentially problematic environmental conditions (e.g., unsignaled transitions, low-attention periods) and (c) information about any potentially emerging concerns.

Consistency During Major Transition Periods

There are several critical points throughout the first third of the lifespan associated with transitions across environments and major task requirements. Transition planning is important for all children with disabilities; however, the likelihood of resistance to change, social skills deficits, and poor skill generalization make individuals with ASDs particularly vulnerable during times of transition (Forest et al., 2004; Luce & Dyer, 1995). The first significant transition that a child with

an ASD is likely to encounter is from in-home or preschool intervention services to kindergarten (Forest et al.). The next is from elementary to middle school and high school. Variables such as the changing of classrooms, increased requirements for independence, presence of new peers, etc., can be overwhelming to an individual with an ASD. Furthermore, many teachers, rather than one primary teacher, are likely to have instructional responsibility for the student. The stressors associated with this transition can be detrimental for both the student and his family, creating risks for increased anxiety, problem behavior, and decline in academic performance unless effective planning and transition management occurs (Schall, Cortijo-Doval, Targett, & Wehman, 2006; Stoner et al., 2007). The next major transition point is from the school environment to a triad of typical providers for adult services – supported employment or college, residential supports, and mental health services (Moxon & Gates, 2001; Van Bergeijk et al., 2008). All major transition points will serve as an assessment of how well previous environments prepared an individual (e.g., targeting meaningful skills, programming for maintenance and generalization, managing anxiety about impending changes) for subsequent environments.

Transition planning for individuals with ASDs creates unique training challenges associated with the transfer of services from one system to another, that is, the most knowledgeable individuals about the client's work in a different organization or location than the individuals who need the training. Employees of the new service agency may not have the same familiarity with ASDs, behavioral interventions, data collection, training, and supervisory infrastructures as the prior providers. Each environment is also likely to have its own hierarchical power structure that should be identified and targeted to ensure optimal support for behavioral programming. For example, in some school settings special education teachers operate independently with proximal support from their in-class aides and distal support from their principal. In other settings, the principal may exert a more direct influence upon educational services.

To facilitate effective training, the practitioner should consider the following recommendations. First, meet with the receiving providers 6 months to 1 year in advance to determine the required skill sets and social or noise tolerance levels for the client, and likely levels of direct support available in the new environment.

This information should be incorporated into the annual behavioral goals for the client (e.g., can work independently for 15 min in an environment with four other individuals), minimizing the need for the new providers to teach these skills during the transition period. When possible, teach pivotal skills that will allow the client to manage more of their environment and individual needs (e.g., self-management, requesting assistance or attention) (Koegel, Koegel, & McNerney, 2001; Lee, Simpson, & Shogren, 2007; Reichle, Dropik, Alden-Anderson, & Haley, 2008). Second, create a brief communication document that clearly describes information about (a) the important ASD characteristics of the consumer (e.g., rituals, social aloofness, use of PECS or sign language), (b) the prior program, (c) the skills that have been targeted to facilitate success in the new environment and the level of progress on those skills, (d) the current behavioral challenges, and (e) the behavioral supports that have proven effective. Third, create accompanying training materials that can be delivered either by the prior practitioner (if the new agency is willing) or by an identified partner at the new agency. Use video extensively to demonstrate critical aspects of behavioral supports and attempt to anticipate questions of the new care providers. Fourth, schedule a series of pretransition visits to the new setting so the client can meet the new care providers. View these visits as gradual exposure to stimuli that are potentially aversive; thus, these visits should be brief, social demands should be kept to a minimum, and highly preferred stimuli should be available. Subsequent visits can focus on establishing for the client important aspects of the routine (e.g., opening the locker, finding the bathroom and classrooms, putting on a work uniform) using visual supports (e.g., activity schedules, written task analyzes) and live demonstration of implementation of behavior management strategies and instructional procedures for care providers.

Summary and Conclusions

Certain features of ASDs and the behavioral interventions that have proved effective in treating them create unique training issues that practitioners should be prepared to address. Most practitioners have extensive experience in curriculum and instruction and management of problem behavior, but less education and experience in organizational and training issues. However, those organizational and systems issues can have a substantial impact on the quality of services for individuals with ASDs who are particularly vulnerable to problems of inconsistency, imprecision, and unexpected change. The information and resources provided in this chapter should guide practitioners to relatively simple but useful strategies to facilitate workforce management and training, development of effective detection and reporting systems to prevent problem behavior and rituals, and improved quality assurance and procedural consistency across environments and during important transition periods.

References

Abernathy, W. B. (1996). *The sin of wages: Where the conventional pay system has led us, and how to find a way out.* USA: PerfSys Press.

Alvero, A. M., & Austin, J. (2004). The effects of observing on the behavior of the observer. *Journal of Applied Behavior Analysis, 37,* 457–468.

Alvero, A. M., Bucklin, B. R., & Austin, J. (2001). An objective review of the effectiveness and essential characteristics of performance feedback in organizational settings. *Journal of Organizational Behavior Management, 21*(1), 3–29.

Austin, J. (2000). Performance analysis and performance diagnostics. In J. Austin & J. E. Carr (Eds.), *Handbook of applied behavior analysis* (pp. 321–349). Reno, NV: Context Press.

Belfiore, P. J., Fritts, K. M., & Herman, B. C. (2008). The role of procedural integrity: Using self-monitoring to enhance discrete trial instruction (DTI). *Focus on Autism and Other Developmental Disabilities, 23,* 95–102.

Campion, J. E. (1972). Work sampling for personnel selection. *Journal of Applied Psychology, 56,* 40–44.

Daniels, A. C., & Daniels, J. D. (2004). *Performance management: Changing behavior that drives organizational effectiveness.* Atlanta, GA: Performance Management Publications.

Davis, B. J., Smith, T., & Donahoe, P. (2002). Evaluating supervisors in the UCLA treatment model for children with autism: Validation of an assessment procedure. *Behavior Therapy, 31,* 601–614.

Dickinson, A. M., & Gillette, K. L. (1993). A comparison of the effects of two individual monetary incentive systems on productivity: Piece rate pay versus base pay plus incentives. *Journal of Organizational Behavior Management, 14,* 3–82.

Eckerman, D. A., Lundeen, C. A., Steele, A., Fercho, H., Ammerman, T., & Anger, W. K. (2002). Interactive training versus reading to teach respiratory protection. *Journal of Occupational Health Psychology, 7,* 313–323.

Eskildsen, J. K., & Dahlgaard, J. J. (2000). A causal model for employee satisfaction. *Total Quality Management, 11,* 1081–1094.

Flannery, K. B., & Horner, R. H. (1994). The relationship between predictability and problem behavior for students with severe disabilities. *Journal of Behavioral Education, 4,* 157–156.

Flannery, K. B., O'Neill, R., & Horner, R. H. (1995). Including predictability in functional assessment and individual program development. *Education and Treatment of Children, 18,* 499–509.

Fleming, R. K., Oliver, J. R., & Bolton, D. M. (1996). Training supervisors to train staff: A case study in a human service organization. *Journal or Organizational Behavior Management, 16*(1), 3–25.

Forest, E. J., Horner, R. H., Lewis-Palmer, T., Todd, A. W., & McGee, G. (2004). Transitions for young children with autism from preschool to kindergarten. *Journal of Positive Behavior Interventions, 6,* 103–112.

Green, G. (1996). Early behavioral intervention for children with autism: What does research tell us? In C. Maurice, G. Green & S. C. Luce (Eds.), *Behavioral intervention for young children with autism: A manual for parents and professionals* (pp. 29–44). Austin, TX: Pro-Ed.

Hirschfield, R. R., Schmitt, L. P., & Bedeian, A. G. (2002). Job-content perceptions, performance-reward expectancies, and absenteeism among low-wage public-sector clerical employees. *Journal of Business and Psychology, 16,* 553–564.

Iwata, B. A., Pace, G. M., Dorsey, M. F., Zarcone, J. R., Vollmer, T. R., Smith, R. G., et al. (1994). The functions of self-injurious behavior: An experimental-epidemiological analysis. *Journal of Applied Behavior Analysis, 27,* 215–240.

Johnson, E., & Hastings, R. P. (2002). Facilitating factors and barriers to the implementation of intensive home-based behavioural intervention for young children with autism. *Child: Care, Health and Development, 28,* 123–129.

Koegel, R. L., Koegel, L. K., & McNerney, E. K. (2001). Pivotal areas in intervention for autism. *Journal of Clinical Child Psychology, 30,* 19–32.

Komaki, J. L., Desselles, M. L., & Bowman, E. D. (1989). Definitely not a breeze: Extending an operant model of effective supervision to teams. *Journal of Applied Psychology, 74,* 522–529.

Lakin, C. K., & Larson, S. A. (1992). Satisfaction and stability of direct care personnel in community-based residential services. In J. W. Jacobson, S. N. Burchard & P. J. Carling (Eds.), *Community living for people with developmental and psychiatric disabilities* (pp. 244–262). Baltimore, MD: Johns Hopkins University Press.

Larson, S. A., & Hewitt, A. S. (eds). (2005). *Staff recruitment, retention, and training strategies for community human services organizations.* Baltimore, MD: Brookes Publishing.

LeBlanc, L. A., & Fisher, W. W. (October, 1997). A preliminary examination of the relation between "insistence on sameness" and maladaptive behavior in individuals with autism. In M. H. Charlop-Christy (Chair), *Procedures for treating young children with autism.* Symposium presented at the Southern California Association for Behavior Analysis and Therapy, Pasadena, CA.

Leblanc, M., Ricciardi, J. N., & Luiselli, J. K. (2005). Improving discrete trial instruction by paraprofessional staff through an abbreviated performance feedback intervention. *Education and Treatment of Children, 28,* 76–82.

Lee, S., Simpson, R. L., & Shogren, K. A. (2007). Effects and implications of self-management for students with autism: A meta-analysis. *Focus on Autism and Other Developmental Disabilities, 22,* 2–13.

Love, J. R., Carr, J. E., Almason, S. M., & Petursdottir, A. I. (in press). Early and intensive behavioral intervention for autism: A survey of clinical practices. *Research in Autism Spectrum Disorders, 3,* 421–428.

Luce, S. C., & Dyer, S. C. (1995). Providing effective transitional programming to individuals with autism. *Behavioral Disorders, 21,* 36–52.

Mackintosh, N. J. (1974). *The psychology of animal learning.* London: Academic Press.

Macurik, K. M., O'Kane, N. P., Malanga, P., & Reid, D. H. (2008). Video training of support staff in intervention plans for challenging behavior: Comparison with live training. *Behavioral Interventions, 23,* 143–163.

Mager, R. F. (1997). *Analyzing performance problems: Or, you really oughta wanna – How to figure out why people aren't doing what they should be, and what to do about it.* Atlanta, GA: CE Publishers.

McCord, B. E., Thomson, R. J., & Iwata, B. A. (2001). Functional analysis and treatment of self-injury associated with transitions. *Journal of Applied Behavior Analysis, 34,* 195–210.

Moxon, L., & Gates, D. (2001). Children with autism: Supporting the transition to adulthood. *Educational and Child Psychology, 18,* 28–40.

Murphy, G., Macdonald, S., Hall, S., & Oliver, C. (2000). Aggression and the termination of "rituals": A new variant of the escape function for challenging behavior? *Research in Developmental Disabilities, 21,* 43–59.

Parsons, M. B., & Reid, D. H. (1995). Training residential supervisors to provide feedback for maintaining staff teaching skills with people who have severe disabilities. *Journal of Applied Behavior Analysis, 28,* 317–322.

Parsons, M. B., Reid, D. H., & Green, C. W. (1996). Training basic teaching skills to community and institutional support staff for people with severe disabilities: A one-day program. *Research in Developmental Disabilities, 17,* 467–485.

Podsakoff, P. M., & Schriesheim, C. A. (1985). Field studies of French and Raven's bases of power: Critique, reanalysis, and suggestions for future research. *Psychological Bulletin, 97,* 387–411.

Reid, D. H. (1998). *Organizational behavior management and developmental disabilities services: Accomplishments and future directions.* Binghamton, NY: Haworth Press.

Reid, D. H., & Green, C. W. (1990). Staff training. In J. L. Matson (Ed.), *Handbook of behavior modification with the mentally retarded* (2nd ed., pp. 71–90). New York: Plenum Press.

Reid, D. H., & Parsons, M. B. (1996). A comparison of staff acceptability of immediate versus delayed verbal feedback in staff training. *Journal of Organizational Behavior Management, 16,* 35–47.

Reid, D. H., & Parsons, M. B. (2007). *Positive behavior support training curriculum* (2nd ed.). Washington, DC: AAIDD.

Reid, D. H., Parsons, M. B., Lattimore, L. P., Towery, D. L., & Reade, K. K. (2005). Improving staff performance through clinician application of outcome management. *Research in Developmental Disabilities, 26,* 101–116.

Reid, D. H., Rotholz, D. A., Parsons, M. B., Morris, L., Braswell, B. A., Green, C. W., et al. (2003). Training human service supervisors in aspects of PBS: Evaluation of a statewide, performance-based program. *Journal of Positive Behavior Interventions, 5*, 35–46.

Reese, R. M., Richman, D. M., Belmont, J. M., & Morse, P. (2005). Functional characteristics of disruptive behavior in developmentally disabled children with and without autism. *Journal of Autism and Developmental Disorders, 35*, 419–428.

Reese, R. M., Richman, D. M., Zarcone, J., & Zarcone, T. (2003). Individualizing functional assessments for children with autism: The contribution of perseverative behavior and sensory disturbances to disruptive behavior. *Focus on Autism and Other Developmental Disabilities, 18*, 89–94.

Reichle, J., Dropik, P. L., Alden-Anderson, E., & Haley, T. (2008). Teaching a young child with autism to request assistance conditionally: A preliminary study. *American Journal of Speech-Language Pathology, 17*, 231–240.

Schall, C., Cortijo-Doval, E., Targett, P. S., & Wehman, P. (2006). Applications for youth with autism spectrum disorders. In P. Wehman (Ed.), *Life beyond the classroom: Transition strategies for young people with disabilities* (4th ed., pp. 535–575). Baltimore, MD: Brookes Publishing.

Schepis, M. M., & Reid, D. H. (1994). Training direct service staff in congregate settings to interact with people with severe disabilities: A quick, effective and acceptable program. *Behavioral Interventions, 9*, 13–26.

Schreibman, L., Whalen, C., & Stahmer, A. C. (2000). The use of video priming to reduce disruptive behavior in children with autism. *Journal of Positive Behavioral Interventions, 2*, 3–11.

Smith, T. (2001). Discrete trial training in the treatment of autism. *Focus on Autism and Other Developmental Disabilities, 16*, 86–92.

Smith, T., Donahoe, P. A., & Davis, B. J. (2001). The UCLA treatment model. In S. L. Harris & J. S. Handleman (Eds.), *Preschool education programs for children with autism* (2nd ed., pp. 23–39). Austin, TX: Pro-Ed.

Sterling-Turner, H. E., & Jordan, S. S. (2007). Interventions addressing transition difficulties for individuals with autism. *Psychology in the Schools, 44*, 681–690.

Stoner, J. B., Angell, M. E., House, J. J., & Brock, S. J. (2007). Transitions: Perspectives from the parents of young children with autism spectrum disorder (ASD). *Journal of Developmental and Physical Disabilities, 19*, 23–39.

Symes, M. D., Remington, B., Brown, T., & Hastings, R. P. (2006). Early intensive behavioral intervention for children with autism: Therapists' perspectives on achieving procedural fidelity. *Research in Developmental Disabilities, 27*, 30–42.

Tidmarsh, L., & Volkmar, F. (2003). Diagnosis and epidemiology of autism spectrum disorders. *The Canadian Journal of Psychiatry, 48*, 517–525.

Van Bergeijk, E., Klin, A., & Volkmar, F. (2008). Supporting more able students on the autism spectrum: College and beyond. *Journal of Autism and Developmental Disorders, 38*, 1359–1370.

Wage Rates:...And Could We Care Less? (n.d.) Retrieved December 21, 2008, from http://www.afscme.org/publications/2261.cfm.

Williams, T. C., & Zahad, H. (1996). Computer-based training versus traditional lecture: Effect on learning and retention. *Journal of Business and Psychology, 11*, 297–310.

Wilson, P. G., Reid, D. H., & Korabek-Pinkowski, C. A. (1991). Analysis of public verbal feedback as a staff management procedure. *Behavioral Residential Treatment, 6*, 263–277.

Chapter 14
Parent Training Interventions for Children with Autism Spectrum Disorders

Lauren Brookman-Frazee, Laurie Vismara, Amy Drahota, Aubyn Stahmer, and Daniel Openden

A number of parent training programs for parents of children with ASD have been developed. An overview and rationale for why parent training for ASD differs from other childhood groups will be described. An overview of the major parent training methods used for ASD, the research to support them, and the effects achieved will be discussed.

Background of Parent Training Interventions

Development of Parent Training Interventions

Since the 1960s, parent training (PT) (also referred to as parent education) interventions have been developed and tested for a variety of childhood problems including disruptive behavior disorders (Eyberg, Nelson, & Boggs, 2008), attention deficit hyperactivity disorder (Pelham & Fabiano, 2008), anxiety (Barrett & Shortt, 2003), developmental disabilities (Feldman & Werner, 2002), and autism spectrum disorders (ASD) (National Research Council, 2001; New York State Department of Health, 1999). The goals of these intervention models are typically to reduce specific childhood behavior problems, to improve disorder specific skills (e.g., communication, social skills), and/or to enhance parenting skills and competence.

The research on PT for disruptive behavior disorders (DBD) and conduct problems is probably the most well-developed, as a number of different PT models meet criteria for well-established (Parent Management Training Oregon Model) or probably efficacious (e.g., Parent–Child Interaction Therapy, The Incredible Years Parent Training model, Triple P Positive Parenting Program) treatments for these disorders according to established criteria for evidence-based practices (Eyberg et al., 2008). This body of DBD PT research is particularly relevant to ASD PT as the areas of similarities and differences between PT interventions for the two populations highlight unique aspects of the development of ASD PT interventions. In the following sections we highlight key findings of a recent systematic review of DBD and ASD PT empirical research published between 1995 and 2005 (Brookman-Frazee, Stahmer, Baker-Ericzén, & Tsai, 2006) to provide context for the development of current ASD PT interventions.[1]

Roots in Operant Conditioning

Parenting interventions for DBD and ASD are both rooted in the development of operant conditioning procedures. In the 1960s, researchers began using these procedures to reduce disruptive behaviors and encourage prosocial development in children with DBD (e.g., Ferster, 1961; Ferster & Simons, 1966; Patterson & Brodsky, 1966) and ASD researchers used similar

L. Brookman-Frazee (✉)
Child and Adolescent Services Research Center (CASRC), University of California-San Diego, 3020 Children's Way, MC 5033, San Diego, CA, 92123, USA
e-mail: lbrookman@ucsd.edu

[1] Portions of this section are adapted from: Brookman-Frazee, L., Stahmer, A., Baker, M., & Tsai, K. (2006). Parenting interventions for children with autism spectrum and disruptive behavior disorders: Opportunities for cross-fertilization. *Clinical Child and Family Psychology Review, 9,* 181–200.

J.L. Matson (ed.), *Applied Behavior Analysis for Children with Autism Spectrum Disorders*,
DOI 10.1007/978-1-4419-0088-3_14, © Springer Science+Business Media, LLC 2009

strategies to reduce behavioral excesses and improve behavioral deficits (e.g., communication and engagement) in children with ASD (Ferster, 1961; Ferster & Demyer, 1962; Lovaas, Baer, & Bijou, 1965; Lovaas, Freitag, Gold, & Kassorla, 1965; Lovaas & Simmons, 1969). In our review of current empirical research for both populations, all DBP PT studies included some operant conditioning procedures and almost three quarters of ASD studies did, suggesting that these strategies remain important components of contemporary PT models.

Rationale for Including Parents

Although the development of DBD and ASD PT interventions were both influenced by the development of operant conditioning procedures, the rationale for including parents in a child's intervention differed. For DBD, research on parent–child interaction patterns significantly influenced the development of the parent training interventions seen in current research. The extensive body of research involving observations of families that demonstrated coercive interaction patterns which promoted childhood aggression and suppressed prosocial behaviors was particularly important (see Patterson, 1982, for review). Dysfunctional parenting practices have been identified as directly related to child psychopathology (Patterson, Reid, & Dishion, 1992).

While early psychoanalytic explanations for ASD cited parenting practices as a possible cause of "autistic" symptoms (Bettelheim, 1967), research has debunked these notions (e.g., Schreibman, 2005) and, in fact, professionals may be wary of implicating any negative parenting practices in the cause of ASD by targeting parenting practices in treatment protocols. Instead, parents were initially included in ASD PT as co-therapists to assist with the generalization and maintenance of behavior changes in individual child treatment (Koegel, Schreibman, Britten, Burke, & O'Neill, 1982; Lovaas, Koegel, Simmons, & Long, 1973).

The distinct rationales for including parents in child intervention are reflected in the content of current PT interventions for the two groups. In our review, we found that all the DBD PT studies reviewed indicated that a main goal of intervention was, at least in part, to improve parenting practices (some studies also targeted child problem solving or child social skills). In contrast, the goal of a majority of the ASD

studies was to instruct parents in methods for teaching children specific skills (communication, social) or to instruct them to systematically determine the functions of disruptive behaviors through functional assessment procedures.

Role of Parent Psychosocial Functioning

Although the role of parent factors is highly relevant to both populations, it has been conceptualized differently in the development of PT intervention models for ASD and DBD. Parental stress and depression in parents of children with ASD have often been discussed as a result of raising a child with a disability (Moes, 1995), while environmental stressors and parental psychopathology have been associated with increased child symptomatology in children with DBD (Patterson et al., 1992). The results of our review of current PT empirical research were consistent with these conceptual differences. ASD interventions were much more likely to explicitly state that parents are active collaborators in designing interventions for their children (e.g., Brookman-Frazee, 2004) and address stress as a reaction to the child issues and reductions in stress as an important collateral effect of intervention (Koegel, Bimbela, & Schreibman, 1996), while DBD interventions were more likely to explicitly target parent factors such as stress, depression, and marital problems as a structured part of their PT/PE program that are suggestive of causal attributes to child issues (e.g., Kazdin & Whitley, 2003).

Research Methodology

Early research in both DBD and ASD employed similar research methodologies which consisted primarily of highly structured and controlled single-subject experimental designs. In current research, however, studies involving the two populations use different methodologies. We found that a majority of ASD studies employed single-subject designs, while DBD studies were conducted as randomized, controlled trials. The challenges associated with conducting RCTs include low base rates of ASD, heterogeneity of the population, the developmental nature of the disorder, ethical considerations of placing children in a control condition, and the potential contamination of the control group as parents are often informed about various intervention approaches (Lord et al., 2005; Schopler, 2005). Despite these challenges, there may be advantages of a clinical trial methodology including methodological rigor and clear examination of the effects of the independent variable. Experts have suggested a sequence for ASD treatment research in which single-subject designs are used first to determine treatment efficacy and RCTs could be used in subsequent studies to further investigate the efficacy (Lord et al., 2005; Smith et al., 2007). Current efforts are using RCT methodology in the investigation of ASD PT interventions (e.g., UC MIND Institute, University of Washington, University of Michigan).

Overview of Current ASD Parent Training Research and Practice

In this section, we focus on the current research and practice of ASD PT interventions. Specifically, we briefly review (1) the content of common PT interventions, (2) delivery of PT interventions, and (3) the documented benefits associated with the various models.

Content of Parent Training Interventions

The content of PT interventions refers to the specific intervention strategies or approach that the parent is taught to deliver to the child. The intervention approach is likely determined by the characteristics of the child (e.g., developmental level), targeted goals, and family characteristics (e.g., learning style, child-rearing practices, interaction preferences, cultural background).

Discrete Trial Training (DTT)

There is a growing interest in examining the impact of parent-implemented discrete trial training. One of the earliest studies to examine parent involvement in DTT (Lovaas et al., 1973) demonstrated the importance of including parents as agents of change in extending and maintaining the behavioral gains made by their children during intervention. Subsequent studies have also illustrated that structured parent training DTT

programs can effectively teach sophisticated behavioral procedures and concepts (i.e., prompting, fading, shaping, chaining, reinforcement, punishment, data collection, generalization, and maintenance) in working with children with autism (e.g., Anderson, Avery, DiPietro, Edwards, & Christian, 1987; Harris, 1983; Koegel, Glahn, & Nieminen, 1978; Smith, Buch, & Gamby, 2000). While numerous studies have demonstrated parents' ability to acquire the skills necessary to teach their children, generalization, or the parents' skill level in transferring their child's learning objectives to other behaviors, has been noted as a weakness in this PT intervention approach (Baker, 1989; Koegel et al., 1978). Recently, Crockett, Fleming, Doepke, and Stevens (2007) examined two parents' implementation of DTT procedures to enhance generalization of untrained child skills and overall cost-effectiveness. The primary investigation demonstrated control of the training program over parents' correct use of DTT and generalized effects of training to multiple functional child skills. While results such as these are encouraging, systematic replications with more participants are needed to strengthen and build upon training procedures to enhance generalization. The teaching practices of DTT emphasize the importance of a structured and adult-guided learning environment in the early stages of teaching children with autism (Smith, Donahoe, & Davis, 2001); however, an important goal for behavioral PT programs is to equip parents with an effective way of teaching their children the many skills they will need to live optimally in their daily environments. Within this general framework, there has been a search for intervention approaches that can produce generalized improvements and target core areas that may impact many broad areas of functioning. Behavioral PT approaches encompassing more naturalistic teaching procedures may help to address this need.

Naturalistic Behavioral Methods

The desire to improve the efficiency of behavioral interventions and response generalization led to the development of naturalistic behavioral intervention methods that are less structured, provided in natural context, and involve intrinsically related rewards. There are multiple naturalistic behavioral methods, including incidental teaching (Hart & Risley, 1968), milieu teaching (Hancock & Kaiser, 2002), and pivotal response training (Koegel, O'Dell, & Koegel, 1987). For this discussion, we focus on pivotal response training which was developed to target pivotal responses that result in widespread improvements on other non-targeted areas, representing an efficient method to produce generalized improvements (Koegel, Koegel, & Brookman, 2003). This approach is a widely used intervention and was specifically developed for PT (National Research Council, 2001).

To date, a number of pivotal responses have been identified. These include child motivation, self-management, self-initiations, and responsivity to multiple cues (Koegel, Koegel, & McNerney, 2001; Koegel, Koegel, Shoshan, & McNerney, 1999; Schreibman & Koegel, 2005). Most of the PT research, however, has focused on targeting two pivotal areas, motivation and responsivity to multiple cues. Intervention procedures targeting these areas are naturalistic strategies, designed to be implemented in a child's natural environment throughout a family's daily routines using real-life, developmentally appropriate toys and materials. This intervention approach was first referred to as the natural language paradigm (NLP: Koegel, O'Dell, et al., 1987) and later referred to as pivotal response training (PRT: Schreibman, Kaneko, & Koegel, 1991). PRT teaches parents to implement strategies to increase a child's motivation to engage in verbal communication, appropriate social interactions, and engagement in learning interactions from the natural environment (Koegel et al., 2003). Typically, clinicians provide parents with immediate and specific feedback on their implementation of the procedures described in written materials (Koegel et al., 1989), while the parent directly interacts with his or her child. These procedures include: (1) following the child's choice in the selection of toys and activities; (2) reinforcing clear attempts; (3) interspersing maintenance with acquisition tasks; (4) responsivity to multiple cues; and (5) the use of contingent natural and direct reinforcers.

Early studies comparing parent-implemented NLP/PRT to parent-implemented analogue, discrete trial procedures documented superior gains in child communication skills, greater generalization of treatment gains, more positive parent–child interactions, and greater reductions in problems behavior in the NLP/PRT conditions (Koegel et al., 1996; Schreibman et al., 1991). More recent PT research continues to utilize similar naturalistic behavioral procedures to target child communication and social skills (e.g., Charlop-Christy & Carpenter, 2000; Gillett & LeBlanc, 2007).

Naturalistic behavioral methods, such as PRT, may be particularly appropriate for a PT model as they are intended to be incorporated more like an interaction style that a parent uses throughout the day, rather than a direct teaching method that may potentially burden a family by requiring a great deal of time to be set aside to teach individual target behaviors (Koegel & Koegel, 2006; National Research Council, 2001; Wetherby & Woods, 2006). The attention to the unique developmental needs of young children, in addition to embedding teaching opportunities throughout meaningful daily activities and routines, points to the appropriateness of naturalistic behavioral models when addressing the needs of young children with autism (Koegel, Koegel, Fredeen, & Gengoux, 2008).

Integrated Developmental and Behavioral Methods

While behavioral interventions have been widely effective in addressing the symptoms and learning needs of preschool and school-aged children (Levy, Kim, & Olive, 2006), there is a pressing need to determine what type of changes or modifications in these intervention programs might be necessary to promote permanent, meaningful developmental growth in infants and toddlers (Boulware, Schwartz, Sandall, & McBride, 2006; Volkmar, Chawarska, & Klin, 2005; Wetherby & Woods, 2006), especially given the focus on early identification and diagnosis (Osterling, Dawson, & Munson, 2002). For example, researchers may need to adapt behavioral protocols to address specific developmental needs, such as the importance of teaching prelinguistic social communicative skills (e.g., joint attention, imitation) or to consider other realistic constraints (e.g., sleep schedules, feeding times).

The integration of developmental methods in behavioral intervention programs uses teaching strategies consistent with the principles of applied behavior analysis in treating the symptoms associated with ASD and concomitant delays; however, these approaches use typical developmental sequences as the content of their interventions and developmental theory as the guiding principle of their approach (Rogers & Ozonoff, 2006). Similar to naturalistic behavioral programs, developmental approaches are child-directed in that opportunities for teaching are arranged within the child's natural environment to elicit child initiations. The adult then follows the child's lead by responding to the child's behavior and modeling, imitating, or expanding on the child's response. There is a strong focus on enhancing the child's relationship with others in the intervention and as such, social engagement, reciprocity, and shared affect represent a major priority of the adult–child interactions. Additionally, these approaches emphasize the development of the full range of interpersonal communicative behaviors, including eye contact, shared affect, intentional vocalization, and manual gestures, as well as speech, to achieve reciprocal communicative exchanges in interactions involving objects and social games. Although developmental interventions for ASD have not been studied as rigorously as behavioral treatments, empirical support is beginning to accumulate. Currently, a few published interventions exist, including two randomized controlled trials, which demonstrated efficacy with infants and toddlers at risk for ASD (e.g., Mahoney, Boyce, Fewell, Spiker, & Wheeden, 1998; Mahoney & Perales, 2005; Strain & Hoyson, 2000).

There are a few integrated developmental and behavioral methods, including the developmental social-pragmatic (DSP) curriculum developed by Ingersoll and Dvortcsak (2006), and the Early Start Denver Model (ESDM: Rogers, Dawson, Smith, Winter, & Donaldson, in press). We focus our discussion on the ESDM, a manualized approach to PT designed to precede intensive early intervention services for toddlers at risk for ASD, aged 12–36 months (described in Vismara, Colombi, & Rogers, in press). The ESDM is a developmental, individualized, and relationship-based model to address the unique social-emotional needs of infants and toddlers with ASD and their families. The three main goals of intervention in the ESDM are: (a) having the child participate in coordinated, interactive social interactions to build social attention, imitation, and symbolic communication skills; (b) increasing the child's reward value of social experiences with others by teaching within child-preferred activities and reading the child's cues and nonverbal behavior during play; and (c) developing joint activity routines in which the child and partner co-construct and participate in play activities together so that the child can understand, predict, and complete the routine while the adult "fills in" the learning deficits to build skills that include teaching,

imitation, communication, flexible toy play, and awareness of social partners.

The ESDM curriculum draws extensively from two existing methods that have received empirical support for improving skill acquisition in very young children with ASD. The first approach, the Denver Model developed by Rogers and colleagues was shown to accelerate learning across a variety of developmental domains (Rogers & DiLalla, 1991; Rogers, Hall, Osaki, Reaven, & Herbison, 2001; Rogers, Herbison, Lewis, Pantone, & Reis, 1986; Rogers & Lewis, 1989; Rogers, Lewis, & Reis, 1987). The Denver Model focuses on building an affectively warm and supportive environment to facilitate social engagement, reciprocity, and shared affect between children and adults. There is also a strong focus on approaching language development from a communication science orientation, addressing the social function of language (i.e., pragmatics) and the development of nonverbal communication and imitation as the precursors to verbal language. The second model is Pivotal Response Training which is described earlier.

Cognitive-Behavioral Methods

Incorporating PT into interventions directed for school-age children and adolescents (rather than toddlers and preschoolers) with ASD and comorbid psychiatric disorders has been of increasing interest to researchers (Anderson & Morris, 2006; Chalfant, Rapee, & Carroll, 2007; Reaven & Hepburn, 2003, 2006; RUPP Autism Network, 2007; Sofronoff, Attwood, & Hinton, 2005; Sze & Wood, 2007). A recent review of the trajectory of development in adolescents with ASD indicates that as children with ASD age, their symptoms of ASD (particularly communication deficits) may become less obvious to observers despite the continued pervasive impairments in their social skills and comprehension (Seltzer, Shattuck, Abbeduto, & Greenberg, 2004). Simultaneously, the prevalence of comorbid psychiatric diagnoses increases as children with ASD age (Simonoff et al., 2008). Internalizing disorders (anxiety and depression), for example, are common among children and adolescents with ASD, affecting 22–84% of the population (de Bruin, Ferdinand, Meester, de Nijs, & Verheij, 2007; Ghaziuddin, Weidmer-Mikhail, & Ghaziuddin, 1998; Green, Gilchrist, Burton, & Cox, 2000; Kim, Szatmari, Bryson, Streiner,

& Wilson, 2000; Leyfer et al., 2006). The additional impairment in a child's social, family, and academic functioning associated with co-occurring psychiatric problems frequently merits intervention. Thus, as children with ASD age and associated psychiatric problems may emerge, the focus of interventions is to teach children strategies to cope with challenges that are commensurate with their cognitive and verbal abilities.

It is suggested that youth with a primary diagnosis of an ASD and comorbid diagnosis of anxiety or depression are likely to be especially responsive to learning cognitive coping strategies through interventions such as Family Cognitive-Behavioral Therapy (FCBT). In this intervention model, emphasis is placed on teaching children and adolescents cognitive coping strategies such as self-monitoring, emotion identification and recognition, cognitive restructuring, and problem solving. Through discussion and questioning, therapists and children identify maladaptive cognitions (e.g., "I can't brush my teeth or take a shower in the morning because I will be late for school, get detention, not get into college, and not have any chance to become an astronaut."), question the validity of the identified cognitions ("If I am late for school, will I really get detention, and if I do get detention, will that make it impossible to get into college?"), and correct the cognitive distortions ("Even if I get detention, I will probably be able to get into college."). These coping skills are learned early in treatment; tests of the "new" cognitions are planned and practiced in the treatment room and then gradually transferred into more naturalistic settings until the child is able to master the skill in the actual setting and across settings. Through this series of steps, clinicians provide immediate feedback, positive regard, and reinforcement to continue or increase children's motivation to persist and finally habituate.

In vivo exposure involves implementing strategies that have been practiced with the clinician but in real-life situations that have previously been avoided (e.g., joining a game of tag on the playground). Exposures begin with situations that are only slightly challenging, and then, building on successes, increase in difficulty until mastery and generalization are evident. This is an optimal area for parent involvement and training because the focus of in vivo exposures is to gain mastery outside of the treatment room and where children would benefit most from developing their skills. Compared to traditional

social and communication skills training and treatment of psychiatric disorders done in the treatment room – which rarely generalizes to daily life – in vivo exposure techniques place training and practice in the actual situations where generalization is desired through the involvement of parents, thus improving the chances of youth's spontaneous use of the skills in these environments after training is complete.

Parental involvement in these interventions has been found to enhance treatment effectiveness for typically developing children (Cobham, Dadds, & Spence, 1998; Mendlowitz et al., 1999), and emerging evidence suggests the same for children and adolescents with ASD (Reaven & Hepburn, 2006; Sofronoff et al., 2005; Sze & Wood, 2007; Wood et al., in press). Parent involvement is important for a number of reasons. First, child noncompliance with intervention goals may be inadvertently sustained by parents who are uncertain or inconsistent with efforts to manage and oversee their children's intervention adherence (RUPP Autism Network, 2007). As a result of the deficits in motivation associated with ASD, parents may provide unnecessary reassurance and assistance with feared situations, further promoting a sense of dependency in their children (Seligman, 1972). Further, training parents to implement cognitive-behavioral strategies outside of the treatment room allows children to achieve mastery in varied settings with varied individuals, and treatment gains are likely to be maintained.

The *Building Confidence FCBT* is an example of an FCBT intervention targeting children with ASD that includes a PT component. The *Building Confidence FCBT* is an enhanced intervention targeting the development of social and independent skills and reducing anxiety disorders by systematically facing feared stimuli (Drahota, in review; Wood et al., in press). In the PT component of this intervention, parents are provided with a rationale for targeting autonomy-supporting behaviors and communication skills by emphasizing the importance of these skills in their child's adaptive functioning and development into adulthood. Further, reasons for which parents have not focused attention on specific skills, such as independent daily living skills, are discussed (e.g., parents have had previous difficulty teaching independent daily living skills to their children; they find it much easier to complete the task for their child) (Koegel & Egel, 1979).

Once parent motivation has been addressed, a plan for developing children's skills is developed.

Parents are taught to support their children's attempts at courageous behavior, social skills, and independence through autonomy-supporting behaviors and communication skills. Autonomy-supporting behaviors include "respecting the child's struggle"; parents are trained to withhold assistance and provide their children time to figure out their own solutions – allowing their child to learn through trial and error. Additionally, communication skills such as "giving choices" (e.g., "Do you want to wait 1 minute before starting your bath, or would you prefer 2 minutes?") (Dyer, Dunlap, & Winterling, 1990; Shogren, Faggella-Luby, Bae, & Wehmeyer, 2004) are taught. Finally, parents are trained to provide immediate positive feedback or reinforcement to their children when reasonable attempts or mastery are made in order to increase their children's motivation to try again.

LeBlanc, 2007; Ingersoll & Dvortcsak, 2006; Schreibman & Koegel, 2005). A meta-analysis of PT components found that requiring parents to practice their new skills with their children during the PT session was associated with larger effects of intervention than programs without these constructs, regardless of other program content or delivery approaches (Kaminski, Valle, Filene, & Boyle, 2008). Others have emphasized the practice-with feedback as a key method to effectively teach parents new skills and ensure parent mastery, suggesting that feedback needs to be succinct, frequent, immediate, and more positive than corrective (Ingersoll & Dvortcsak, 2006; Kaiser & Hancock, 2003; Kaminski et al., 2008). Related, Ingersoll and Dvortcsak (2006) warn against spending too much time on modeling, rather than having a parent practice skills.

Delivering Parent Training Interventions

While much of the ASD PT research emphasizes the *content* of PT programs discussed above, *how* parents are taught is equally important. PT format and characteristics of PT participants are key aspects of PT delivery.

Individual Family Format

There are a number of advantages of an individual (one-on-one) teaching model (Kaiser & Hancock, 2003). It allows the teaching strategies and interventions strategies to be tailored to the individual child and his or her family. Further, it allows for more emphasis on active teach strategies (practice-with feedback) which facilitates learning. Individual sessions also provide flexibility in the location of teaching in a child's home which can facilitate maintenance and generalization of parent skill, while sessions in the clinic can provide a distraction-free environment which may facilitate the initial acquisition of parent (and child) skills.

A common approach to teaching parents specific intervention strategies in individual PT (as opposed to in a group) is to combine (1) review of written materials and introduction to techniques, (2) modeling or demonstrating new procedures, and (3) in vivo practice with immediate clinician feedback/coaching (Gillett &

Group Format

Group models and combined group–individual models have also been used in PT programs. The advantages of a group model are that it is less time-intensive and cost-efficient than the individual model. Group teaching formats typically include (1) didactic instruction (2) modeling (typically through videotape exemplars), (3) role-playing, and (4) group problem solving and discussion (Ingersoll & Dvortcsak, 2006). An example of a research study utilizing a group PT format is presented in the case example section.

Characteristics of Parent Participants

The targeted learners in PT intervention are typically the child's primary caregivers. This may include a child's mother, father, grandparents, or other family members. Until recently, participants in most of the PT research studies have been mothers. However, there is growing research on teaching fathers (e.g., Seung, Ashwell, Elder, & Valcante, 2006). Probably more important than which parent participates is that they are motivated and committed to learning new skills (Kaiser & Hancock, 2003). Further, it is important that at least one parent attend all sessions to increase consistency and facilitate learning. Another important consideration when determining who should participate in a PT program is parental stress. Although research demonstrates reductions in child-related stress (related to child's behavior or symptoms) following participation in a PT program (e.g., Moes, 1995), studies have also documented that parents who are experiencing clinical levels of parent-related stress (including depression, marital discord, or health issues) do not benefit as much as parents who do not demonstrated clinically elevated stress (Robbins, Dunlap, & Plienis, 1991).

Characteristics of Effective Parent Educators

Until recently, there has been a significantly greater focus on the content of PT programs than on who provides the intervention. This is an important consideration because clinicians are frequently trained to provide intervention directly to children, rather than on strategies to teach parents to delivery intervention. Kaiser and Hancock (2003) highlight key prerequisite skills of parent educators and suggest that clinicians be explicitly taught these skills. These include mastery and conceptual understanding of the intervention procedures, responsive and collaborative teaching style, fluency in presentation of content and providing immediate feedback, and ability to individualize intervention and evaluate progress. Ingersoll and Dvortcsak (2006) highlight other interactions skills that are important when working with families. For example, they stress the importance of building rapport with parents by acknowledging parental feelings (e.g., guilt, frustration), listening to parents' concerns, and avoiding alliance with one parent or another when working with more than one. In addition, research has compared the impact of two clinician interaction approaches on the PT process (Brookman-Frazee, 2004 – summarized in case example section below).

Benefits of Parent Training

Efficiency of Services

Research findings support the benefits of PT in terms of increasing the quantity and availability of intervention (Iacono, Chan, & Waring, 1998; Koegel, Koegel, & Schreibman, 1991; Koegel et al., 1996; McClannahan, Krantz, & McGee, 1982), while requiring less time for child gains than clinician-implemented intervention

(Koegel et al., 1982). Recent research on an intensive, short-term PT model demonstrates that once parents are trained to deliver intervention strategies to their child, they can effectively train other family members and service providers (Symon, 2005).

Child Improvements

Research has demonstrated that parents of children with ASD can effectively implement behavioral interventions strategies with a high degree of fidelity (Koegel, Symon, & Koegel, 2002; Koegel et al., 1996; Koegel et al., 1991; Laski, Charlop, & Schreibman, 1988). They learned to use techniques that led to reductions in problem behaviors (Frea & Hepburn, 1999; Koegel, Koegel, & Surratt, 1992; Moes & Frea, 2002; Sofronoff, Leslie, & Brown, 2004), increased child functional communication skills (Koegel, Koegel, Harrower, & Carter, 1999; Koegel et al., 2002; Laski et al., 1988; McGee, Morrier, & Daly, 1999; McGee, Paradis, & Feldman, 1993), increased child joint attention skills (Rocha, Schreibman, & Stahmer, 2007; Vismara & Lyons, 2007), developed play skills (Stahmer, 1995; Stahmer & Schreibman, 1992), improved social skills (Sofronoff et al., 2004), and reduced sleep problems (Weiskop, Richdale, & Matthews, 2005).

Parent–Child Interactions and Family Functioning

In addition to expanding the skills acquired by children and parents' delivery of specific intervention strategies, numerous other positive effects on the family have been documented following PT programs. Early ASD PT research documented positive impacts of PT on parent–child interactions. For example, in a study comparing the impacts of parent versus clinician-implemented intervention, Koegel et al. (1992) found that children who received the PT intervention were more responsive to their parents' questions and directions. Likewise, parents of children with ASD have demonstrated increased positive affect (R.L. Koegel et al., 1996; Schreibman et al., 1991), reduced stress (Moes, 1995), and reported more time for leisure activities (Koegel, Schreibman, Johnson, O'Neil, & Dunlap, 1984) following participation in a PT program in pivotal response interventions. In other PT models, reductions in maternal depression (Blackledge & Hayes, 2006; Bristol, Gallagher, & Holt, 1993) and increased parent self-efficacy (Sofronoff & Farbotko, 2002) have been observed.

Examples of Recent Parent Training Research

PT Content Example #1: Early Start Denver Model

As described earlier, The ESDM PT intervention was designed as a follow up to diagnosis that would support parents and stimulate child progress as families wait for more intensive services to begin. In a preliminary study of the feasibility and impact of a parent coaching model, that include twelve 1-h per week sessions designed to begin just after the diagnosis of autism, the following outcomes were examined: (a) whether parents could learn and apply the same intervention skills that therapists use within the short time frame of the program to engage, communicate with, and teach their young children; (b) what immediate changes in children's social communicative behaviors would occur as a result of their parents' implementation of these teaching techniques; and (c) whether changes in parents' and children's behavior maintain over time. After 12 continuous weeks of intervention, four additional 1-h sessions were scheduled across a period of 3 months to assess maintenance and generalization of child and parent outcome measures. The four follow-up visits also included a generalization probe with a new therapist to examine the child's transfer of behaviors to an unfamiliar person.

Participants

The study involved the first eight families of children recently diagnosed or determined at significant risk of autism, between 9 months and 36 months of age, who were referred to the program. Two of the families were Latino; the remaining four were Caucasian. The families represented a range of educational socio-economic and marital statuses.

Procedures

Following the completion of baseline measures, individual training sessions were conducted once weekly for 1 h, over 12 weeks, in a treatment room at a university-based research center. The first 10–15 min were spent observing the parent and child in play in order to provide new information and feedback about the previous sessions (e.g., the parent's technique use, the child's behavior) and to collect data on parent's acquisition of teaching techniques and on child behaviors. New information was introduced verbally, using a detailed parent manual to highlight ten therapy strategies (Rogers, Vismara, & Colombi, in preparation) that are consistent with the ESDM teaching practices: (a) increasing the child's attention and motivation; (b) sensory social routines; (c) dyadic engagement; (d) nonverbal communication; (e) imitation; (f) joint attention; (g) speech development; (h) Antecedent-Behavior-Consequence relationship (ABC's of learning); (i) prompting, shaping, and fading techniques; and (j) functional assessment of behavior. Each strategy was the focus of one session in which the parent was taught to deliver the techniques during play or other every-day routines (e.g., meals, bed time, bath time), as well as in different contexts (e.g., grandparents' home, park, grocery store, church). The therapist modeled the procedures with the child in addition to coaching and providing specific feedback during parent–child interactions. Handouts adapted to the parent's reading level were also given and summarized after the practice session.

Results

Parents who completed the program (two families terminated at week 8 due to illness and at week 10 due to the start of the child's intensive in-home intervention program, respectively) acquired the ESDM intervention techniques between the fifth and sixth hours of intervention and maintained their fidelity throughout the remaining sessions, as well as during four follow up visits across a 3-month period. Children showed improvements in the number of spontaneous vocalizations, imitative behaviors, and in overall engagement and initiations during interactions with their parents and with therapists in weekly sessions. Children were not observed to exhibit high rates of problem behavior (e.g., screaming, throwing, biting) or noncompliance during any phase of this study. The low level of disruptive behaviors may have been prevented by the use of motivational components (i.e., reinforcing child attempts, child-preferred activities, stimulus variation, and direct response-reinforcer relationships) within naturalistic play routines, as indicated by prior research (Dunlap & Koegel, 1980; Koegel, Dyer, & Bell, 1987; Koegel, O'Dell, & Dunlap, 1988; Koegel & Williams, 1980). Further, child gains were maintained during interactions with parents and with unfamiliar therapists during the 3-month period of follow up visits (see Vismara et al., in press for findings).

Implications

This study provides preliminary support for the use of a brief and economical 12-week intervention designed for the early diagnostic process. Specifically, using early short-term, specific developmental-behavioral curriculum can lead to rapid acquisition of intervention techniques and immediate improvement in children. It suggests that a condensed parent coaching program may be a cost-effective model in terms of minimizing the need for additional parent education services and/or requiring fewer hours of direct child services. In addition, the model provides an essential support for families in the confusing and emotional period just after diagnosis, and can serve as a tool to instill in parents the necessary skills and confidence to encourage development in their child with autism.

A multi-site randomized controlled study examining the impact of the ESDM parent-coaching program compared to community intervention programs on child development for 12–24 month olds with ASD is currently underway. This study includes a larger group of participants from a wider range of socio-economic and ethnic backgrounds. An examination of how effective this parent coaching model is translated to community early intervention providers and support states in providing coordinated services to young children (birth to 3 years) is also underway. Future research will identify the type of support and length of intervention necessary for parent coaching skills to transmit meaningful, permanent developmental growth in infants and toddlers at risk for ASD.

PT Content Example #2: Building Confidence – Family Cognitive-Behavioral Therapy

Several case studies and exploratory clinical trials have suggested that cognitive behavioral therapy (CBT) may lessen anxiety symptoms in children with ASD (e.g., Chalfant et al., 2007; Reaven & Hepburn, 2003; Sze & Wood, 2007). Sofronoff et al. (2005) evaluated two variants of a 6-week CBT program in group-therapy format for children with Asperger syndrome, focusing on emotion recognition and cognitive restructuring. While participating children were not diagnosed with anxiety disorders at pretreatment per se, parent-report measures showed declines in child anxiety symptoms in the CBT groups compared to a waitlist group at post-treatment. Additionally, a 16-week group-therapy CBT intervention tested by Chalfant and colleagues targeted children with ASD and concurrent anxiety disorders, finding that the children in the immediate treatment group had significant reductions in anxiety as compared with the waitlist group. However, study of clinicians, rather than independent evaluators, administered the posttreatment diagnostic interviews, and fidelity checks were not conducted. Thus, while CBT may be a promising intervention modality for the ASD population, methodological characteristics of the extant studies preclude conclusions about efficacy (e.g., Chambless & Hollon, 1998). Further, concerns regarding generalization and maintenance persist when considering CBT without parental involvement.

Research is currently underway at the University of California, Los Angeles, examining the impacts of one model of family cognitive-behavioral therapy (FCBT) on children with a primary diagnosis of Asperger syndrome or high-functioning autism and a comorbid anxiety disorder. Initial findings from this randomized, controlled trial are summarized below (Drahota et al., in preparation; Wood et al., in press).

Participants

The intent-to-treat sample included 40 high-functioning children with a primary ASD diagnosis and a comorbid anxiety disorder, ranging in age from 7 years to 11 years, and their primary parent (e.g., the parent primarily responsible for overseeing the child's daily activities).

As expected, 67.5% of the child participants were male. Children's ethnic background included Caucasian (48%), Asian (15%), Latino/a (13%), African–American (2%), and multiple (two or more) ethnic backgrounds (22%). Eighty percent of the primary caregivers were mothers, with a majority having graduated from college (62.5%). Socio-economic status of participating families ranged from below $40,000 (27%) to over $90,000 (49%).

Procedures

Following an intake assessment, eligible families were randomly assigned to either the immediate treatment condition or a 3-month waitlist condition. Families assigned to the immediate treatment condition began the *Building Confidence* FCBT, consisting of 16 weekly treatment sessions, each lasting approximately 90 min, and involving an individual child session, individual parent session, and a family session. The PT components of the intervention focused on supporting in vivo exposures, using positive reinforcement, and using communication skills to encourage children's independence and autonomy in daily routines. Further enhancements to the PT components of the manual were designed to address friendship skill deficits through parental "social coaching"; encourage independence in adaptive self-help skills by teaching parents principles of task analysis, suppressing their child's circumscribed interests and stereotypes, and developing a rewards system; and using contingency management procedures to address relevant behavioral problems (failure to follow directions, aggression, and teasing/disrespectful language). Parents were given written materials, engaged in didactic discussions and role play with the therapist, and were provided in vivo coaching to enhance their competence and mastery of these skills and to increase parental adherence to the treatment techniques outside of the therapy room.

A posttreatment assessment was conducted at the termination session for the families in the immediate treatment condition. Families in the waitlist condition were re-assessed 3 months after the intake assessment, after which the FCBT treatment was provided.

Results

In terms of anxiety outcomes, results indicate that 92.9% of the treatment completers in the immediate treatment condition met criteria for positive treatment response, compared to only 9.1% of the children in the waitlist condition. Additionally, 64.3% of the treatment completers did not meet criteria for any anxiety disorder diagnosis at posttreatment. For the intent-to-treatment sample, 76.5% of the children in the immediate treatment condition met criteria for a positive treatment response, whereas only 8.7% of the children in the waitlist condition did so. Further, clinician severity rating scores were lower in the immediate treatment group than in the waitlist group at posttreatment/post-waitlist, with an effect size of 2.46, a large effect (Wood et al., in press). In addition to reductions in anxiety, children in the immediate treatment condition significantly increased their personal and global independent daily living skills and increased their total social skills and responsible social behaviors, and parents significantly reduced their over-involvement in their child's personal self-care tasks (e.g., bathing, grooming) when compared with children and parents in the waitlist condition (Drahota et al., in preparation).

In addition to the primary outcomes, parents were able to learn the procedures and implement them with fidelity. Evaluation of therapist progress notes indicates that 90% of the home-based practice assignments were implemented (e.g., homework was done and reward systems were followed) by parents. When examining the quality of the home-based practice assignments, 83% of the weekly home-based assignments were completed correctly and consistently (e.g., at or above 75% accuracy and completeness). Finally, parent satisfaction with the *Building Confidence* FCBT was assessed at posttreatment. Parents reported a high level of satisfaction with the program, endorsing feeling "satisfied" to "very satisfied" with the quality of the treatment and their child's progress, that their child was "improved" or "much improved," and that their optimism toward their child's future increased.

Implications

Despite the high levels of comorbidity encountered in this group, children randomized to the immediate treatment group had primary outcomes comparable to those of typically developing children (children without ASD) enrolled in previous clinical trials of family-based CBT for anxiety disorders (e.g., Barrett, Dadds, & Rapee, 1996; Wood, Piacentini, Southam-Gerow,

Chu, & Sigman, 2006). This study provides initial support for the feasibility and efficacy of this FCBT model for treating co-morbid disorders, such as anxiety, as well as increasing the adaptive functioning of children with ASD. Parental involvement was emphasized to address the generalization problems inherent in previous child-focused interventions for ASD. These results provide empirical support for including parents in CBT and suggest that parents can use these techniques in naturalistic settings with a high level of fidelity.

PT Delivery Format Example #1: Parent–Professional Partnership Model of PT in Pivotal Response Training

The importance of active parent–professional collaboration and partnership has been discussed extensively in recent literature on providing comprehensive interventions for children with disabilities (Lucyshyn, Dunlap, & Albin, 2002; Seligman & Darling, 1997; Singer, Goldberg-Hamblin, Peckham-Hardin, Barry, & Santarelli, 2002), but limited empirical data exist to support the use of this model of PT. Therefore, the purpose of the Brookman-Frazee (2004) study was to extend the PT research by assessing a parent–professional partnership approach to teaching Pivotal Response Training strategies. Specifically, a repeated reversals design was used to compare a parent/clinician partnership PT model to a purely clinician-directed model on measures of observed parent–child interactions, including parental stress and confidence, child affect (i.e., happiness and interest), and child responding and engagement.

Participant Families

Three boys with autism and their mothers participated in the study which was conducted at the University of California, Santa Barbara Autism Research and Training Center. The mothers were all the primary caregivers of their children. There was no selection criteria based on the gender of the children or parents. The first three families who met the selection criteria were included in the study. The boys ranged in age from 2 years 5 months to 2 years 10 months at the

beginning of the study and were at least 1 year delayed in their communication skills as measured on the Vineland Adaptive Behavior Scales.

PT Content: Pivotal Response Training (PRT)

The specific naturalistic procedures are described in the preceding section. PT sessions occurred either in the child's home or in a clinic. The strategies to increase the child's motivation to engage in social communication were taught to the parent through review of written materials and in vivo coaching practice-with-feedback approach. The type of teaching interactions (e.g., verbal instruction provided to the parent) and specific targeted child behaviors varied according to the following PT conditions:

"Partnership" PT Condition

This condition was characterized by a collaborative interaction between the parent and clinician and could be initiated by either the clinician or the parent. The clinician engaged the parent throughout the session by eliciting input or providing her a choice on specific opportunities for language and implementation of intervention. Examples of clinician instructions include, "It looks like Johnny is interested in playing with the Play Doh. What would you like to have him say here in order to play with the Play Doh?" or "It looks like Jason wants to play with the ball. There are a number of different ways to incorporate a language opportunity here. For example, maybe he could say 'ball' or 'throw' for you to throw it to him. What would you like him to say?'" The parent also initiated the partnership by spontaneously choosing intervention opportunities or target behaviors and the clinician followed the parent's lead.

"Clinician-Directed" PT Condition

This condition was characterized by the clinician primarily choosing specific target behaviors, intervention activities, or opportunities for language without eliciting parent input into the specific implementation of intervention procedures or giving the parent a choice in the specific manner of implementing of the procedures.

Examples of clinician instructions to the parent include, "It looks like Johnny is interested in the Play Doh. Let's have him label the color that he wants." Or "It looks like Johnny wants the ball. Have him say 'ball' before you throw it to him.

Results

The results of this investigation demonstrate that forming a collaborative relationship between clinicians and parents in PT programs positively affects parent–child teaching interactions. Specifically, the mothers in this study were observed to demonstrate lower levels of observed stress and higher levels of observed confidence during the partnership condition compared to the clinician-directed condition. Likewise, children demonstrated more positive affect, higher levels of responding, and appropriate engagement when parents were partners in the intervention process. Overall, the effect sizes were medium to large across outcome measures.

Implications

The results of this study provide initial empirical support for a parent–professional partnership model of PT and provide direction and promise for incorporating partnerships in parent–professional relationships. The results of this study provide direction on *how* to implement and foster partnerships in PT programs through the types of instructions that the parent educator gives to the parent throughout the session. This study demonstrates that the subtle differences in the types of instructions yielded significant effects on the parent–child teaching interactions. Potentially, actively eliciting parent input during the PT sessions capitalizes on parents' expertise of their children. It is possible that these procedures used may be useful in increasing participation in educational and clinical programs for families from diverse cultural backgrounds, establishing more effective relationships with resistant parents, increasing treatment success, and decreasing attrition rates among parents participating in PT programs. The findings also suggest that explicitly training parent educators on how to most effectively teach parents is warranted.

PT Delivery Format Example #2: Group PT in Pivotal Response Training

The call for effectively translating evidence-based interventions into community practice is substantially magnified for children with ASD due to the many families in need of services. The purpose of the Openden (2005) study was to extend the PT research by evaluating a four-day group PT workshop for parents with children with ASD. Specifically, a randomized, controlled trial was used to assess the effects of the workshop on parents' ability to implement the motivational procedures of PRT for teaching social communication and the associated effects on their children's production of functional verbalizations.

Participant Families

Thirty-two families who primarily resided in rural/remote areas participated in the study. Primary caregivers were eligible to participate in the study if they had a child diagnosed with an ASD between the ages of 2 years and 8 years and no previous training in PRT. Pre-intervention videotape probes of parents interacting with their children while trying to elicit language were collected and scored for fidelity of implementation of the motivational procedures of PRT. Primary caregivers were matched on fidelity of implementation scores and then randomly assigned into either treatment or waitlist control conditions.

Group Parent Education Workshop

The workshops were conducted at two California Regional Centers. Each workshop included seven to ten primary caregivers and was held for 5 h per day over four consecutive days (20 h total). The first of the four days included didactic instruction, video modeling of the motivational procedures of PRT, role play with toys to practice implementation of the techniques, and questions and discussion. At the end of the first day of the workshop, each parent was instructed to return home and videotape their implementation of PRT with their child for 15 min.

Following questions and discussion on the second day of the workshop, each parent showed their videotape and received individualized feedback from the workshop presenter on their implementation of the PRT procedures (as well as from the other parents). At the end of the second day, each parent was again instructed to make a videotape implementing PRT, but with the feedback provided in the workshop. The third and fourth days of the workshop were identical to the second day; thus, each parent received feedback on their implementation of the procedures – and observed the feedback given to every other parent – for three consecutive days. Following the final day of the workshop, parents were asked to make a post-intervention videotape according to the same standardized instructions they received for the pre-intervention probe: 15 min of engaging their children in typical play interactions while attempting to elicit as much language as possible. The post-intervention videotapes were used to assess parent's fidelity of implementation of the PRT procedures and to assess the children's progress.

Results

Analyses showed significant differences between treatment and control groups on the four dependent measures at posttest: fidelity of implementation of PRT motivational procedures, parent positive affect, child responsivity to language opportunities, and functional verbal utterances produced by the child.

Implications

The results of this study provide initial evidence of training parents of children with ASD to implement the motivational procedures of PRT for teaching social communication within a group workshop format. Training parents in a group workshop format has important implications for PT as well as for the dissemination of evidence-based practices for families with children with ASD. First, most of the ASD PT research, and specifically those studies that have taught parents to implement PRT, has been limited to training one parent–child dyad at a time. While the current study did not directly compare single parent–child dyad training versus group parent training, the data indicated that training parents in groups of seven to ten was indeed efficacious. That is, parents were not only able to learn to implement intervention procedures

correctly, but also able to do so with enough intensity to produce changes in their children within a fairly brief period of time (four days), though additional research is needed to examine long-term impact. These findings are consistent with the large body of literature on group PT for families with other disabilities and suggest that group PT may be an effective way to help meet the growing demand for evidence-based intervention for families with children with ASD.

A second implication of this study is that group PT workshops may be an effective mechanism for intervention delivery to families living in rural or remote locations, in which many of the families in the current study resided. These families face an even greater challenge of identifying service providers with sufficient training in autism interventions (Koegel et al., 2002; Symon, 2001, 2005). Thus, group PT workshops may serve as a cost-effective format for delivering treatment to these families who live geographically distant from an intervention center.

Finally, similar group workshops could be developed that include a team of service providers and parents to ensure coordination of care across providers and ongoing, wraparound support for families. For instance, this model has been adapted for training teams of intervention providers and parents toward province-wide dissemination and implementation of PRT in Nova Scotia, Canada (Bryson et al., 2007). In a team-based group workshop model that includes parents and professionals, the professionals can be trained to support the families in the workshop as well as additional families, thereby further addressing the shortage of trained providers and the growing number of families in need or services.

Current Parent Training Practices in Community Settings

It is clear that several research-based methods for teaching parents to facilitate developing in their children with autism have been developed in laboratory settings. While knowledge about the efficacy of treatments for children with ASD conducted in controlled settings is increasing at a rapid rate, the effectiveness and transportability of these treatments to diverse community populations and settings are less clear (NAMHC, 2001; National Research Council, 2001; Rogers &

Vismara, 2008; Stahmer, 2007). Although there has recently been a strong emphasis on implementation of research-based interventions in real world settings, few studies have examined whether or not services systems are using these treatments. Stahmer, Collings, and Palinkas (2005) examined provider self-reports of the use of both evidence-based and non–evidence-based interventions in community settings. Service providers' reports indicate that both evidence- and non–evidence-based techniques are often combined and/or modified based on child characteristics, personal preferences, and external factors (e.g., parent requests, availability of training, financial resources). Additionally, in most cases the interventions have not been tested on the populations of concern within community programs. The diversity of the populations served in communities seems to stand in stark contrast to the populations of children studied in traditional clinical research (Shirk, 2001). In order to understand the effectiveness of research-based interventions in community settings there appears to be a need to examine more diverse children and families, including broader diagnostic profiles, larger age ranges, and race/ethnic diversity. Specifically, given the multiple and complex needs of children in community programs, and possible barriers to use of research-based interventions in community settings there are significant questions about the degree to which providers are attempting to implement these interventions and whether children and families will demonstrate the same level of positive outcomes as those in research settings. Efforts to examine the feasibility of transferring research-based, university-delivered intervention approaches to community settings are underway and will shed critical information as to the type of delivery systems and teaching modalities required for effective dissemination (Vismara, Rogers, Stahmer, & Griffith, 2008).

There is some research to suggest that parents are receiving some sort of education or training as part of their children's intervention programs. A few researchers have surveyed families of children with autism regarding service use throughout the county (Mandell, Morales, & Levi, in review; Thomas, Morrissey, & McLaurin, 2007; Wood, Stahmer, & Conn, 2004). Up to 50% of families (range = 36–50) indicated that parent training, education, or support was part of their program. In a survey of 80 early intervention providers (teachers and Part C program providers) in Southern California regarding service provision, 96%

of practitioners reported active parent involvement in intervention programs (Stahmer, 2007). Providers in toddler programs were significantly more likely to provide parent education (100%) than providers in preschool programs (78%). Ninety percent of in-home providers indicated that they worked with both parent and child during home visits. However, the depth and quality of the use of parent involvement remains a critical question. For example, for many families this involvement was observation of the child's program (34%). Only 39% of parents received opportunities to practice techniques with feedback. So, it appears that programs are attempting to use PT, but whether or not they teach parent research-based intervention strategies is not clear.

It is also important to examine community programs that are using research-based interventions to examine their effectiveness in these settings. Many research-based parent training programs, while effective, are also time-consuming, costly and some parents continue to have difficulty learning and implementing the techniques (Cordisco, Strain, & Depew, 1988; Mahoney & Perales, 2003; Schreibman & Koegel, 1996; Stahmer & Gist, 2001). In the service system, parent education programs are rarely covered by insurance. In Southern California, the San Diego Regional Center for the Developmentally Disabled (service system for individuals with developmental disabilities) does fund some PT, however it is typically brief (e.g., 12–15 h total).

Research has been conducted on a specific Southern California community program offering a condensed parent education program using research-based intervention, Pivotal Response Training (described above). This program consists of 12 weeks of one-on-one manualized training for the parent which includes PRT and general behavioral strategies. Parents review reading material, observe a trained therapist working with their child, and receive direct feedback on their interactions with the child. A preliminary assessment of the effectiveness of this community-based parent education PRT intervention and whether specific child variables are associated with its effectiveness was conducted (Baker-Ericzén, Stahmer, & Burns, 2007). One hundred fifty-eight families with children with ASD participated. Children were heterogeneous with regards to age, gender, and race/ethnicity. Results indicated that all children showed significant improvements in adaptive functioning as total sample of children significantly improved from pre- to post-intervention on measures of Communication, Daily Living Skills, Socialization, Motor Skills, and Adaptive Behavior Composite domains of the Vineland Adaptive Behavior Scales. However, younger children (3 year old or younger) showed the least impairment at intake and the most improvement at post-intervention. The positive effect of PRT PT remained when examining only Hispanic families (35% of the sample). This is one of the first large-scale community studies of PRT which included a diverse sample. This particular study did not include a measure of fidelity of implementation which limits our understanding of the relationship between accurate implementation and child progress. However, a subset of families in the program have had assessments of treatment integrity (see below).

Parents enrolled in PT programs often report that opportunities for social support are lacking in their communities and that additional support would reduce stress and increase their ability to focus on the teaching techniques (Feldman & Werner, 2002; Gallagher, Beckman, & Cross, 1983). Therefore, in a quasi-experimental design, Stahmer and Gist (2001) compared two groups of parents with children ages 2–5 who had recently been diagnosed with an ASD. The first group ($n = 11$) received the 12 week parent training program as described above. In the comparison group ($n = 11$) parents also attended a parent support group. For half of the parents, a parent support and information group offered in conjunction with the parent education program. The parent information/support group did not discuss the PT techniques at all. The purpose of this investigation was twofold: (a) to assess the effectiveness of the accelerated parent education program and (b) to examine the effects of providing disorder-specific support and information to parents participating in a parent education program. Both technique mastery (fidelity of implementation) and improvements in child performance were assessed. Results indicated that parents who participated in the parent information/support group met fidelity of implementation criteria significantly more often than parents who did not participate in the support group. Furthermore, the range in levels of skill mastery, defined as appropriate use of all of the PRT strategies during 75% of the intervals scored, was much greater in individual parents who did not participate in the parent support group than parents who did participate. In fact, of the 11 families who participated in the parent information support group only 3

did not reach criteria ($M = 75$, range = 68–86). This is quite different than the control group in which seven of the parents did not reach criteria for skill mastery ($M = 60$, range = 29–78). The majority of parents in both groups improved in their use of the techniques with only two parents (of the 22 educated) using PRT techniques less than 50% of the intervals. The children of parents who demonstrated greater mastery of the techniques had better outcomes. These children increased their use of language significantly more than the group of children whose parents did not meet criteria for the techniques to criterion even though their average language use was the same before training.

These data provide some support for the use of PRT as a parent education protocol in community settings, even when the program is accelerated. Although there are limitations to these studies because both were quasi-experimental, it is clear that children can improve and parents can learn these techniques in community programs. In addition, it may be that family functioning mediates child outcomes, especially in parent education programs. It also indicates that when moving research-based programs into service setting there are necessary modifications that must be made to ensure the effectiveness of the program. Shortening the sessions had a clear affect on fidelity of implementation for these parents, which was improved by the addition of a parent information support group. This type of adaptation was not apparent through PRT work in the research setting. If parent education programs require this much adaptation to move them into a service system with a trained researcher implementing/overseeing the intervention, the adaptations necessary to translate early intervention research programs to larger service systems may be even greater. Studying these adaptations may assist researchers in adapting their line of research and program development to be better suited to service system environments.

Implications and Future Directions

Overall, the research suggests that PT is a feasible and effective intervention method for children with ASD of varying ages and functioning levels (National Research Council, 2001). Many parents want to learn and be involved in their children's development and because this approach is cost-efficient and increases the number of hours of teaching, many programs now include a PT component (Koegel et al., 2008). PT research conducted on PT programs for other childhood disorders such as disruptive behavior disorders and conduct problems highlight key future directions for ASD PT research (Brookman-Frazee et al., 2006). For example, more research is needed to understand rates of attrition in PT programs to better understand how to serve families that may be benefiting from these models. Additionally, more research is needed on the impact of parent factors (especially depression and stress) on PT intervention implementation and outcome and the impact of PT intervention on parent factors. Further, more information is required to systematically individualize PT content and format for the individual needs of the child and family. The specific manner in which parents are included and participate in the intervention process deserves attention, as does individualizing the parent education content to be sensitive to different family needs and circumstances. Not all parents may progress or learn from traditional behavioral parent education programs (Forehand & Kotchick, 2002), and some parents may require additional assistance or support in order to be more effective interventionists for their children (Corcoran, 2000). Factors, such as marital discord, parental depression, severe child behavioral problems, inadequate social support, may interfere with families benefiting from traditional parent training (Stern, 2000; Webster-Stratton & Reid, 2003). Thus, researchers must continue to examine specific strategies and program components (e.g., directive vs. nondirective) to be incorporated into the process of parent training that may be more effective for families who have not responded to traditional parent education approaches. Future studies concentrating on how best to integrate concrete behavioral procedures while emphasizing parental empowerment and family support will be especially critical for parents of children with autism. In the area of community practice, additional research is needed to address how to most effectively implement research-based PT interventions into "usual care" community settings, such as how to most efficiently train community-based providers and how to reach families that may be less motivated than those who participate in university-based intervention studies.

References

Anderson, S. R., Avery, D. L., DiPietro, E. K., Edwards, G. L., & Christian, W. P. (1987). Intensive home-based early intervention with autistic children. *Education and Treatment of Children, 10*, 352–366.

Anderson, S., & Morris, J. (2006). Cognitive behaviour therapy for people with asperger syndrome. *Behavioural and Cognitive Psychotherapy, 34*, 293–303.

Baker, B. L. (1989). *Parent training and developmental disabilities*. Washington, DC: American Association on Mental Retardation.

Baker-Ericzén, M. J., Stahmer, A. C., & Burns, A. (2007). Child demographics associated with outcomes in a community-based pivotal response training program. *Journal of Positive Behavior Interventions, 9*, 52–60.

Barrett, P. M., Dadds, M. R., & Rapee, R. M. (1996). Family treatment of childhood anxiety: A controlled trial. *Journal of Consulting and Clinical Psychology, 64*, 333–342.

Barrett, P. M., & Shortt, A. L. (2003). Parental involvement in the treatment of anxious children. In A. E. Kazdin & J. R. Weisz (Eds.), *Evidence-based psychotherapies for children and adolescents* (pp. 101–119). New York: Guilford Press.

Bettelheim, B. (1967). *The empty fortress: Infantile autism and the birth of the self*. Oxford, England: Free Press of Glencoe.

Blackledge, J. T., & Hayes, S. C. (2006). Using acceptance and commitment training in the support of parents of children diagnosed with autism. *Child & Family Behavior Therapy, 28*, 1–18.

Boulware, G., Schwartz, I. S., Sandall, S. R., & McBride, B. J. (2006). Project DATA for toddlers: An inclusive approach to very young children with autism spectrum disorder. *Topics in Early Childhood Special Education, 26*, 94–105.

Bristol, M. M., Gallagher, J. J., & Holt, K. D. (1993). Maternal depressive symptoms in autism: Response to psychoeducational intervention. *Rehabilitation Psychology, 38*, 3–10.

Brookman-Frazee, L. (2004). Using parent/clinician partnerships in parent education programs for children with autism. *Journal of Positive Behavior Interventions, 6*, 195–213.

Brookman-Frazee, L., Stahmer, A., Baker-Ericzén, M. J., & Tsai, K. (2006). Parenting interventions for children with autism spectrum and disruptive behavior disorders: Opportunities for cross-fertilization. *Clinical Child and Family Psychology Review, 9*, 181–200.

Bryson, S. E., Koegel, L. K., Koegel, R. L., Openden, D., Smith, I. M., & Nefdt, N. (2007). Large scale dissemination and community implementation of pivotal response treatment. *Research and Practice for Persons with Severe Disabilities, 32*, 142–153.

Chalfant, A. M., Rapee, R., & Carroll, L. (2007). Treating anxiety disorders in children with high functioning autism spectrum disorders: A controlled trial. *Journal of Autism and Developmental Disorders, 37*, 1842–1857.

Chambless, D. L., & Hollon, S. D. (1998). Defining empirically supported therapies. *Journal of Consulting and Clinical Psychology, 66*, 7–18.

Charlop-Christy, M. H., & Carpenter, M. H. (2000). Modified incidental teaching sessions: A procedure for parents to increase spontaneous speech in their children with autism. *Journal of Positive Behavior Interventions, 2*, 98–112.

Cobham, V. E., Dadds, M. R., & Spence, S. H. (1998). The role of parental anxiety in the treatment of childhood anxiety. *Journal of Consulting and Clinical Psychology, 66*, 893–905.

Corcoran, J. (2000). Family treatment of preschool behavior problems. *Research on Social Work Practice, 10*, 547–588.

Cordisco, L. K., Strain, P. S., & Depew, N. (1988). Assessment for generalization of parenting skills in home settings. *Journal of the Association for Persons with Severe Handicaps, 13*, 202–210.

Crockett, J. L., Fleming, R. K., Doepke, K. J., & Stevens, J. S. (2007). Parent training: Acquisition and generalization of discrete trials teaching skills with parents of children with autism. *Research in Developmental Disabilities, 28*, 23–36.

de Bruin, E. I., Ferdinand, R. F., Meester, S., de Nijs, P. F. A., & Verheij, F. (2007). High rates of psychiatric co-morbidity in PDD-NOS. *Journal of Autism and Developmental Disorders, 37*, 877–886.

Drahota, A., Wood, J. J., Sze, K. M., & Van Dyke, M. (in review). Effects of cognitive behavioral therapy on daily living skills in children with high-functioning autism and concurrent anxiety disorders.

Dunlap, G., & Koegel, R. L. (1980). Motivating autistic children through stimulus variation. *Journal of Applied Behavior Analysis, 13*, 619–627.

Dyer, K., Dunlap, G., & Winterling, V. (1990). Effects of choice making on the serious problem behaviors of students with severe handicaps. *Journal of Applied Behavior Analysis, 23*, 515–524.

Eyberg, S. M., Nelson, M. M., & Boggs, S. R. (2008). Evidence-based psychosocial treatments for children and adolescents with disruptive behavior. *Journal of Clinical Child and Adolescent Psychology, 37*, 215–237.

Feldman, E. A., & Werner, S. E. (2002). Collateral effects of behavioral parent training on families of children with developmental disabilities and behavior disorders. *Behavioral Interventions, 17*, 75–83.

Ferster, C. B. (1961). Positive reinforcement and behavioral deficits of young children. *Child Development, 32*, 437–456.

Ferster, C. B., & Demyer, M. K. (1962). A method for the experimental analysis of the behavior of autistic children. *American Journal of Orthopsychiatry, 32*, 89–98.

Ferster, C. B., & Simons, J. (1966). Behavior therapy with children. *Psychological Record, 16*, 65–71.

Forehand, R., & Kotchick, B. A. (2002). Behavioral parent training: Current challenges and potential solutions. *Journal of Child and Family Studies, 11*, 377–384.

Frea, W. D., & Hepburn, S. L. (1999). Teaching parents of children with autism to perform functional assessments to plan interventions for extremely disruptive behaviors. *Journal of Positive Behavior Interventions, 1*, 112–116.

Gallagher, J. J., Beckman, P. J., & Cross, A. H. (1983). Families of handicapped children: Sources of stress and its amelioration. *Exceptional Children, 50*, 10–19.

Ghaziuddin, M., Weidmer-Mikhail, E., & Ghaziuddin, N. (1998). Comorbidity of Asperger syndrome: A preliminary report. *Journal of Intellectual Disability Research, 42*, 279–283.

Gillett, J. N., & LeBlanc, L. A. (2007). Parent-implemented natural language paradigm to increase language and play in children with autism. *Research in Autism Spectrum Disorders, 1*, 247–255.

Green, J., Gilchrist, A., Burton, D., & Cox, A. (2000). Social and psychiatric functioning in adolescents with Asperger syndrome compared with conduct disorder. *Journal of Autism and Developmental Disorders, 30*, 279–293.

Hancock, T. B., & Kaiser, A. P. (2002). The effects of trainer-implemented Enhanced Milieu Teaching on the social communication of children with autism. *Topics in Early Childhood Special Education, 22*, 39–54.

Harris, S. L. (1983). *Families of the developmentally disabled.* New York: Pergamon Press.

Hart, B. M., & Risley, T. R. (1968). Establishing use of descriptive adjectives in the spontaneous speech of disadvantaged preschool children. *Journal of Applied Behavior Analysis, 1*, 109–120.

Iacono, T. A., Chan, J. B., & Waring, R. E. (1998). Efficiency of a parent-implementation early language intervention based on collaborative consultation. *International Journal of Communication Disorders, 33*, 281–303.

Ingersoll, B., & Dvortcsak, A. (2006). Including parent training in the early childhood special education curriculum for children with autism spectrum disorders. *Journal of Positive Behavior Interventions, 8*, 79–87.

Kaiser, A. P., & Hancock, T. B. (2003). Teaching parents new skills to support their young children's development. *Infants and Young Children, 16*, 9–21.

Kaminski, J. W., Valle, L. A., Filene, J. H., & Boyle, C. L. (2008). A meta-analytic review of components associated with parent training program effectiveness. *Journal of Abnormal Child Psychology, 36*, 567–589.

Kazdin, A. E., & Whitley, M. K. (2003). Treatment of parental stress to enhance therapeutic change among children referred for aggressive and antisocial behavior. *Journal of Consulting and Clinical Psychology, 71*, 504–515.

Kim, J. A., Szatmari, P., Bryson, S. E., Streiner, D. L., & Wilson, F. J. (2000). The prevalence of anxiety and mood problems among children with autism and Asperger syndrome. *Autism, 4*, 117–132.

Koegel, R. L., Bimbela, A., & Schreibman, L. (1996). Collateral effects of parent training on family interactions. *Journal of Autism and Developmental Disorders, 26*, 347–359.

Koegel, R. L., Dyer, K., & Bell, L. K. (1987). The influence of child-preferred activities on autistic children's social behavior. *Journal of Applied Behavior Analysis, 20*, 243–252.

Koegel, R. L., & Egel, A. L. (1979). Motivating autistic children. *Journal of Abnormal Psychology, 88*, 418–426.

Koegel, R. L., Glahn, T. J., & Nieminen, G. S. (1978). Generalization of parent-training results. *Journal of Applied Behavior Analysis, 11*, 95–109.

Koegel, R. L., & Koegel, L. K. (2006). *Pivotal response treatments for autism: Communication, social, and academic development.* Baltimore, MD: Paul H. Brookes Publishing Co., Inc.

Koegel, R. L., Koegel, L. K., & Brookman, L. I. (2003). Empirically supported pivotal response interventions for children with autism. In A. E. Kazdin & J. R. Weisz (Eds.), *Evidence-based psychotherapies for children and adolescents* (pp. 341–357). New York, NY: Guilford Press.

Koegel, L. K., Koegel, R. L., Fredeen, R. M., & Gengoux, G. W. (2008). Naturalistic behavioral approaches to treatment. In K. Chawarska, A. Klin & F. R. Volkmar (Eds.), *Autism spectrum disorders in infants and toddlers: Diagnosis, assessment, and treatment* (pp. 207–241). New York: Guilford Press.

Koegel, L. K., Koegel, R. L., Harrower, J. K., & Carter, C. M. (1999). Pivotal response intervention I: Overview of approach. *Journal of the Association for Persons with Severe Handicaps, 24,* 174–185.

Koegel, R. L., Koegel, L. K., & McNerney, E. K. (2001). Pivotal areas in intervention for autism. *Journal of Clinical Child Psychology, 30,* 19–32.

Koegel, R. L., Koegel, L. K., & Schreibman, L. (1991). Assessing and training parents in teaching pivotal behaviors. *Advances in Behavioral Assessment of Children and Families, 5,* 65–82.

Koegel, L. K., Koegel, R. L., Shoshan, Y., & McNerney, E. (1999). Pivotal response intervention II: Preliminary long-term outcome data. *Journal of the Association for Persons with Severe Handicaps, 24,* 186–198.

Koegel, R. L., Koegel, L. K., & Surratt, A. (1992). Language intervention and disruptive behavior in preschool children with autism. *Journal of Autism and Developmental Disorders, 22,* 141–153.

Koegel, R. L., O'Dell, M. C., & Dunlap, G. (1988). Producing speech use in nonverbal autistic children by reinforcing attempts. *Journal of Autism and Developmental Disorders, 18,* 525–538.

Koegel, R. L., O'Dell, M. C., & Koegel, L. K. (1987). A natural language teaching paradigm for nonverbal autistic children. *Journal of Autism and Developmental Disorders, 17,* 187–199.

Koegel, R. L., Schreibman, L., Britten, K., Burke, J. C., & O'Neill, R. E. (1982). A comparison of parent training to direct child treatment. In R. L. Koegel, A. Rincover & A. I. Egel (Eds.), *Educating and understanding autistic children.* San Diego, CA: College Hill- Press.

Koegel, R. L., Schreibman, L., Good, A., Cerniglia, L., Murphy, C., & Koegel, L. K. (1989). *How to teach pivotal behaviors to children with autism: A training manual.* Santa Barbara, CA: University of California.

Koegel, R. L., Schreibman, L., Johnson, J., O'Neil, R. E., & Dunlap, G. (1984). Collateral effects of parent-training on families with autistic children. In R. F. Dangel & R. A. Polster (Eds.), *Behavioral parent-training: Issues in research and practice* (pp. 358–378). New York: The Guilford Press.

Koegel, R. L., Symon, J. B., & Koegel, L. K. (2002). Parent education for families of children with autism living in geographically distant areas. *Journal of Positive Behavior Interventions, 4,* 88–103.

Koegel, R. L., & Williams, J. A. (1980). Direct versus indirect response-reinforcer relationships in teaching autistic children. *Journal of Abnormal Child Psychology, 8,* 537–547.

Laski, K. E., Charlop, M. H., & Schreibman, L. (1988). Training parents to use the Natural Language Paradigm to increase their autistic children's speech. *Journal of Applied Behavior Analysis, 21,* 391–400.

Levy, S., Kim, A., & Olive, M. L. (2006). Interventions for young children with autism: A synthesis of the literature. *Focus on Autism and Other Developmental Disabilities, 21,* 55–62.

Leyfer, O. T., Folstein, S. E., Bacalman, S., Davis, N. O., Dinh, E., Morgan, J., et al. (2006). Comorbid psychiatric disorders in children with autism: Interview development and rates of disorders. *Journal of Autism and Developmental Disorders, 36,* 849–861.

Lord, C., Wagner, A., Rogers, S., Szatmari, P., Aman, M., Charman, T., et al. (2005). Challenges in evaluating psychosocial interventions for autistic spectrum disorders. *Journal of Autism and Developmental Disorders, 35,* 695–708.

Lovaas, O. I., Baer, D. M., & Bijou, S. W. (1965). Experimental procedures for analyzing the interaction of symbolic social stimuli and children's behavior. *Child Development, 36,* 237–247.

Lovaas, O. I., Freitag, G., Gold, V. J., & Kassorla, I. C. (1965). Recording apparatus and procedure for observation of behaviors of children in free play settings. *Journal of Experimental Child Psychology, 2,* 108–120.

Lovaas, O. I., Koegel, R., Simmons, J. Q., & Long, J. S. (1973). Some generalization and follow-up measures on autistic children in behavior therapy. *Journal of Applied Behavior Analysis, 6,* 131–166.

Lovaas, O. I., & Simmons, J. Q. (1969). Manipulation of self-destruction in three retarded children. *Journal of Applied Behavior Analysis, 2,* 143–157.

Lucyshyn, J. M., Dunlap, G., & Albin, R. W. (2002). *Families and positive behavior support: Addressing problem behavior in family contexts.* Baltimore, MD, US: Paul H. Brookes Publishing.

Mahoney, G., Boyce, G., Fewell, R. R., Spiker, D., & Wheeden, C. A. (1998). The relationship of parent-child interaction to the effectiveness of early intervention services for at-risk children and children with disabilities. *Topics in Early Childhood Special Education, 18,* 5–17.

Mahoney, G., & Perales, F. (2003). Using relationship-focused intervention to enhance the social-emotional functioning of young children with autism spectrum disorders. *Topics in Early Childhood Special Education, 23,* 77–89.

Mahoney, G., & Perales, F. (2005). The impact of relationship focused intervention on young children with autism spectrum disorders: A comparative study. *Journal of Developmental and Behavioral Pediatrics, 26,* 77–85.

Mandell, D. S., Morales, K. H., & Levy, S. E. (in review). A latent class model of treatment use among children with autism spectrum disorders.

McClannahan, L., Krantz, P., & McGee, G. (1982). Parents as therapists for autistic children: A model for effective parent training. *Analysis and Intervention in Developmental Disabilities, 2,* 223–252.

McGee, G. G., Morrier, M. J., & Daly, T. (1999). An incidental teaching approach to early intervention for toddlers with autism. *Journal of the Association for Persons with Severe Handicaps, 24,* 133–146.

McGee, G. G., Paradis, T., & Feldman, R. S. (1993). Free effects of integration on levels of autistic behavior. *Topics in Early Childhood Special Education, 13,* 57–67.

Mendlowitz, S. L., Manassis, K., Bradley, S., Scapillato, D., Miezitis, S., & Shaw, B. F. (1999). Cognitive-behavioral group treatments in childhood anxiety disorders: The role of parental involvement. *Journal of the American Academy of Child & Adolescent Psychiatry, 38,* 1223–1229.

Moes, D. (1995). Parent education and parenting stress. In R. L. Koegel & L. K. Koegel (Eds.), *Teaching children with autism: Strategies for initiating positive interactions and improving learning opportunities* (pp. 79–93). Baltimore, MD: Paul H Brookes Publishing.

Moes, D., & Frea, W. D. (2002). Contextualized behavioral support in early intervention for children with autism and their families. *Journal of Autism and Developmental Disorders, 32,* 519–533.

National Advisory Mental Health Council. (2001). *Blueprint for change: Research on child and adolescent mental health. A report by the National Advisory Mental Health Council's*

Workgroup on Child and Adolescent Mental Health Intervention Development and Deployment. Bethesda, MD: National Institutes of Health/National Institute of Mental Health.

National Research Council. (2001). *Educating children with autism*. Washington, DC: National Academy Press, Division of Behavioral and Social Sciences and Education, Committee on Educational Interventions for Children with Autism.

New York State Department of Health Early Intervention Program. (1999). *Clinical practice guideline: The guideline technical report. Autism/pervasive developmental disorders, assessment and intervention for young children (age 0-3 years)*. Albany, NY: NYS Department of Health.

Openden, D. (2005). *Pivotal Response Treatment for multiple families of children with autism: Effects of a 4-day group parent education workshop*. Unpublished dissertation.

Osterling, J., Dawson, G., & Munson, J. (2002). Early recognition of 1-year-old infants with autism spectrum disorder versus mental retardation. *Development and Psychopathology, 14*, 239–251.

Patterson, G. R. (1982). *Coercive family process: A social learning approach (Vol. 3)*. Eugene, OR: Castalia.

Patterson, G. R., & Brodsky, G. (1966). A behaviour modification programme for a child with multiple problem behaviours. *Journal of Child Psychology and Psychiatry, 9*, 277–295.

Patterson, G. R., Reid, J. B., & Dishion, T. J. (1992). *Antisocial boys*. Eugene, OR: Castalia.

Pelham, W. E., & Fabiano, G. A. (2008). Evidence-based psychosocial treatments for attention-deficit/hyperactivity disorder. *Journal of Clinical Child and Adolescent Psychology, 37*, 184–214.

Reaven, J., & Hepburn, S. (2003). Cognitive-behavioral treatment of obsessive-compulsive disorder in a child with Asperger syndrome. *Autism, 7*, 145–164.

Reaven, J., & Hepburn, S. (2006). The parent's role in the treatment of anxiety symptoms in children with high-functioning autism spectrum disorders. *Mental Health Aspects of Developmental Disabilities, 9*, 73–80.

Research Units on Pediatric Psychopharmacology [RUPP] Autism Network. (2007). Parent training for children with pervasive developmental disorders: A multi-site feasibility trial. *Behavioral Interventions, 22*, 179–199.

Robbins, F. R., Dunlap, G., & Plienis, A. J. (1991). Family characteristics, family training, and the progress of young children with autism. *Journal of Early Intervention, 15*, 173–184.

Rocha, M. L., Schreibman, L., & Stahmer, A. C. (2007). Effectiveness of training parents to teach joint attention in children with autism. *Journal of Early Intervention, 29*, 154–172.

Rogers, S. J., Dawson, G., Smith, C. M., Winter, J. M., & Donaldson, A. L. (in press). *Early Start Denver Model intervention for young children with autism manual*. Seattle, WA: University of Washington.

Rogers, S. J., & DiLalla, D. (1991). A comparative study of the effects of a developmentally based instructional model on young children with autism and young children with other disorders of behavior and development. *Topics in Early Childhood Special Education, 11*, 29–48.

Rogers, S. J., & Lewis, H. (1989). An effective day treatment model for young children with pervasive developmental disorders. *Journal of the American Academy of Child & Adolescent Psychiatry, 28*, 207–214.

Rogers, S. J., Lewis, H. C., & Reis, K. (1987). An effective procedure for training early special education teams to implement a model program. *Journal of the Division of Early Childhood, 11*, 180–188.

Rogers, S. J., Hall, T., Osaki, D., Reaven, J., & Herbison, J. (2001). The Denver model: A comprehensive, integrated, educational approach to young children with autism and their families. In J. S. Handleman & S. L. Harris (Eds.), *Preschool education programs for children with autism* (2nd ed., pp. 95–134). Austin, TX: Pro-Ed.

Rogers, S. J., Herbison, J., Lewis, H., Pantone, J., & Reis, K. (1986). An approach for enhancing the symbolic, communicative, and interpersonal functioning of young children with autism and severe emotional handicaps. *Journal of the Division of Early Childhood, 10*, 135–148.

Rogers, S. J., & Ozonoff, S. (2006). Behavioral, educational, and developmental treatments for autism. In S. O. Moldin & J. L. R. Rubenstein (Eds.), *Understanding autism: From basic neuroscience to treatment* (pp. 443–473). Boca Raton, FL: CRC Press.

Rogers, S. J., & Vismara, L. A. (2008). Evidence-based comprehensive treatments for early autism. *Journal of Clinical Child and Adolescent Psychology, 37*, 8–38.

Rogers, S. J., Vismara, L. A., & Colombi, C. (in preparation). *The Early Start Denver Model parent manual*. Davis, CA: University of California.

Schopler, E. (2005). Comments on "Challenges in evaluating psychosocial intervention for autistic spectrum disorders" by Lord et al. *Journal of Autism and Developmental Disorders, 35*, 709–711.

Schreibman, L. (2005). *Science and fiction of autism*. Cambridge, MA: Harvard University Press.

Schreibman, L., Kaneko, W. M., & Koegel, R. L. (1991). Positive affect of parents of autistic children: A comparison across two teaching techniques. *Behavior Therapy, 22*, 479–490.

Schreibman, L., & Koegel, R. L. (1996). Fostering self-management: Parent-delivered pivotal response training for children with autistic disorder. In E. D. Hibbs & P. S. Jensen (Eds.), *Psychosocial treatments for child and adolescent disorders* (pp. 525–552). Washington, DC: American Psychological Association.

Schreibman, L., & Koegel, R. L. (2005). Training for parents of children with autism: Pivotal responses, generalization, and individualization of interventions. In E. D. Hibbs & P. S. Jensen (Eds.), *Psychosocial treatments for child and adolescent disorders: Empirically based strategies for clinical practice* (2nd ed., pp. 605–631). Washington, DC: American Psychological Association.

Seligman, M. E. P. (1972). Learned helplessness. *Annual Review of Medicine, 23*, 407–412.

Seligman, M., & Darling, R. B. (1997). *Ordinary families, special children: A systems approach to childhood disability* (2nd ed.). New York, NY: Guilford Press.

Seltzer, M. M., Shattuck, P., Abbeduto, L., & Greenberg, J. S. (2004). Trajectory of development in adolescents and adults with autism. *Mental Retardation and Developmental Disabilities Research Reviews, 10*, 234–247.

Seung, H. K., Ashwell, S., Elder, J. H., & Valcante, G. (2006). Verbal communication outcomes in children with autism after in-home father training. *Journal of Intellectual Disability Research, 50*, 139–150.

Shirk, S. R. (2001). The road to effective child psychological services: Treatment processes and outcome research. In J. Hughes & A. M. La Greca (Eds.), *Handbook of psychological services for children and adolescents* (pp. 43–59). London: Oxford University Press.

Shogren, K. A., Faggella-Luby, M. N., Bae, S. J., & Wehmeyer, M. L. (2004). The effect of choice-making as an intervention for problem behavior: A meta-analysis. *Journal of Positive Behavior Interventions, 6*, 228–237.

Simonoff, E., Pickles, A., Charman, T., Chandler, S., Loucas, T., & Baird, G. (2008). Psychiatric disorders in children with autism spectrum disorders: Prevalence, comorbidity, and associated factors in a population-derived sample. *Journal of the American Academy of Child & Adolescent Psychiatry, 47*, 921–929.

Singer, G. H. S., Goldberg-Hamblin, S. E., Peckham-Hardin, K. D., Barry, L., & Santarelli, G. E. (2002). Toward a synthesis of family support practices and positive behavior support. In J. M. Lucyshyn, G. Dunlap & R. W. Albin (Eds.), *Families and positive behavior support: Addressing problem behavior in family contexts. Family, community & disability* (pp. 155–183). Baltimore, MD: Paul H Brookes Publishing.

Smith, T., Buch, G. A., & Gamby, T. E. (2000). Parent-directed, intensive early intervention for children with pervasive developmental disorder. *Research in Developmental Disabilities, 21*, 297–309.

Smith, T., Donahoe, P. A., & Davis, B. J. (2001). The UCLA young autism project. In J. S. Handleman & S. L. Harris (Eds.), *Preschool education programs for children with autism* (pp. 23–39). Austin, TX: Pro-Ed.

Smith, T., Scahill, L., Dawson, G., Guthrie, D., Lord, C., Odom, S., et al. (2007). Designing research studies on psychosocial interventions in autism. *Journal of Autism and Developmental Disorders, 37*, 354–366.

Sofronoff, K., Attwood, T., & Hinton, S. (2005). A randomised controlled trial of a CBT intervention for anxiety in children with Asperger syndrome. *Journal of Child Psychology and Psychiatry, 46*, 1152–1160.

Sofronoff, K., & Farbotko, M. (2002). The effectiveness of parent management training to increase self-efficacy in parents of children with Asperger syndrome. *Autism, 6*, 271–286.

Sofronoff, K., Leslie, A., & Brown, W. (2004). Parent management training and Asperger syndrome: A randomized controlled trial to evaluate a parent based intervention. *Autism, 8*, 301–317.

Stahmer, A. C. (1995). Teaching symbolic play skills to children with autism using pivotal response training. *Journal of Autism and Developmental Disorders, 25*, 123–141.

Stahmer, A. C. (2007). The basic structure of community early intervention programs for children with autism: Provider descriptions. *Journal of Autism and Developmental Disorders, 37*, 1344–1354.

Stahmer, A. C., Collings, N. M., & Palinkas, L. A. (2005). Early intervention practices for children with autism: Descriptions from community providers. *Focus on Autism and Other Developmental Disabilities, 20*, 66–79.

Stahmer, A. C., & Gist, K. (2001). Enhancing parent training through additional support services. *Journal of Positive Behavior Interventions, 3*, 75–82.

Stahmer, A. C., & Schreibman, L. (1992). Teaching children with autism appropriate play in unsupervised environments using a self-management treatment package. *Journal of Applied Behavior Analysis, 25*, 447–459.

Stern, J. (2000). Parent training. In J. R. White & A. S. Arthur (Eds.), *Cognitive-behavioral group therapy: For specific problems and populations* (pp. 331–360). Washington, DC: American Psychological Association.

Strain, P. S., & Hoyson, M. (2000). The need for longitudinal intensive social skill intervention: LEAP follow-up outcomes for children with autism. *Topics in Early Childhood Special Education, 20*, 116–122.

Symon, J. B. (2001). Parent education for autism: Issues in providing services at a distance. *Journal of Positive Behavior Interventions, 3*, 160–174.

Symon, J. B. (2005). Expanding interventions for children with autism: Parents as trainers. *Journal of Positive Behavior Interventions, 7*, 159–173.

Sze, K. M., & Wood, J. J. (2007). Cognitive behavioral treatment of comorbid anxiety disorders and social difficulties in children with high-functioning autism: A case report. *Journal of Contemporary Psychotherapy, 37*, 133–143.

Thomas, K. C., Morrissey, J. P., & McLaurin, C. (2007). Use of autism related services by families and children. *Journal of Autism and Developmental Disorders, 37*, 818–829.

Vismara, L. A., Colombi, C., & Rogers, S. J. (2009). Can 1 hour of therapy lead to lasting changes in young children with autism? *Autism, The International Journal of Research and Practice, 13*, 93–115.

Vismara, L. A., & Lyons, G. L. (2007). Using perseverative interests to elicit joint attention behaviors in young children with autism: Theoretical and clinical implications for understanding motivation. *Journal of Positive Behavior Interventions, 9*, 214–228.

Vismara, L. A., Rogers, S. J., Stahmer, A., & Griffith, E. (2008). Partners in Autism Research Studies (PAIRS): A university-community alliance program. *7th Annual International Meeting for Autism Research*. London, England.

Volkmar, F., Chawarska, K., & Klin, A. (2005). Autism in infancy and early childhood. *Annual Review of Psychology, 56*, 315–336.

Webster-Stratton, C., & Reid, M. J. (2003). The incredible years parents, teachers and children training series: A multifaceted treatment approach for young children with conduct problems. In A. E. Kazdin & J. R. Weisz (Eds.), *Evidence-based psychotherapies for children and adolescents* (pp. 224–240). New York: Guilford Press.

Weiskop, S., Richdale, A., & Matthews, J. (2005). Behavioural treatment to reduce sleep problems in children with autism or Fragile X syndrome. *Developmental Medicine and Child Neurology, 47*, 94–104.

Wetherby, A. M., & Woods, J. J. (2006). Early social interaction project for children with autism spectrum disorders beginning in the second year of life: A preliminary study. *Topics of Early Childhood Special Education, 26*, 67–82.

Wood, J. J., Drahota, A., Sze, K., Har, K., Chiu, A., & Langer, D. A. (2009). Cognitive behavioral therapy for anxiety in children with autism spectrum disorders: A randomized, controlled trial. *Journal of Child Psychology and Psychiatry, 50*, 224–234.

Wood, J. J., Piacentini, J. C., Southam-Gerow, M., Chu, B. C., & Sigman, M. (2006). Family cognitive behavioral therapy for child anxiety disorders. *Journal of the American Academy of Child & Adolescent Psychiatry, 45*, 314–321.

Wood, H., Stahmer, A. C., & Conn, J. (2004, February). *Provision and funding of early intervention programs for children with autism*. Paper presented at the California Association for Behavior Analysis, San Francisco, CA.

Index